Obesity

The Regulation of Weight

Obesity

The Regulation of Weight

Pauline S. Powers, M.D.

Assistant Professor
Department of Psychiatry
University of South Florida College of Medicine
Tampa, Florida

WILLIAMS & WILKINS
Baltimore/London

The Publishers have made every effort to trace the copyright holders for borrowed material. If they have inadvertently overlooked any, they will be pleased to make the necessary arrangements at the first opportunity.

Made in the United States of America

Library of Congress Cataloguing in Publication Data

Powers, Pauline S
Obesity: the regulation of weight.

Includes index.
1. Obesity—Psychological aspects. 2. Obesity. I. Title. [DNLM: 1. Obesity. WD210 P888o]
RC552.025P68 616.3′98 78-31620
ISBN 0-683-06953-5

Composed and printed at the
Waverly Press, Inc.
Mt. Royal and Guilford Aves.
Baltimore, Md. 21202, U.S.A.

To
Irwin Lunianski

Foreword

Caesar's comment "Let me have men about me that are fat; yon Cassius hath a lean and hungry look; such men are dangerous" may have reflected the attitudes of Rome, but in the present-day Western world, obesity does not receive that sort of glowing testimonial. Fat people are traditionally jolly, as witness Santa Claus, but obesity is too frequently associated with hypertension, diabetes, atherosclerotic heart disease, gallstones, gout, and perhaps endometrial carcinoma to be really admirable. Furthermore, in a culture which admires physical fitness and leanness, the fat person is cosmetically out of step.

Having said this, it would seem fairly easy to define obesity and to explore the reasons for developing and maintaining it. As Dr. Powers points out, however, none of these matters is easily determined. Even the definition of obesity is complicated. Total body weight above a certain arbitrary limit is not necessarily obesity. Football players and others in excellent athletic condition may be "overweight but not overfat." Nor is a total gain in weight significant since it may start from a pathologically low point. Correspondingly, the total *loss* in weight is not a good criterion for evaluating the status of the patient with anorexia nervosa. For the obese patient, the use of skinfold measurement is probably the most practical diagnostic tool, and Dr. Powers gives clear and succinct directions as to its use.

The questions of the distribution of fat, the number and structure of fat cells, the possible correlation with endocrinological problems, and even the speculation of the existence of a "ponderostat" in the hypothalamus receive in this book thoughtful attention and a wide range of references in the literature.

The psychological and socioeconomic aspects of obesity deserve—and receive—special consideration. Dr. Powers feels that obesity is increasing and that those elements obviously affect the incidence. In less affluent countries, the poor are seldom obese, for "only in an affluent country can the poor afford to be obese."

The amount of tolerable fat depends to some extent on the usefulness of it in culturally determined activities. Polynesians who needed to store fat for long sea voyages were required to be obese; conversely, Zulus who need to outrun gazelles have only 3% of fat content by weight. In our society a woman of average height with this fat content would weigh about 83 pounds.

There are religious, ethnic, and other cultural factors which modify the situation. As Dr. Powers encapsulates the picture, "the woman most likely to be thin is a fourth generation American who has high intelligence, a graduate school education, was an only child of an upper middle-class family who herself is now in the upper class and is Episcopalian with a thin, upwardly mobile husband. The man most likely to be fat is in his 50's, in a median income group (although studies disagree on this point), has a fat wife, is Jewish, from a large family with several siblings, with a high school education and in a socioeconomic class below his parents."

The psychological aspects of obesity are especially troublesome and interesting. Even hunger and satiety are subjective entities, and there is a sex difference in the irritability experienced as a concomitant of hunger. More women than men reported tenseness when experiencing even ordinary hunger. Further, preoccupation with food and eating may continue even after the obesity itself is no longer a problem. A similar situation obtains in the companion eating disturbances subsumed under the (actually erroneous) label of anorexia nervosa.

These elements bear on the treatment procedures used in dealing with obese patients, and Dr. Powers considers all of them in her very complete exposition of the possibilities and difficulties. Probably the most important initial consideration must be the appraisal of the motivation of the patient and the family of the patient for real weight reduction. Not only do patients have a distorted body image concept which renders their appreciation of weight loss questionable, but also families do get involved in the treatment process in a way which may be fatal to a successful outcome. Families, for many reasons, may wish to sabotage (or, as they might put it, not be involved in) therapy. Although they verbalize concern for and sympathy with the patient, in actuality they find some resolution of the family difficulties in the maintenance of the patient's fatness.

Drugs have been recommended for weight reduction. They lend themselves, as do some "Fat Farms," to a great deal of charlatanism and exploitation of these unfortunate people. They are, as Dr. Powers points out, seductive in that they provide a ready, non-demanding solution to the problem and further fit into our expectation that better living can be acquired through chemistry. Her analysis of the drugs available and their disappointing ability to provide easy solutions to the problem is a very valuable part of the book. She is equally cautious about recommending the surgical procedures which have been used.

The psychological treatment modalities are legion, and they have varying reported success rates. The problems mentioned above come into focus when they are related to the bread-and-butter matter of trying to look after these disturbed and unhappy people. Aversion conditioning, hypnosis, professionally directed and self-help group therapies, psychoanalysis, etc., have all been suggested and to some degree have helped. Stunkard and his co-workers have noted that psychoanalysis has resulted in improvements in patients who were in psychoanalysis and happened to be obese, but when this was mentioned at a recent meeting there was a snide wisecrack that when the patients had paid for their psychoanalyses, they couldn't afford food. The serious and significant thing is that the improvement in self-image apparently resulted in the ability to lose weight.

It is wise of Dr. Powers to encompass in this book the problems of over-eating and under-eating as though they are etiologically related which, of course, they are. Our patients with anorexia nervosa have repeatedly admonished us that they are not anorectic in the sense that they have no desire for food; they are dysorectic in the sense that they are preoccupied with food and use eating and non-eating as coping devices rather than as aids to nutrition. In this section of the book she has included, for the sake of completeness, Pica, Rumination, and the Eating Disorders associated with Disturbances of Sleep (the Klein-Levin and Pickwickian syndromes).

For the conditions grouped under the Anorexia Nervosa umbrella, she offers very practical classification and treatment suggestions. It has apparently become obvious that the "classical" anorexia nervosa described by Morton in 1689 is only one form of this fascinating illness; it is now designated as "primary anorexia nervosa" to distinguish it from other varieties and those related and similar eating disorders which derive from schizophrenia and the various neuroses.

A very significant—and hitherto poorly recognized—difficulty in the treatment of these patients is the tremendous benefit they derive from maintaining their emaciated state. Obviously, some of them are incapable of recognizing their body image as abnormal, but many of them are supported in their illness by friends and relatives who either regard them as admirable for their Vogue-model or ballerina contours or actually reward them for maintaining their illness. A mini-survey at the University of California at Santa Barbara revealed that while friends and relatives were concerned, they tended to regard the appearance of these patients as "attractive," "fashionable," etc. Dr. Powers comments on a patient with anorexia nervosa who derived great satisfaction from posing for life classes in sculpture, and we know another who, with the threat of a recurrence of the difficulty, has been able to achieve almost round-the-clock attention from her father, in addition to a whole series of glamorous trips abroad. The secondary gains in these situations are so blatant that eliminating them would seem to be an obvious and essential part of successful therapy, yet they have been inadequately emphasized in the past.

Dr. Powers has backed up her clinical discussions with much-needed biological, biochemical, and physiological data which have seldom been brought together in such an encyclopedic way. The over-fat and the over-lean patients, as well as their therapists, will be grateful for so complete an exposition.

C. H. Hardin Branch
Staff Psychiatrist
Student Health Service
University of California at Santa Barbara
Emeritus Clinical Professor of Psychiatry
University of Southern California

Preface

The goal of this book is to present the currently available information needed to offer the most effective treatment to obese patients. Primary care physicians including internists, family practitioners, pediatricians and psychiatrists are bombarded daily with new information about obesity. It is the aim of this book to provide a basic core of information about what is known and is not known about the etiology, effects, treatment and prevention of obesity. Thus, it is hoped that the practicing physician will be able to evaluate new data about obesity and integrate relevant aspects of this information into the day to day care of patients. Prevention and the cultural resistances to prevention are emphasized because current treatment modalities have thus far failed to make significant inroads into a national problem that is reaching epidemic proportions.

For most obese individuals, several factors converge to produce the symptom of obesity. It is the author's belief that attention to the multicausal nature of this condition may well improve effectiveness of treatment.

Pauline S. Powers

Acknowledgments

My heartfelt thanks to my husband Henry and our daughter Jessica who now both know more than they ever wanted to about obesity. Kathy Anello was of invaluable assistance in preparing the manuscript. Ursula Mahlendorf contributed valuable advice and assistance in the selection of some of the illustrations. George Maring kindly lent his original art work to illustrate the relationship one anorexia nervosa patient had with the world. Paul Montecalvo prepared most of the original illustrations. Finally, several faculty members at the University of South Florida offered useful criticism and advice.

Contents

CHAPTER

1

Definition and Classification of Obesity

DIFFICULTIES IN DEFINITION AND CLASSIFICATION

Obesity is the most prevalent, chronic, medical condition in our society and is directly or indirectly associated with a wide variety of diseases that collectively account for 15–20% of the mortality rate. In developed countries, approximately 35% of the adult population is obese, and there are indications that the prevalence is increasing. The medical and psychological literature on obesity is voluminous and confusing, and the lay literature on obesity ranges from the rational to the nonsensical. It is difficult for both the physician and the obese patient to choose clinically relevant data from this morass of information.

Part of the difficulty is that various studies define obesity in different ways, making comparison of results difficult. An increase in readily available, high-calorie, high-fat foods and a change to a more sedentary life style are among the cultural factors that contribute to the rising rate of obesity. Endocrine, metabolic, and psychological factors have also been implicated in the pathogenesis of obesity.

Another major problem is the classification of obesity. Obesity for which a specific cause cannot be found accounts for 95–97% of obese patients, and it has often been assumed that these patients are a homogeneous group. Many classification systems have been devised to subtype the obese population into groups that have some common characteristics. Although certain of these classification systems have provided useful information in evaluating various etiologies and treatments, it is well to remember that obesity is not an all-or-none condition and that the presence of some fat content is normal.

NECESSITY OF FAT FOR EVOLUTION

The metabolic ability to store energy in the form of fat represents a major evolutionary step forward. Immobile animals or those confined to water did not need to store energy for motility. To move around out of the water required a capacity to store energy, and fat synthesis is an effective mechanism to achieve this capacity. In man, for example, there are two major ways of storing energy. Small amounts of carbohydrates (78–80 g) are stored for energy reserves in the form of glycogen; in an emergency, glycogen can be catalyzed to glucose and then to lactate with the production of energy without the use of oxygen. For each gram of glycogen stored, 3–4 g of water must also be stored. Fat, however, can be stored with virtually no water. A 180-pound man with 30 pounds of fat would weigh 900 pounds if the energy in fat were stored as glycogen![1] Clearly, locomotion and, hence, survival would be drastically impaired at such weights. In one sense, then, fat synthesis has been paramount to survival and the evolutionary development of man.

VARIATION OF "NORMAL" FAT CONTENT

The amount of fat content that is normal depends, in part, on the environment. For example, Polynesians who made the Kon Tiki trip weighed an average of 250 pounds; since the trip involved 3 months of near starvation, a high content of stored energy in the form of fat was highly adaptive. At the other extreme are the Zulu tribe who must outrun the gazelle; their fat content is only 3% by weight. Zulus store just enough energy to be able to catch the gazelle, yet not impair their capacity to run. In our society, a woman of average height with only 3% fat content would weigh approximately 83 pounds and would probably be diagnosed as having anorexia nervosa. Although the Polynesians and Zulus are extreme examples, they highlight some of the difficulties in defining normal fat content.

The major methods of determining fat content and lean body mass will be outlined in the following discussion. Classification schemes which offer promise in elucidating the etiology of various obesities will be described as well as some of the practical, behavioral classification systems that have been used with some success in eating disorder clinics.

DETERMINATION OF BODY COMPOSITION

Body composition has been determined by a variety of direct and indirect methods. The only direct method is analysis of carcass composition and Bray[2] notes that this has been performed on but eight adult cadavers in the last 50 years. Indirect methods have included anthropometric measurements (for example, weight, height, and skinfold measurements), measurement of body density, dilutional techniques, and radiographic and ultrasound techniques. Each method has its disadvantages and only a few are applicable to the clinical situation. Various terms are utilized in evaluating the extent of obesity, and some terms are erroneously used interchangeably in studies of obesity, particularly those evaluating different methods of treatment.

DIFFERENCE BETWEEN OBESITY AND OVERWEIGHT

Obesity means an excess of body fat. Overweight means the body weight is in excess of some arbitrary standard. Although persons who are grossly overweight (above 250 pounds) are usually also overfat, at weights closer to the standard weights, this is not necessarily the case. Not only are some overweight persons actually underfat but, conversely, some underweight subjects are actually overfat. Since it may be that some of the dire consequences of obesity are actually related to an excess of fat rather than an excess of muscle or other body constituents, it is important that measures that estimate body fat, rather than just weight, be used whenever possible.

One dramatic example of the difference between overweight and obesity was demonstrated in a study of football players in 1942.[3] Seventeen professional football players whose average weights were well over 200 pounds were evaluated. Even in relation to his height, and even when he is considered in the "large frame" class, the 6-foot 200-pound lineman is at least 10% overweight by the usual ideal weight tables. However, these men had a greater than average specific gravity, indicating a lower than average fat content. Therefore, these football players who were overweight were actually underfat! Admittedly, this is an extreme example, and many people who weigh over 200 pounds are actually obese as well as overweight. However, a normal-weight, very sedentary person may actually be obese,[4] and this may be a greater public health hazard. To identify patients who fall into this latter category requires more sophisticated techniques than measurement of height and weight.

DETERMINATION OF BODY FAT FROM TOTAL BODY WEIGHT

Lean body mass (LBM) includes body solids and intracellular and extracellular water, and excludes body fat. Strictly speaking, LBM is defined as that fraction of body weight that is required to contain total body water at the percentage normally found in lean tissues. Since adipose tissue is assumed to be anhydrous, *fat-free body* and lean body mass are usually used synonymously (Fig. 1.1). Fat-free tissue is approximately 72% water.[5] Based on the two assumptions that adipose tissue is anhydrous and that lean body mass is 72% water, lean body mass in normal subjects can be calculated by

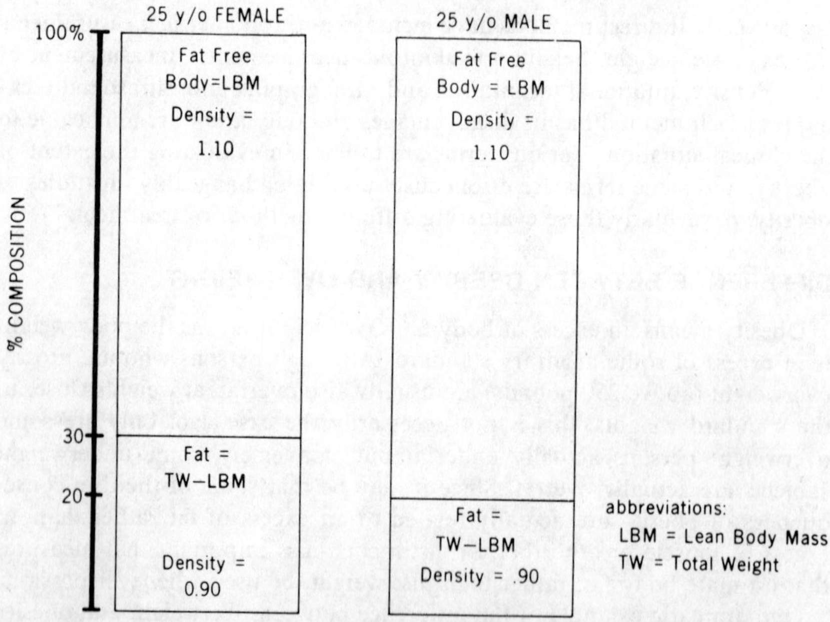

Figure 1.1. Fat content. Approximately 30% of the female body is fat and 20% of the male body.

this formula:

$$\text{LBM} = \text{total body water} \div 0.72$$

Therefore, a close approximation of body fat is:

$$\text{body fat} = \text{total weight} - \text{LBM}$$

or:

$$\text{body fat} = \text{total weight} - \text{total body water} \div 0.72$$

Total body water has been calculated using tritiated water (^3H_2O).[6] In this dilutional technique, a known volume of a known concentration of tritiated water is injected intravenously, and after equilibration (2–3 hours), blood samples are drawn and the concentration of tritium in the blood sample is determined. If the tritiated water equilibrates in the space termed total body water, then the volume of that space can be easily calculated using this formula:

$$(\text{concentration of injected } ^3H_2O) \times (\text{volume injected}) = (\text{total body water}) \times (\text{concentration of } ^3H_2O \text{ in blood sample}).$$

Figure 1.2 illustrates this principle.

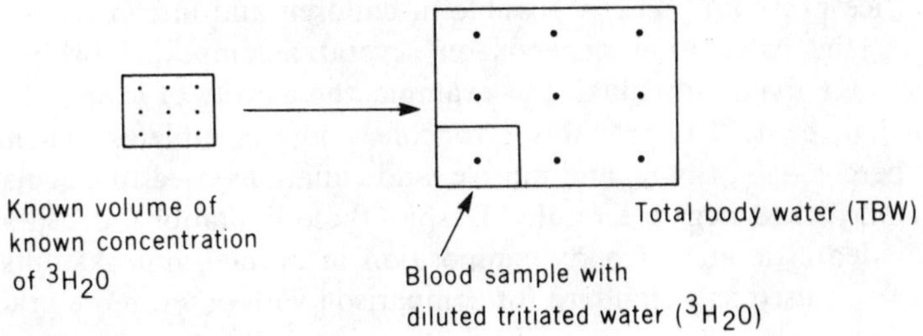

(Concentration injected ^3H_2O) (Volume injected) = (TBW) (Concentration ^3H_2O in sample)

Figure 1.2. Isotope dilution method used to determine total body water (adapted with permission from Bray,[2] p. 17).

There is a variety of problems with calculating body fat utilizing these methods. First, the assumption that lean body mass is 72% water is probably only true for healthy young adults. In infants, water content of lean body mass is probably higher than 72%,[7] and in the elderly it is probably less than 72%. Second, for routine clinical evaluation, measurement of total body water using any of the available dilutional techniques is impractical. However, these methods of calculating body fat are useful for establishing standards against which other methods can be compared.

DENSITOMETRY

The measurement of density is another technique that has been used to evaluate body composition. The basic principle of this method is that an object submerged in water displaces its own weight. If two objects of equal volume but different densities are submerged, the more dense object will displace a greater volume of water. Then, the density of each object can be calculated either by weighing the object before and after submersion or by measuring the volume of water displaced. In evaluation of body fat content, it is known that body fat is less dense than lean body mass. The density of fat at 36° C is approximately 0.9007[8] and the density of the non-fat body has been estimated to be 1.10.[4] Since fat is less dense than lean body mass, the greater the proportion of fat in the body, the smaller is the body density. Therefore, measurement of body density by underwater weighing provides an estimate of body fat. Various equations have been devised to estimate percentage of fat using body density measurements.[9] In using these equations, corrections must be made for residual lung volume which varies among individuals.

The difficulty with densitometry is that it is a method that is impractical as an office procedure and impossible in children and infirm adults. Furthermore, the calculation depends on several assumptions likely to be incorrect in a given individual. For example, the density of lean body mass estimated to be 1.10 is probably erroneously low in athletes that have a greater percentage of bone and muscle, and equations used to calculate fat content may yield negative results. Despite these limitations, densitometry has provided estimates of body composition in normal young adults and, again, can be used as a standard for comparison with other, more practical, methods.

In summary, densitometry and dilutional techniques have been used to estimate body composition in healthy young non-obese adults. In women, approximately 30% of the body is fat, whereas in men 20% of the body is fat.

ANTHROPOMETRIC METHODS OF MEASUREMENT

CRITERIA FOR VALID MEASURES

Anthropometric methods widely used to evaluate obesity include measurements of height, weight, skinfold thicknesses, and various body circumferences. There are two major requirements for any valid anthropometric measurement. The first is that a good index of obesity should have a low correlation with height since there is no *a priori* reason to assume that shorter individuals tend to be more or less obese than taller individuals. The second requirement for a good index of obesity is that it should correlate well with one of the accepted laboratory measurements of fat content, such as densitometry. In addition, to be clinically useful, the method selected should not only be a valid indicator of body fat, but should be reliable. Ideally, ancillary personnel should be able to replicate the measurement accurately.

W/H^2 BEST RELATIVE WEIGHT INDEX

There are three major types of relative weight indices. The first type includes weight (W) height (H) relationships such as W/H, W/H^2, or W^3/H. The second type is the "percentage overweight" for individuals of the same sex, height, and age; the standard weights used are those listed in the tables of the Metropolitan Life Insurance Company.[10] The third type involves calculating the fat-free mass (FFM) from regression equations.[6] Given an individual's weight (W) and height (H):

Men: $0.72\ FFM = 0.297W + 19.5H - 14.013$
Women: $0.72\ FFM = 0.184W + 34.5H - 35.270$

Body fat is then determined by subtracting the fat-free mass from body weight:

$$\text{body fat} = \text{body weight} - \text{fat-free mass (LBM)}$$

The problem with these equations is that generally they have not been extensively tested in groups with varying degrees of obesity.

Of the relative weight indices, weight divided by height squared (W/H^2) appears to be the most valid and reliable index of obesity.[11, 12] Other things being equal, W/H^2 (also termed the *body mass index*) shows the least correlation with height and the highest correlation with independent measures of body fat. Various relative weight indices were compared in 245 men and 324 women between the ages of 17 and 74.[12] W/H^2 correlated best with body fat estimated by densitometry. However, skinfold measurements were compared with the various relative weight indices, and skinfold measures were the most valid. If skinfold calipers are not available, W/H^2 is currently the best available index of obesity for clinical use. It does tend, however, to overestimate fat content in very lean individuals.

INACCURACY OF PONDERAL INDEX

The ponderal index[13] is the cube root of weight divided by height ($W^{0.33}/H$) and was devised to compare weight, a 3-dimensional entity, with height, a linear 1-dimensional measurement. The inverse of the ponderal index ($H/W^{0.33}$) was promulgated by Sheldon and colleagues in the somatotype studies,[14] and therefore is widely known. However, the ponderal index has been found to be highly correlated with height, and therefore, fails the first criterion for a valid index of obesity. For example, Keys and colleagues[11] cite the example of a 60-kg, 1.70-m tall man who gains 15 kg. He gains 25% in weight; the value of W/H changes in the same proportion, his body mass index (W/H^2) changes from 20.76 to 25.95, i.e. it increases by 25% also. But his ponderal index changes only from 2.3029 to 2.4807, an increase of only 7.7%. Therefore, the ponderal index, or its inverted form, is not independent of height.

SKINFOLD MEASUREMENTS

Of all the various indirect measures of body fat, the skinfold measurement offers the greatest promise in terms of validity, reliability, and practicality. About half the total body fat is deposited in the subcutaneous tissues and is readily available for observation and measurement. The body fat is deposited in a single sheet of tela adiposa which, in many parts of the body, is only loosely attached to the underlying tissue. Therefore, sometimes observation alone is sufficient to determine that the person is obese and in doubtful cases the physician can pinch the skin between the thumb and forefinger in various places and settle the question. The skinfold calipers were devised to put the manual pinching method on a more systematic basis that allows for comparison with other laboratory means of determining body fat.

SKINFOLD MEASUREMENTS THAT INDICATE OBESITY

There are marked age and sex differences in the distribution and amount of subcutaneous fat. For infants, children, and adolescents, relatively few broad epidemiological studies have been undertaken using skinfold measurements as the means of evaluating fat content. However, data from several studies[15–18] have been used to establish approximate upper limits of normal in children and adults. Table 1.1 shows the triceps skinfold thicknesses that usually indicate obesity.

The values for infants and children up to 5 years of age are less certain than for older children because they are derived from cross-sectional data, much of which is poorly controlled. Also, the "normal" fat content of infants and very young children is not known. Furthermore, this table is based on data drawn from an American population wherein obesity was defined as having a triceps skinfold measurement greater than one standard deviation from the mean. By definition, therefore, 16% of the population was defined as obese. Since longitudinal data for children are sketchy, it is not known with certainty if a higher body fat content in very early life portends later obesity. This table, then, is a very approximate guide for determining obesity at different ages. It has the great advantage of being independent of height or body frame.

Equations utilizing measurements of various fatfolds and circumferences have been derived to calculate actual fat content.[19] A nomogram has been devised for determining percentage of fat and body density from two fatfold measurements.[20] Although not necessary for most clinical work, these equations and nomograms will be useful in research and epidemiological surveys.

SKINFOLD THICKNESS VARIATIONS IN MEN AND WOMEN

There are sex differences in subcutaneous fat distribution which affect skinfold thickness. In adult men approximately 11% of body weight is subcutaneous tissue. In adult women approximately 18% of body weight is subcutaneous tissue.[21] These differences are reflected in skinfold measurements that are larger in non-obese women than in non-obese men. Sex differences in the distribution of subcutaneous fat are pronounced at puberty and afterwards, but have been detected even at birth.

In newborn girls skinfold thickness over the hips is significantly greater than in boys and this difference persists even during the period of weight loss from the 2nd to the 5th postnatal day.[22]

CALIPERS AVAILABLE FOR SKINFOLD MEASUREMENT

Although skinfold measurement is in itself a very simple procedure, it must be performed under standard conditions to be valid. The two major

Table 1.1
Upper limits of normal triceps skinfold measurements. Measurements over these values suggest obesity.

AGE	MALES		FEMALES
BIRTH		10 MM	
3 MONTHS		11 MM	
6 MONTHS		14 MM	
9 MONTHS		15 MM	
12 MONTHS	15 MM		16 MM
2 YEARS	14		15
3 YEARS	13		14.5
4 YEARS	12.5		14
5 YEARS	12		14
6 YEARS	12		14
7 YEARS	12		15
8 YEARS	12.5		16
9 YEARS	13		18
10 YEARS	15		19
11 YEARS	17		20
12 YEARS	18		21
13 YEARS	18		21
14 YEARS	17		21
15 YEARS	15		23
16 YEARS	14.5		24
17 YEARS	15		24
18 YEARS	16		25
19 YEARS	17		27
20 YEARS	17		28
21 YEARS	17		28
22 YEARS	18		28
23 YEARS	18		28
24 YEARS	19		28
25 YEARS	20		29
26 YEARS	20		29
27 YEARS	21		29
28 YEARS	22		29
29 YEARS	22		29
30-50 YEARS	23		30

instruments available for measuring skinfolds are the Harpenden caliper and the Lange caliper. The Lange caliper (Fig. 1.3) is the only one commercially produced in the United States. Its current cost is approximately $120.00. The Harpenden caliper is produced in England and is slightly more expensive. Certain plastic calipers (for example, the Ponderax) have inadequate springs and incorrect tension. An Arthrogauge is in the testing phase; it is a flat sheet of plastic with notches for accomodating different size fatfolds. Currently, however, either the Lange caliper or Harpenden caliper is the most useful since standards for obesity have been established with these instruments.

TRICEPS SKINFOLD VS. OTHER SITES

Selection of the skinfold site remains controversial. The skinfold overlying the main point of the triceps of the left arm has been used most frequently in large epidemiological studies, and most available studies establishing the upper limits of normal at different ages are based on this measurement. The triceps skinfold has the great advantage of easy accessability, not requiring that the patient disrobe. Other sites have been used including points over the

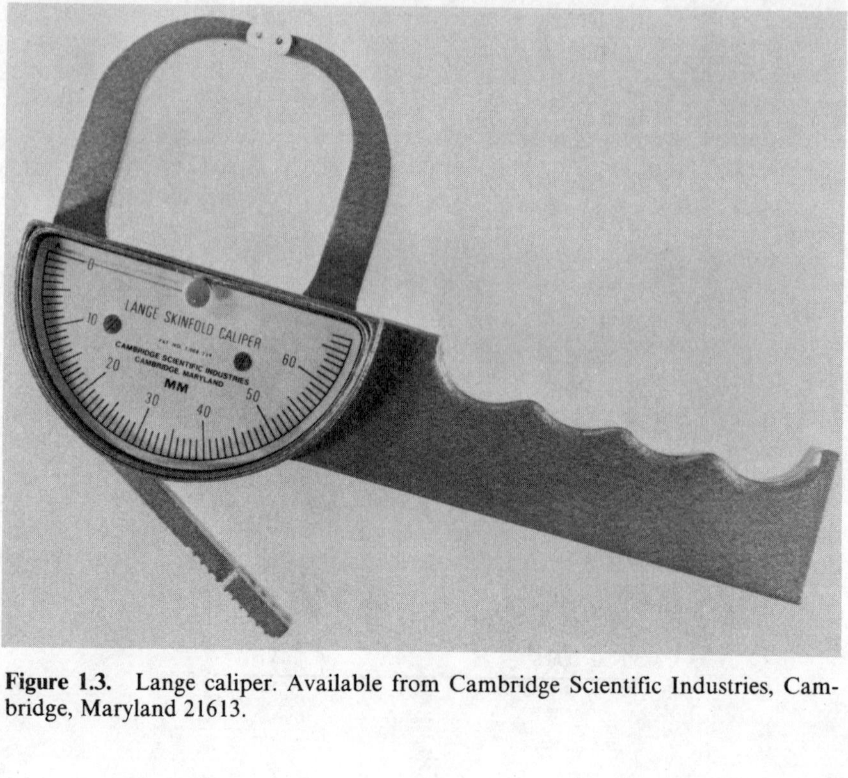

Figure 1.3. Lange caliper. Available from Cambridge Scientific Industries, Cambridge, Maryland 21613.

biceps muscle, above the iliac crest, immediately under the costal margin, and close to the umbilicus.

In studies on the distribution of subcutaneous fat, Edwards[23, 24] selected 53 sites as representative of the body and offering good repeatability. When the measurements of these 53 sites are totaled, the average for young women of average height and weight is 640 mm. For men, the total of all 53 skinfold measurements is 412 mm. This is but another demonstration that fat content in women is greater than in men, but for clinical purposes measurement of 53 sites is impractical.

The major problem with the triceps skinfold is that accurate determination of the midpoint of a left triceps is difficult, and an error in placement of the caliper can result in markedly skewed readings. Some investigators have recommended that the subscapular skinfold be used because fat is distributed more uniformly; therefore, placement of the caliper is not as critical and measurements are most easily reproduced, even by relatively inexperienced investigators. However, in terms of validity, the triceps skinfold measurement correlates more closely with density values obtained from underwater weighings than does the subscapular skinfold measurement.[15, 25] Some studies[26, 27] show a higher correlation between density values and the subscapular skinfold measurement than between density values and the triceps skinfold measurement. However, the subjects were from general non-obese populations.

The triceps skinfold measurement is the best to select if only one measurement is to be made. If measurement of two sites is feasible, the triceps and subscapular skinfolds are the best choices.

PROCEDURE FOR MEASUREMENT OF SKINFOLDS

The skinfold caliper to be used should be calibrated to exert a pressure of about 10 g/mm^2 and the pressure should be constant over a range of openings from 2–40 mm. The Lange caliper has a jaw surface which consists of a mobile flat metal piece, and care is required to prevent misalignment. The contact surface between the jaw of the caliper and the skin should be from 20–40 mm. Readings are made to the nearest 0.5 mm.

Measurement of the triceps skinfold is as follows (see Fig. 1.4 *A* and *B*). A small mark is made on the left upper arm halfway between the tip of the olecranon and the tip of the acromial process with the arm flexed at a 90 degree angle. On young children this midpoint often appears higher than expected and is not necessarily at the point of the widest arm circumference. A line is drawn vertically above the olecranon to cross the midpoint. The subject's arm then hangs straight and relaxed for the measurement. The examiner uses his left thumb and index finger to grasp and lift the triceps skinfold parallel with the long axis of the arm about ½ inch proximal to the

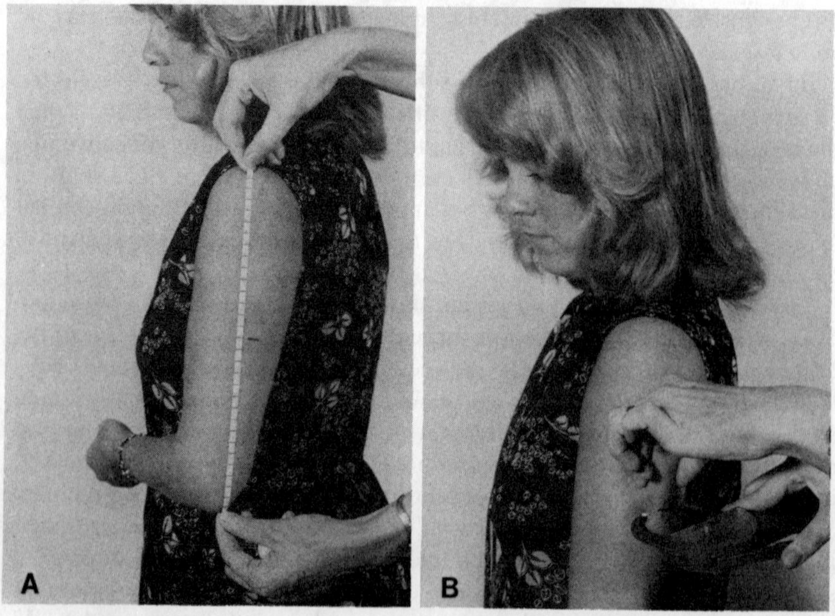

Figure 1.4. Procedure for determining triceps skinfold measurement.

cross mark. The calipers are applied to the fold below the fingers so that the pressure at the point measured is exerted by the caliper tips, not the fingers. If the deep fatfold appears anchored to the intermuscular septum, or if the main bulk of the triceps muscle is not directly felt with the thumb and forefinger just deep to the fatfold, the position should be rechecked as it is probably too medial or too lateral. In infants, the muscle-subcutaneous fat interface must be clearly identified because the calipers are often placed too deep. The dial should be read 2–3 seconds after the caliper tips are placed on the fatfold. Two readings at the selected site are made and the average recorded.

Whenever feasible, the subscapular fatfold can also be measured. Again, the left side should be used. The fatfold below the tip of the scapula is located and the same procedure followed. Precise localization of the site for this measurement is less critical than for the triceps fatfold measurement.

SOURCES OF MEASUREMENT ERRORS

Measurement of skinfolds, particularly the triceps fatfold, is subject to a number of technical errors.[28] These include: use of the wrong arm, incorrect measurement of the mid-arm point, and incorrect placement of the caliper tips. The common errors are itemized in Table 1.2. One group[29] found a

Table 1.2
Errors in triceps skinfold measurement (adapted from Zerfas et al[28]).

- Wrong arm (should be left)
- Midpoint of arm or posterior plane incorrectly measured or marked
- Arm not loose by side during measurement
- Examiner not comfortable
- Finger-thumb pinch or caliper placement too deep (muscle) or too superficial (skin)
- Caliper jaws not at marked site
- Reading done too early or too late (should be 2 to 3 seconds)
- At time of reading, pinch not maintained or caliper handle not fully released

wide variability in recorded triceps fatfold measurements among three observers who measured skinfold thickness in 21 subjects three times. Therefore, careful attention to detail by experienced observers is necessary for reliable clinical use with obese patients.

OTHER MEASUREMENT METHODS

Some investigators have measured various diameters to estimate body fatness. Measurement of the mid-upper arm circumference has been widely used in developing countries, primarily to evaluate undernutrition in children.[30] However, mid-upper arm circumference could easily be used to evaluate obesity. The mid-point of the left upper arm is obtained in the same way as for the triceps skinfold measurement. The tape is applied to the skin around the entire arm at a snug tension but not so tightly applied as to cause an indentation. This method has the advantage of requiring very inexpensive equipment (less than $1.00 as compared to $120.00 for the Lange caliper).

Steinkamp and colleagues[31] have found close correlations between measurements of several body diameters and densitometry. In their investigation, they used 20 measurements including height and weight, 14 different diameters and circumferences, and 4 skinfold measurements. Correlation of these 20 anthropometric measures with density estimates of body fat was high, r = 0.98. However, measurement of these circumferences is time-consuming and must be replicated precisely for accurate estimates of body fat. Therefore, the method of measuring several body diameters and circumferences is not in wide clinical use.

Ultrasound and radiographic techniques have been used to estimate fat content. Soft x-rays can be useful in assessing the thickness of subcutaneous fat. Since fat is less dense than muscle and other components of lean body mass, fat is more opaque on x-rays. Estimates of body fat from skinfold measurements were found to correlate highly with estimates of fat from x-rays.[32] However, radiation dose limits the usefulness of this technique. Hawes and colleagues[33] have compared estimates of fat content using ultrasound, radiography, skinfold, and thigh circumference measurements over the greater trochanter and iliac crest. There are close correlations between radiography and skinfold or circumference measures. The authors conclude that ultrasound may provide the safest, most valid estimates of subcutaneous fat.

In summary, probably the single most valid clinical method of assessing obesity is the triceps skinfold measurement. It is much more likely to assess actual fat content than are any of the relative weight charts, even those which attempt to incorporate an estimate of somatotype. Its major drawback is that expertise is required to obtain reliable readings.

CLASSIFICATION OF OBESITY

A number of schemes for classifying obesity have been devised. The following discussion will emphasize those which are the most useful clinically and those which may prove useful in understanding the etiology or pathogenesis of obesity. The plethora of classification systems reflects both our lack of knowledge about obesity and the fact that there are probably several different types of obesity which have different causes. Some of the proposed systems reflect the widespread judgmental attitude toward obesity. For example, Zondek[34] divided obesity into three types: elementary (gluttony), endocrine (thyroid, pituitary, genital, pineal, pancreatic), and localized (lipomatosis). Classifying the most common form of obesity as the elementary or gluttony type intensifies the negative attitude toward the obese patient and serves little useful purpose. The major classification schemes to be discussed include the anatomical, descriptive, and etiological methods.

HYPERCELLULAR VS. NORMOCELLULAR OBESITY

The anatomical classification of obesity into hypercellular and normocellular types is based on the work of Hirsch and Knittle[35] and Bjorntörp.[36] Obese subjects are classified as normocellular if they have the normal number of fat cells and as hypercellular if the number of fat cells is increased. Since all fat people have enlarged adipocytes, both types are "hypertrophic."

The theoretical basis underlying this classification system is discussed fully in Chapter 7, but, briefly, is as follows. Fat cell number normally increases rapidly during the last trimester of fetal life, during the first 6 months of infancy, and during adolescence from approximately ages 11–13. There is a continuing increase in fat cell number during all of childhood, but the rate of increase is less than at these three periods. Fat cells probably continue to increase after age 13, but at a slower rate until the late teens or early 20's when the normal complement of fat cells has been attained. After this time, most increase in adipose tissue is due to an increase in fat cell size rather than in the number of fat cells. Several studies have found that most massively obese patients had the onset of obesity during childhood. Other studies have found that with weight reduction by diet or exercise there is a decrease in fat cell size but not in fat cell number. Therefore, an abnormal increase in number of fat cells during childhood and adolescence has been thought to predispose to later obesity which is likely to be very resistant to treatment. The implication is that obesity which starts in childhood, particularly at these critical periods, will result in an increased number of fat cells and that weight loss in later life will only result in a decrease in the size of fat cells, not a decrease in the number of cells. Therefore, the metabolic machinery for maintaining this increased number of fat cells would be present even when the individual was slim. This might well predispose to reaccumulation of the weight that was lost, a notoriously common occurrence in obese patients.

JUVENILE ONSET: CONSTITUTIONAL VS. SYMPTOMATIC

A second classification scheme described by Court[37, 38] and Bray[39] is based on the assumption that certain forms of obesity may be due to genetic or constitutional factors. Court describes constitutional and symptomatic obesity, both of which start in childhood, but which have very different courses.

Constitutional obesity usually starts in infancy and is often familial. When these children's weights are plotted on growth charts, the weight gain runs parallel to, but above, the normal growth pattern (Fig. 1.5). These youngsters usually have good social, school, and emotional adjustment. Triglyceride levels are normal, as are free fatty acids and glycerol levels. These children usually do not eat more than slim children although they may be less active. It may be very difficult for these children to lose weight and sustain the weight loss since they would have to maintain a severely restricted diet or consistently increase their physical activity. Court postulates that the constitutionally obese youngsters may have a high physiological set point as postulated by Nisbett (see Chapter 5), and attempts to lose weight may result in a chronic state of starvation. Active treatment of these youngsters may actually be harmful since weight loss may be physiologically extremely difficult and the child may be criticized unduly when failure occurs. In these youngsters the best treatment may be to help the child adjust to his body habitus and counsel the family to accept the youngster as he is.

Symptomatic obesity is a symptom of an underlying physical or emotional disorder. It may begin any time in childhood and there may be precipitating factors. Obesity may occur rapidly and there is usually no relationship to the

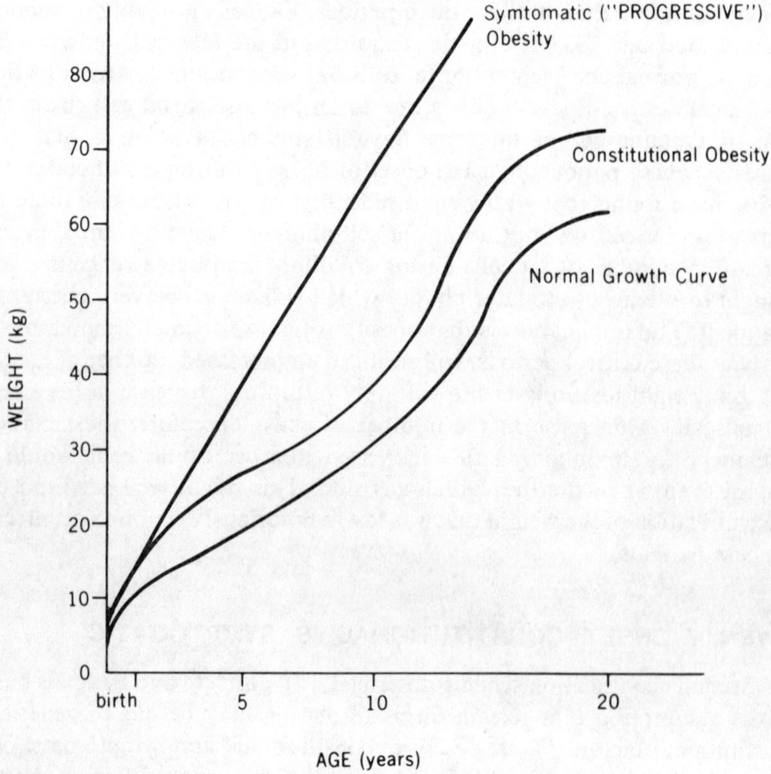

Figure 1.5. Constitutional vs. symptomatic obesity.

normal growth curve (see Fig. 1.5). These youngsters usually have school problems and emotional disturbances. This group is markedly less active than their non-obese peers. Also, there is evidence that triglyceride levels are elevated and that free fatty acids and glycerol levels are reduced. Bray[39] describes a variant, which he terms "progressive" obesity, in which the incremental weight gain each year is approximately the same, resulting in weights as high as 300 pounds or more. To increase their weight each year, these progressively obese patients are probably continually eating more than their body requires.

Classifying most obese youngsters as either "constitutional" or "symptomatic" is undoubtedly an oversimplification. However, it does emphasize the facts that not all obese children have severe emotional disturbances and that treatment can be detrimental.

REGULATORY VS. METABOLIC OBESITY

A third method of classifying obesity is based on mechanisms of development of obesity (i.e. pathogenesis). This method, based primarily on animal studies, has been promulgated by Jean Mayer.[40] "Regulatory obesities" are those in which the primary disorder is impairment of the mechanisms regulating food intake, and "metabolic" obesities are those in which there is an inborn or acquired error in the metabolism of tissues.

Animals that have bilateral destruction of the ventromedial nucleus of the hypothalamus (VMN) and that subsequently become obese have "regulatory" obesity, according to this classification system. Patients with craniopharyngiomas that destroy parts of the hypothalamus and become obese also have a type of "regulatory" obesity. In these two examples, the distinction between etiology and pathogenesis is important. In the experimental animal with VMN destruction, the cause of obesity is trauma, and in the human example the cause is tumor growth. However, the pathogenesis in both examples is the same: the VMN, the so-called satiety center, is not functioning, and food intake is not correctly regulated.

The "metabolic obesities" are best exemplified by genetically obese rodents. At this writing, at least 13 varieties of rodents with a genetic predisposition to obesity have been identified. Perhaps the best known is the fatty rat described by Zucker[41] in which obesity is transmitted by an autosomal recessive trait. There are various endocrine and metabolic abnormalities in these fatty rats which are probably not all due to hyperphagia (excessive food intake). For example, Zucker fatty rats pair-fed the same amounts as normal lean rats have an increased fat cell size as well as elevated serum insulin. The exact etiology of these obesities has yet to be identified, but it is probably a biochemical alternation in nuclear DNA, resulting in defective coding of an enzyme involved in lipolysis or lipogenesis. Initially, Mayer classified these obese rodents as an example of "metabolic" obesities on the basis of the pathogenesis. As more is learned about the genetics, the etiology as well as the pathogenesis may be elucidated. Although these rodent studies may not be relevant to the great majority of patients with obesity, there may be some specific subtypes of human obesity that have similar metabolic consequences from genetic defects. The Prader-Willi syndrome and the Laurence-Moon-Bardet-Biedl syndrome in children may be examples.

PSYCHOLOGICAL CLASSIFICATION

Body Image

Body image is a concept that pervades the literature on the psychological aspects of obesity. It refers to one's physical, emotional, and interpersonal view of one's self. Body image is an internal model that has physical and emotional components. The physical aspect is analogous to a 3-dimensional inner blueprint of one's actual size and shape, as well as the spatial relationship between all parts of one's body. The emotional aspect of body image is the sum of all the attitudes one has about one's body. Inaccuracies in the physical aspect of body image may occur in obese patients; some may believe their actual dimensions are larger or smaller than they really are. Also, an obese person may have a negative emotional feeling about his body and believe it is loathesome or grotesque. However, many obese patients do not have disturbances in body image. These individuals gauge their size correctly and consider their bodies attractive to themselves and others.

Probably 40–50% of obese individuals have no disturbance in either the perceptual or attitudinal aspect of body image.[42] However, accurate estimates are difficult to obtain, particularly when patient populations are studied. Medical consultations may be sought more frequently by obese patients with disturbances in body image. Obese subjects who respond to advertisements for research projects may be more prone to abnormalities in body image. In any case, the salient point is that, contrary to cultural expectations, not all obese subjects have disturbances in body image.

Psychological Disturbance in One-Third of Obese

Several classification systems are based on theories of different types of emotional disturbances in obese patients. A common defect of most of these systems is that they are based on biased subject selection. Such theories are derived from intense studies of obese patients who come to psychiatrists for treatment and, therefore, may not be representative of the general obese population. Although it is difficult to determine the amount of emotional disturbance in any population, probably about one-third of the obese population suffers from emotional problems. However, there is apparently little difference in the amount of emotional disturbance when obese and non-obese groups are compared. A broad epidemiological study in 1962[43] reported a slightly higher incidence of emotional disturbance in the obese, and a recent study by Crisp and McGuiness[44] reported slightly less emotional disturbance among the obese patients that they studied than among the non-obese. Furthermore, it is difficult to determine whether the emotional disturbance found is related to the obesity or to other factors. Even when the emotional disturbance seems to be related to the obesity, it is difficult to determine if it is the cause or the consequence of the obesity. Nonetheless, some obese patients do have emotional disturbances and the following classification system may be clinically useful.

Reactive vs. Developmental Obesity (Bruch)

Bruch,[45, 46] a psychiatrist who has been studying the eating disorders for several decades, has divided obesity into three major types: constitutional, reactive, and developmental. *Constitutional obesity*, as noted earlier, is presumably due to genetic or physiological causes and is usually associated with normal personality development. Reactive and developmental obesities, however, are associated with emotional maladjustment.

In *reactive obesity* Bruch postulates that the person overeats in response to tension or anxiety. Eating is thought to somehow compensate for, and relieve, emotional conflict. In addition, the same emotional factors that trigger an increase in food intake may also result in a drastic reduction of physical activity. In these patients, therefore, episodes of depression or grief result in marked increases in weight. Since these patients are also prone to recurrent depressions, a significant amount of weight may be gained over the course of a few years. Bruch believes that this type of obesity is more common in adulthood than in childhood. If it does occur in childhood, clear precipitating factors can usually be identified.

Developmental obesity, like reactive obesity, is associated with emotional problems but begins in childhood and has a more ominous psychological import. Bruch believes that these youngsters grow up in a family setting where they are used by one or both parents as an object to fulfill the needs of the parent and to compensate for failure and frustration in the parent's own life. According to this theory, from birth there are two types of behavior: behavior that originates in the infant and behavior in the infant in response to stimuli. The family producing the disturbed patient does not respond appropriately to cues from the child and overprotects and overfeeds the child in order to meet its own needs.

Generally, the mother plays the dominant role in such families and keeps the obese child close to her by constant and excessive demands. Overfeeding the child comes not from love and caring but comes from the parent's need for continuing symbiotic bonds with the child.

Since feeding is often a response to the parent's emotional needs, rather than to the child's hunger, these obese patients grow up confused about their own body urges and may be unable to distinguish hunger from anxiety or other emotional states. The pathological bond between mother and child is postulated to result in a deficient sense of separateness in these obese patients, thus promoting feelings of helplessness and inadequacy. Bruch thinks that the psychodynamic factors in these youngsters are similar to those in patients with schizophrenia and contends that the core problem, a deficient sense of separateness, is the same.

THIN FAT PEOPLE

"Thin fat people" is a term coined by Bruch[47] to describe obese patients who have lost weight but remain preoccupied with food and weight.

These people, usually women, have succeeded in staying slim but continue to have unresolved emotional conflicts. In fact, their conflicts are often worse when they are slender because overeating may have been a defense that helped them maintain a precarious emotional balance. Characteristically, these "thin fat people" focus the majority of their attention on their appearance and may be very critical of others, particularly members of their own family, who are unable to remain slim. Bruch makes the point that overeating and obesity are complex phenomena and that it is unwise to assume that overweight is an unmitigated evil. Furthermore, she believes that society's harsh negative attitude toward obesity prevents recognition of these "thin fat people." Because they are fashionably thin, their need for medical attention may be overlooked. The psychological cost of slimness in such individuals may be exorbitant. "Thin fat people" and anorexia nervosa patients are similar in that both groups are preoccupied with weight, food, and dieting. However, in anorexia nervosa the preoccupation is more intense and pervades all areas of the patient's life. Also, in anorexia nervosa the patient may be delusional about his/her body size, which is misperceived as larger than it really is. Despite these differences, Bruch believes that anorexia nervosa can be conceptualized as the end stage of the unrealistic preoccupation with weight and size that characterizes our society. "Thin fat people" are closer on the continuum to anorexia nervosa than to the general population.

BINGE-EATING SYNDROME (BULIMIA)

A related but distinct problem is the "binge-eating syndrome," also termed bulimia. It was first described as a distinct entity by Stunkard in 1959[48] and recently has been incorporated into the diagnostic nomenclature for psychiatric conditions.[49] There are three prime characteristics of the syndrome. First, there is impulsive, unpredictable, episodic, uncontrolled, and rapid ingestion of large quantities of food within a short time. Second, the episode terminates when physical discomfort occurs. Self-induced vomiting is common. Third, the episode is followed by feelings of guilt and self-contempt. These patients may or may not have an associated weight problem.

In a group of 20 subjects with the binge-eating syndrome,[50] half were of normal weight using the Metropolitan Insurance Company's height-weight tables. Four subjects had a history of anorexia nervosa.

Differentiating anorexia nervosa and the "binge-eating syndrome" is difficult, and occasionally the two syndromes may merge. Although body image disturbances have been more rigorously studied in anorexia nervosa, probably some patients with bulimia also have perceptual and attitudinal disturbances in body image. Figure 1.6, drawn by a patient with bulimia, but of normal weight, illustrates the point. Also, the obsessive rumination about weight, food, and dieting that occurs in "thin fat people" may be associated with bulimic episodes. In fact, one of the patients described by Bruch[47] could probably be diagnosed as having bulimia. (See Chapter 10 for further details.)

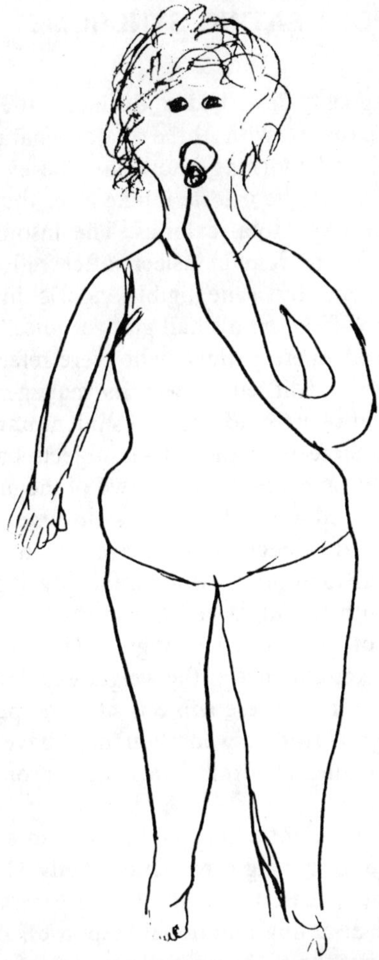

Figure 1.6. DRAW-A-PERSON TEST by patient with bulimia (the "binge-eating syndrome"). She was of normal weight but considered herself grotesquely fat during periods of frequent binges.

In terms of prevalence, the binge-eating syndrome probably accounts for a very small percentage of the obese population. It is apparently an uncommon, but not rare, condition. It is important to identify such patients because there is some evidence[50, 51] that treatment with phenytoin (Dilantin) results in a decrease in the number and severity of the binges in some patients. Nonspecific EEG abnormalities have been identified in approximately one-third of the patients studied,[50] but reduction in binges during treatment with phenytoin was not correlated with improvement in the EEG findings.

NIGHT-EATING SYNDROME

Stunkard and colleagues[52] described a distinct pattern of food intake among certain obese patients with three major characteristics: evening hyperphagia, insomnia, and morning anorexia. The evening hyperphagia was considered present when the caloric intake after the evening meal was greater than 25% of the day's total calories. The insomnia noted was an inability to fall asleep or to remain asleep after retiring. The morning anorexia was characterized by a negligible caloric intake at breakfast, including no more than coffee and a small glass of juice.

This study evaluated 25 obese patients who were referred because of the severity of their obesity, or difficulty with its management. The control group consisted of 38 non-obese graduate and student nurses who had never had a weight problem. Sixteen of the obese subjects had all three of the major criteria of the syndrome, and four had two of the major criteria. None of the control group reported the night-eating syndrome. Although many of the non-obese subjects had a snack after the evening meal, none consumed even close to 25% of their total daily caloric intake during this time.

The obese patients with the night-eating syndrome reported that it was associated with periods of stress and weight gain. The authors conclude that the syndrome is not the consequence of the weight gain but rather a response to stress that occurs in certain obese subjects at some periods of their life. Although the obese subjects studied were thought to have other responses to stress, when the night-eating syndrome was most pronounced, it was in association with stress.

The 20 patients with the night-eating syndrome had a marked incidence of untoward responses during weight reduction. Only 11 of the 20 patients had been able to lose more than one third of their excess weight, and eight of these had associated disabling emotional responses. By contrast, of the five obese subjects without the night-eating syndrome, four had lost significant amounts of weight without an emotional complication. The night-eating syndrome did not occur at all times during the lives of these obese patients, and the authors speculate that weight loss might be attempted during periods when the syndrome was absent and perhaps might obviate the possibility of untoward emotional responses.

In an unpublished report of 26,000 patients in the Eating Disorders Clinic at Johns Hopkins Medical Institutions, Simonson[53] reported that at least three variants of the night-eating syndrome have been detected. In one case, the patient eats little all day ands often believes that there is no harm in eating in the evenings. From about 7:00 to 11:00 p.m. the person may consume up to 5000 calories composed primarily of starches and carbohydrates. These patients may appear frantic to lose weight; yet, paradoxically, they are reported to have poor motivation. In the second case, the mid-evening snacker is relaxed after the problems of the day are over and he/she may unconsciously decide on a food reward at about 10:00 p.m. In this instance, Simonson postulates that the food may be used as a tranquilizer. In the third, the very late-night-eater awakens from sleep and has a snack. Often, these patients will hide the food. The reason for this very late-night-eating pattern is unclear and reportedly resistant to change. Although Simonson's report is interesting, no further details are yet available, and it is not certain that the patients described have the classic night-eating syndrome initially reported by Stunkard.

COMPARISON OF BULIMIA AND NIGHT-EATING SYNDROME

Stunkard[48] has detailed the differences between the night-eating syndrome and bulimia (the binge-eating syndrome). In both, there is a relationship to stress, but in bulimia there is associated self-condemnation and an apparent personal meaning to the binge. The patient with the binge-eating syndrome can often describe the stress that precipitated the binge.

One 24-year-old woman we have seen with the binge-eating syndrome gained 25 pounds while visiting her boyfriend and his family in Syria. There was a hazardous political situation with armed guerrillas in the streets, and the patient's boyfriend had told his parents that he and the patient were already married. In fact, the patient was undecided about whether to marry anyone or not, was afraid to contradict her boyfriend, and didn't speak the language well enough to clarify the situation with his parents, who also forbade her to leave the home for fear she would get lost or hurt. She became angry, yet was unable to extricate herself from this situation and had many uncontrollable binges in which she ate everything available unless she was interrupted by her boyfriend or developed abdominal pain. She was very remorseful after each binge and wrote many letters to her psychiatrist pleading for assistance in controlling her binges. Eventually she married her boyfriend, returned home, and was experiencing less stress and very few binges, but by that time she had gained the 25 pounds.

Patients with the night-eating syndrome may have apparent psychiatric problems and may express concern about their obesity but do not report severe self-condemnation about the evening hyperphagia. In the three case reports of the night-eating syndrome described by Stunkard and colleagues,[48, 52] there were apparent psychiatric problems but a striking absence of self-condemnation about the disordered eating pattern itself.

It is possible that the two conditions differ in the frequency of body image disturbance, but this has not yet been systematically studied. Perhaps bulimia patients are more prone to misperceptions about body size and negative attitudes toward their appearance than are patients with the night-eating syndrome.

SUMMARY

Although there are various classification systems for obesity which overlap each other, it seems likely that certain subtypes are actually separate diseases, e.g., the binge-eating syndrome or the night-eating syndrome. The normocellular-hypercellular concept of obesity has great potential in the prevention of obesity. The "regulatory" and "metabolic" obesities probably occur in pure form only in animals, but animal models can be useful in research that may eventually be applicable to human obesity. Classification systems which include careful descriptions of quantifiable behavior are likely to be very useful clinically.

References

1. Cahill G: Internist's overview of obesity. Lecture at conference: The Management of Obesity. Johns Hopkins Medical Institutions, Feb 13–16, 1978.
2. Bray GA: The Obese Patient. Philadelphia, WB Saunders, 1976, p 5.
3. Welham WC, Behnke AR Jr: The specific gravity of healthy men; body weight divided by volume and other physical characteristics of exceptional athletes and of naval personnel. JAMA 118: 498–501, 1942.
4. Keys AJ, Brozek J: Body fat in adult men. Physiol Rev 33: 245–325, 1953.
5. Pace N, Rathbun EN: Studies on body composition: body water and chemically combined nitrogen content in relation to fat content. J Biol Chem 158: 685–691, 1945.
6. Hume R, Weyers E: Relationship between total body water and surface area in normal and obese subjects. J Clin Pathol 24: 234–238, 1971.
7. Flynn MA, Hanna F, Long CH, et al: Deuterium-oxide dilution as a predictor of body composition in children and pigs. In: Body Composition in Animals and Man. Proceedings of a Symposium May 4–6, 1967, at University of Missouri, Publication No 1598, National Academy of Science, Washington DC, 1968, pp 480–491.
8. Brozek J, Grande F, Anderson JT, Keys A: Densitometric analysis of body composition: revision of some quantitative assumptions. Ann NY Acad Sci 110: 113–140, 1963.
9. Siri WE: Body composition from fluid spaces and density: analysis of methods. University of California Radiation Publication No 3349, 1956.
10. Metropolitan Life Insurance Co: New weight standards for men and women. Stat Bull Metropol Life Ins Co 40: 1–10, 1959.
11. Keys A, Fidanza F, Karvonen MJ, et al: Indices of relative weight and obesity. J Chron Dis 25: 329–343, 1972.
12. Womersley J, Durnin JVGA: A comparison of the skinfold method with extent of overweight and various weight-height relationships in the assessment of obesity. Br J Nutr 38: 271–284, 1977.
13. Livi R: L'indice ponderale o il rapporto tra la statura e il peso. Atti Soc Romana Antrop 5: 125–153, 1897.
14. Sheldon WH, Stephens SS, Tucker CB: The Varieties of Human Physique: An Introduction to Constitutional Psychology. New York, Harper and Row, 1940.
15. Seltzer CC, Mayer J: A simple criterion of obesity. Postgrad Med 38: A101–107, 1965.
16. Tanner JM, Whitehouse RH: Standards for subcutaneous fat in British children. Br Med J 1: 446–450, 1962.
17. Foman SJ: Infant Nutrition. Ed 2. Philadelphia, WB Saunders Co, 1974, pp 35–37.
18. Ten State Nutrition Survey, 1968–70 US Dept HEW Pub (HSM) July 1972, pp 72–78.
19. Durnin JVGA, Womersley J: Body fat assessed from total body density and its estimation from skinfold thickness: measurements on 481 men and women aged from 16 to 72 years. Br J Nutr 32: 77–97, 1974.

20. Sloan SW, Weir JB: Nomograms for prediction of body fat from skinfold measurements. J Appl Physiol 28: 221–222, 1970.
21. Wilmer HA: Quantitative growth of skin in relation to human surface area. Proc Soc Exp Biol Med 43: 386–388, 1940.
22. Huenemann RL: 1. Obesity in six-month-old children: environmental factors associated with preschool obesity. J Am Diet Assoc 64: 480–487, 1974.
23. Edwards DAW: Observations of the distribution of subcutaneous fat. Clin Sci 9: 259–270, 1950.
24. Edwards DAW: Differences in the distribution of subcutaneous fat with sex and maturity. Clin Sci 10: 305–315, 1951.
25. Seltzer CC, Mayer J: Greater reliability of the triceps skinfold over the subscapular skinfold as an index of obesity. Am J Clin Nutr 20: 950–953, 1967.
26. Parizkova J: Total body fat and skinfold thickness in children. Metabolism 10: 794–807, 1961.
27. Young CM, Blondin J, Tensuan R, Fryer JH: Body composition of "older" women thirty to seventy years of age. Ann NY Acad Sci 110: 589–607, 1963.
28. Zerfas AJ, Shorr IJ, Neumann CG: Office assessment of nutritional status. In: Nutrition in Pediatrics. Neumann CG, Jelliffee DB (eds). Pediatr Clin North Am 24: 253–272, 1977.
29. Burkinshaw L, Jones PR, Krupowicz DW: Observer error in skinfold thickness measurements. Hum Biol 45: 273–279, 1973.
30. Jelliffee DB: Assessment of nutritional status of the community. Geneva, WHO Monogr Ser, Vol 53, 1966.
31. Steinkamp RC, Cohen NL, Siri SW, et al: Measures of body fat and related factors in normal adults. I. Introduction and methodology. J Chron Dis 18: 1279–1289, 1965.
32. Garn SM: Roentgenogrammetric determinations of body composition. Hum Biol 29: 337–353, 1957.
33. Hawes SF, Albert A, Healy MJR, Garrow JS: A comparison of soft tissue radiography, reflected ultrasound, skinfold calipers and thigh circumference for estimating the thickness of fat overlying the iliac crest and greater trochanter. Proc Nutr Soc 31: 91A–92A, 1972.
34. Zondek B: Die Krankheitender endokrinen Drüsen. Berlin, 1926, cited in Bray G: The Obese Patient. WB Saunders, Philadelphia, 1976, p 159.
35. Hirsch J, Knittle JL: Cellularity of obese and non-obese human adipose tissue. Fed Proc 29: 1516–1521, 1970.
36. Bjorntörp P: Effects of age, sex and clinical condition on adipose cellularity in man. Metabolism 23: 1091–1102, 1974.
37. Court JM, Dunlop M: Obese from infancy: A clinical entity. In: Recent Advances in Obesity Research. I. Proceeding of the First International Congress on Obesity. Howard A (ed). London, Newman Pub Ltd, 1975, pp 34–36.
38. Court JM: Obesity in childhood. Med J Aust 1: 888–891, 1977.
39. Bray GA: The Obese Patient. Philadelphia, WB Saunders, 1976, p 197.
40. Mayer J, Thomas DW: Regulation of food intake and obesity. Science 156: 328–337, 1967.
41. Zucker LM, Zucker TF: Fatty, a new mutation in the rat. J Hered 52: 275–278, 1961.
42. Stunkard AJ: Obesity. In: Comprehensive Textbook of Psychiatry. Freedman AM, Kaplan HI, Sadock BJ (eds). Baltimore, Williams & Wilkins, 1975, pp 1648–1655.
43. Moore ME, Stunkard A, Strole L: Obesity, social class, and mental illness. JAMA 181: 962–966, 1962.
44. Crisp AH, McGuiness B: Jolly fat: relation between obesity and psychoneurosis in general population. Br Med J 1: 7–9, 1976.
45. Bruch H: Obesity in childhood: physical growth and development of obese children. Am J Dis Child 8: 457–484, 1939.
46. Bruch H: Eating Disorders: Obesity, Anorexia Nervosa and the Person Within. New York, Basic Books, Inc, 1973.
47. Bruch H: Thin fat people. J Am Med Wom Assoc 28: 187–208, 1973.
48. Stunkard AJ: Eating patterns and obesity. Psychiatr Q 33: 284–294, 1959.
49. Diagnostic and Statistical Manual III Draft, prepared by Task Force on Nomenclature and Statistics, American Psychiatric Association, Washington, DC, January 1978.

50. Wermuth BM, Davis KL, Hollister LE, et al.: Phenytoin treatment of the binge-eating syndrome. Am J Psychiatry 134: 1249–1253, 1977.
51. Green RS, Rau JH: Treatment of compulsive eating disturbances with anticonvulsant medication. Am J Psychiatry 131: 428–432, 1974.
52. Stunkard AJ, Grace WJ, Wolff HG: The night-eating syndrome: a pattern of food intake among certain obese patients. Am J Med 19: 78–86, 1955.
53. Simonson M: Classification of obesity. Lecture at Conference: The Management of Obesity. Johns Hopkins Medical Institutions. February 13–16, 1978.

CHAPTER 2

Epidemiology of Obesity

The prevalence of obesity in the general population is increasing, as is obesity among infants and children. Although data regarding the prevalence of obesity, particularly in childhood and adolescence, are contradictory and often rely on recalled evidence of obesity in childhood, it is clear that obesity originating in childhood is more severe and associated with the poorest treatment prognosis. Furthermore, among the common causes of death, the only one that does not occur more often in the obese population than in the lean population is suicide (Table 2.1). One-third of the population is estimated to be overweight with an associated decrease in life expectancy. It has been estimated[1] that if a cure were found for cancer, the life expectancy would be increased by 2 years, but if obesity could be cured the life expectancy would be increased by 4 years.

In the young, obesity is rarely associated with death except in the rare Pickwickian syndrome. This disease is named after Dickens' description of Fat Joe in the *Pickwick Papers* and is associated with hypoventilation, somnolence, and hypercapnia. The hypoventilation may be secondary to decreased compliance of the ponderous thoracic wall and failure to make the increased respiratory effort necessary to move the thorax. Other rare causes of obesity in childhood, such as Fröhlich's disease or Laurence-Moon-Biedl syndrome, may result in an early demise. Although obesity in childhood and adolescence is rarely associated with death, it is often associated with severe psychological trauma. It is during the emotional upheaval of adolescence that one's body image becomes "imprinted" and the obese youngster often views himself as fat and unattractive and may maintain this body image throughout life, even if he becomes thin. Furthermore, obese children and adolescents are often rejected and taunted by their thinner

Table 2.1
Ratio of death rate of obese to standard-risk individuals analyzed as to cause of death. (Reprinted with permission from R. Williams: Textbook of Endocrinology. Philadelphia, W. B. Saunders Co., 1974, p. 914.)

CONDITION	MEN	WOMEN
DIABETES	3.83	3.72
CIRRHOSIS OF LIVER	2.49	1.47
APPENDICITIS	2.23	1.95
BILIARY CALCULI	2.06	2.84
CHRONIC NEPHRITIS	1.91	2.12
CEREBRAL HEMORRHAGE	1.59	1.62
CORONARY DISEASE	1.42	1.75
AUTO ACCIDENTS	1.31	1.20
SUICIDES	0.78	0.73
TUBERCULOSIS	0.21	0.35

peers, and this may adversely affect their self-esteem and subsequent accomplishments.

INCIDENCE AND PREVALENCE AT VARIOUS AGES

BIRTH WEIGHT AND OBESITY

Some studies have evaluated the association of birth weight and obesity. Bauer,[2] in 1929, found that birth weight had been higher among the obese. However, in a later and more extensive study, Bruch[3] found no difference in the birth weights in the obese and the lean; infants who were obese at birth were usually children of chemically or overtly diabetic mothers and these infants lost the extra weight early in extrauterine life.

OBESITY IN INFANCY

The evidence for a significant and increasing prevalence of overweight or obesity in infancy is impressive. In all studies of infants and children, however, it must be remembered that norms for weight have not been clearly established, nor is it known what part of the increased weight in these children is due to an increase in lean body mass and what portion is due to an increase in adipose tissue. In most studies of prevalence, overweight is defined as 10% above the "ideal" body weight given in standard tables and obesity is defined as 20% above the "ideal" weight. In 1966, Asher[4] retrospectively studied 269 children, aged 18 months to 14 years, and 44% were overweight as infants. Of 21 children whose weight was above the 97th percentile in the second half of the 1st year, all were at or above the 50th percentile at 5 years. Eid,[5] again in a retrospective study, evaluated 6, 7, and 8 year olds whose weight and height at 6 weeks, 3 months, and 6 months were known, and found that those who had been overweight in infancy (even as early as 6 weeks) were significantly more likely to be overweight in later childhood. Charney et al.[6] studied 366 subjects, aged 20 to 30, whose weight was known in the first 6 months. Of those above the 90th percentile as infants, 36% were overweight adults, compared to 14% of average and lightweight babies. Those who attained the 90th percentile at least once in the first 6 months were 2.6 times more likely to be overweight.

The estimates of prevalence of obesity in infancy have been recorded as high as 59.6% by Taitz[7]; a substantial number of infants had doubled their birth weights by 6 weeks rather than at 5 or 6 months as recommended in many pediatric textbooks. Shukla et al.[8] studied 300 normal children in Northern England and found 16.7% to be obese and 27.7% overweight, a total of 44.4%. In a 1973 study,[9] 40% of otherwise healthy babies in Britain weighed 15½ pounds at 2 months of age compared with 10% 20 years ago. In summary, more than one-third of babies, at least in Britain, and probably in the entire affluent Western world, are too fat.

The evidence that obesity in infancy portends obesity in later childhood is less impressive than the association between obesity in infancy and obesity in adulthood. A 1958 study[10] of 373 outpatients found that one-third of the adults were overweight, and in one-third of these, obesity dated from childhood. However, the criterion for childhood obesity in this study was being called "fatty" by peers. Also no attempt was made to divide persistence of obesity by time of onset.

OBESITY IN CHILDHOOD

Estimates of obesity in schoolchildren are sparse and vary widely from a low of 6% to a high of 15%. However, most estimates indicate that obesity in schoolchildren is less common than in infants or in adolescents, assuming the definition of obesity in infants to be correct. Taitz,[7] in the study of British schoolchildren, found the prevalence to be 6%. In a 1952 study[11] of suburban Boston schoolchildren, 10% were obese. A study[12] of Iowa children in the 1950's showed 15% of 9-year-old girls and 2% of 9-year-old boys to be obese.

At all ages in this study, fewer boys than girls were overweight, with a maximum percentage of boys overweight at age 13.

There are studies associating childhood obesity with adult obesity. Abraham and Nordsieck[13] in a cross-sectional study of 10- to 13-year-olds, reexamined 120 of these subjects as adults and found 86% of overweight boys were overweight adults as compared to 42% of normal weight boys who became overweight men. Eighty percent of overweight girls were overweight women. Eighteen percent of average weight girls became overweight women. Also, markedly overweight girls and boys were even more likely to become obese adults.

OBESITY IN ADOLESCENCE

Prevalence rates of obesity in adolescence range from 20–30%. To state the situation more graphically, 3 million adolescents in the United States are significantly obese. In evaluating any study of weight during adolescence, it must be remembered that there is normally a huge change in body mass during adolescence. For example, between ages 10 and 18, boys almost double their body mass. Therefore, in the overweight adolescent, it must be clearly known what kind of weight is being gained. In 1971, in a German study reported by Jelliffe and Jelliffe,[9] 23% of adolescent boys and 27% of adolescent girls were fat. In the Iowa study,[12] 45% of the 16-year-old girls and 15% of 16-year-old boys were obese. In the Ten-State Nutrition Study[14] of 1968–1970, 10–30% of a very large group of adolescents were obese. A study by Colley,[15] which defined obesity as a greater than 25-mm triceps skinfold thickness, found obesity in 32.4% of 14-year-old girls and in 3.6% of 14-year-old boys.

Studies of height differences between obese and lean children in adolescence have shown that although the obese may be taller at an earlier age and may enter puberty sooner, their epiphyses also close sooner, and consequently, they are shorter than average adults. One study[16] of 98 obese children revealed that when these youngsters were first measured at ages 4–5, they were taller than average, but after cessation of growth in height, they were shorter than their peers.

Several studies have noted an association between overweight in adolescence and overweight in adulthood. Abraham and Nordsieck's study of children aged 10 to 13, noted above, confirmed this association. Other studies[17, 18] with small numbers of children have emphasized the persistence in adulthood of most obesity cases seen in childhood, and these studies suggest this is particularly true for girls. However, a common defect of all these studies is that they fail to differentiate their findings among subjects in whom obesity started at various ages. For example, it is not known whether obesity at age 9 has a worse prognosis than obesity at age 14.

DO FAT BABIES AND CHILDREN BECOME FAT ADULTS?

In summary, there is clear evidence that obesity in infancy, childhood, or adolescence tends to persist into adulthood and several studies have indicated that obese individuals with early onset of the disease are more refractory to treatment and also have more serious degrees of obesity. There are suggestions that obesity in infancy portends obesity in childhood, and that childhood obesity persists into adolescence, and that adolescent obesity persists into adulthood. However, the link between each of these stages is by no means proven. Furthermore, the studies suggest a relatively high prevalence of obesity in infancy with a decrease in school-age children and a rise again in adolescence. The reasons for these findings are not clear. The factors which account for the significant percentage of lean adults who were once obese youngsters are also not known. Fat babies apparently are more likely to become fat adults, but the factors that mediate this progression are not clearly established.

OBESITY IN ADULTHOOD

In the adult, estimates of prevalence of obesity vary with age and sex.[19] In the third decade, approximately 20% of men are overweight and 10% of women. Approximately 10% of both men and women are obese (20% or more above the "ideal" weight). After the third decade, in women in the United States, these figures continue a steady rise to a high of 45% in the overweight category and a high of 23% in the obese category. In men, aged 50–59, the percentage continues to rise to highs of 29% in the overweight category and 34% in the obese category. However, in the age range 60–69, 28% of men are overweight and 29% are obese. This may reflect an increased mortality rate among obese men, with fewer overweight or obese survivors aged 60–69. It has been wryly noted that there are very few obese men in nursing homes.

OVERALL INCREASE IN OBESITY

There is evidence that obesity is increasing in general. The 1959 Build and Blood Pressure Study,[19] which describes weights of 5 million people, found that men in the United States weigh 1–5 pounds more than previously recorded studies while women weigh 2–6 pounds less. The greatest increase in average weight was found in short men. Compared to previous data, women's weights decreased most in their younger years. In Britain, Jelliffe and Jelliffe[9] found young and middle-aged men 15 pounds heavier than 30 years ago, with only slight increases in height.

FACTORS IN THE EPIDEMIOLOGY OF OBESITY

Numerous factors influence the prevalence of obesity: intelligence, sex, education, sibling position, socioeconomic status, race, culture, religion, and age. Results of some studies are not clear-cut because many of the factors interrelate; for example, intelligence and socioeconomic factors relate to one another.

INTELLIGENCE AND EDUCATION

There have been a few rather poorly controlled studies which have associated obesity with lower intelligence. In an early study by Mullins,[10] for example, low intelligence and lack of education were found among the obese. Mayer,[20] on the other hand, found no correlation between school grades and obesity, except in physical education. In a study of 554 adults, Kriezc[21] found a strong inverse correlation between intelligence quotient and obesity. Among the women, 41.4% of the obese were in the low IQ category, 21.9% of the obese were in the average IQ category, and 10.7% were in the above average IQ category. A similar, but less pronounced, trend was noted among men. Importantly, however, this study did not control for socioeconomic factors.

The Hathaway[12] study suggested that education beyond high school is associated with lower weight and less obesity. However, education beyond high school is also positively correlated with higher socioeconomic status, which is associated with less obesity. Charney et al.'s study[6] of more than 300 patients found that of subjects who had a high school education or less, 33% were overweight or obese adults, as compared to 7% of subjects with a graduate school education.

SOCIOECONOMIC FACTORS

Socioeconomic factors have been shown to be correlated with obesity all over the world, although in different ways. In less affluent countries, there is a direct, positive correlation between rise in mean body weight and rise in socioeconomic status. Only in an affluent country can the poor be obese. The society must be sufficiently wealthy that highly caloric, largely carbohydrate foods are both inexpensive and readily available. With decreasing affluence, the constraint on obesity is lack of food. With increasing affluence, fads and fashions probably have a significant influence. In some cultures, an increase in weight is a highly prized symbol of prestige. In affluent Western societies, in direct contrast, there is a marked, negative correlation between socioeconomic status and obesity, at least in adult women; poor women tend to be fatter and affluent women tend to be leaner.

Stunkard[22, 23] concludes from two broad epidemiological studies,[22, 23] one of 3,344 white schoolchildren and one of 1,660 adults, that at all ages the poor are fatter and the affluent leaner. Silverstone and colleagues[24] found that the prevalence of obesity in women in lower socioeconomic status was nearly twice that found in those of upper socioeconomic status.

Garn et al.,[25] in two broader studies, the Ten-State Nutrition Study and the Pre-School Nutritional Study, involving more than 20,000 people of European, Mexican, African, and Puerto Rican ancestry, found a different pattern. He found that after the first few years of life and into adolescence, the poor are the leanest and the affluent are the fattest; this is true for both boys and girls, whether income or parental occupation is the measure of socioeconomic class. Furthermore, for men, he found this to be true at all ages; the higher the income-to-needs ratio, the fatter they are. In the female, however, Garn found a different pattern. At lower socioeconomic levels girls were leaner, but in adulthood this trend is reversed and the more affluent women are leaner than the impoverished women. In other words, the leaner poor girl becomes the fatter impoverished woman. This is an important finding in terms of recent theories about adipose cell number. Early investigators found that in adult life the number of fat cells is apparently constant. Other investigators have identified three periods when adipose cell number increases (during the last trimester, in the 1st year of life, and during adolescence). It has been theorized that the fat cells laid down in these three periods are never decreased in number (although they may decrease in size) and that the increased adipose cell number in the obese child predisposes him to later obesity. If, in fact, the fat female infant does not become the fat woman, as Garn's study suggests, this theory needs reconsideration. (See Chapter 7 for details.)

DOWNWARD SOCIAL MOBILITY

There are other findings regarding socioeconomic factors in obesity. For example, Stunkard[22] reports obesity to be more prevalent among downwardly socially mobile subjects than among those who remain in the social class of their parents and far more prevalent than among those subjects who were upwardly socially mobile. Furthermore, in Stunkard's findings, the longer one's family had been in this country the less likely the subject was to be obese. This finding was independent of socioeconomic factors. Another factor correlated to obesity and socioeconomic factors is serum and urinary vitamin levels. Obese children tend to have higher levels of vitamins A and C and several of the B vitamins but there is an even stronger positive correlation between income level and elevated serum and urinary vitamins.

RACIAL DIFFERENCES

There are racial differences in level of fatness, even at the same income levels. In the Ten-State Nutrition survey comparing American white children (of European ancestry) and black children (of African ancestry), black males are fatter from age 1–4 and then systematically leaner through late adolescence and beyond. In this study, Americans of Puerto Rican ancestry were fatter than the black or white Americans. Furthermore, several studies have documented differences between American and English children, with American boys and girls fatter than their English age peers, independent of socioeconomic factors. Among Navajo Indians, those who follow the traditional life style are leaner than their age peers who assimilate into the surrounding white culture. Stunkard[22] reported that among the lower socioeconomic group, obesity occurred in decreasing percentages according to the following sequence: Hungarian, Czechoslovakian, German, Italian, Irish, British, Russian and Lithuanian, Puerto Rican, and fourth generation Americans. Among each ethnic group except the Puerto Rican, obesity was higher in women in lower socioeconomic classes than in median socioeconomic classes or upper socioeconomic classes. Furthermore, the number of generations a family has lived in the United States was also correlated with obesity. Among women, the longer her family was in the country, the less likely she was to be obese.

RELIGION

Associations between religion and obesity have also been noted. One study[1] found Lutherans to be more obese than Episcopalians (24% vs. 3%). Stunkard[22] found the prevalence of obesity highest among Jews, less among Roman Catholics, and least among Protestants; among Protestants, prevalence was highest among Baptists, less in Methodists, and least in Lutherans and Episcopalians.

FAMILY

Whitelaw[26] found that obesity is less frequent in persons who have a large number of siblings than in persons with few or no siblings; this finding may well relate to socioeconomic status, a factor which was not controlled. However, Charney et al.,[6] found no correlation between obesity and sibling number after controlling for socioeconomic factors.

Finally, an association between obesity and the weight of one's spouse has also been noted. Lean women usually have lean husbands and vice versa; obese women usually have obese spouses and vice versa. An association between obese pet owners and their pets has even been noted![14]

OVERALL SUMMARY OF EPIDEMIOLOGICAL FACTORS

In summary, the woman most likely to be thin is a fourth generation American who has high intelligence and a graduate school education; she is from an upper middle-class family, who, herself, is now in the upper class, is an Episcopalian, and has a thin, upwardly mobile husband. The man most likely to be fat is in his 50's, is in a median income group (although studies disagree on this point), has a fat wife, is Jewish, has a high school education, and is in a socioeconomic class below that of his parents.

CONSEQUENCES OF OBESITY

"More are slain by suppers than by the sword"—Old proverb[9]

Obesity has been widely reported to predispose to an impressive number of diseases including hypertension, diabetes, coronary artery disease, gout, gallstones, and the Pickwickian syndrome, as well as to produce a damaged body image with consequent psychological maladjustment. There is a continuing debate about the etiological significance of obesity in these diseases, particularly coronary artery disease, and opinions vary regarding the effects of obesity on mortality.

HYPERTENSION

A number of large, well-controlled studies have shown an association between obesity and hypertension (Fig. 2.1). Other studies have shown a relationship between hypertension and coronary artery disease. In determining blood pressure of obese individuals the correct size sphygmomanometer must be used. The auscultatory method produces erroneously high readings on fat arms only when the rubber bag of the sphygmomanometer is short in relationship to the circumference of the arm.[27] The large studies, to be described, utilized the correct size sphygmomanometer.

The Framingham study,[28] designed to delineate factors related to the development of coronary artery disease, includes 5,209 subjects, initially aged 30–62, who have been followed since 1949. With increasing degrees of obesity, there was an associated rise in blood pressure and increase in serum cholesterol. This relationship was more marked in men than in women. The prevalence of hypertension at all ages increased with weight. Furthermore, the rise in blood pressure was clearly related to more exact measures of adiposity, such as triceps skinfold measurement as well as relative weight. Importantly, 60% who lost weight became normotensive.

In a seven-nation, cross-cultural study reported by Keys and colleagues,[29] a clear association between obesity and hypertension was demonstrated. In

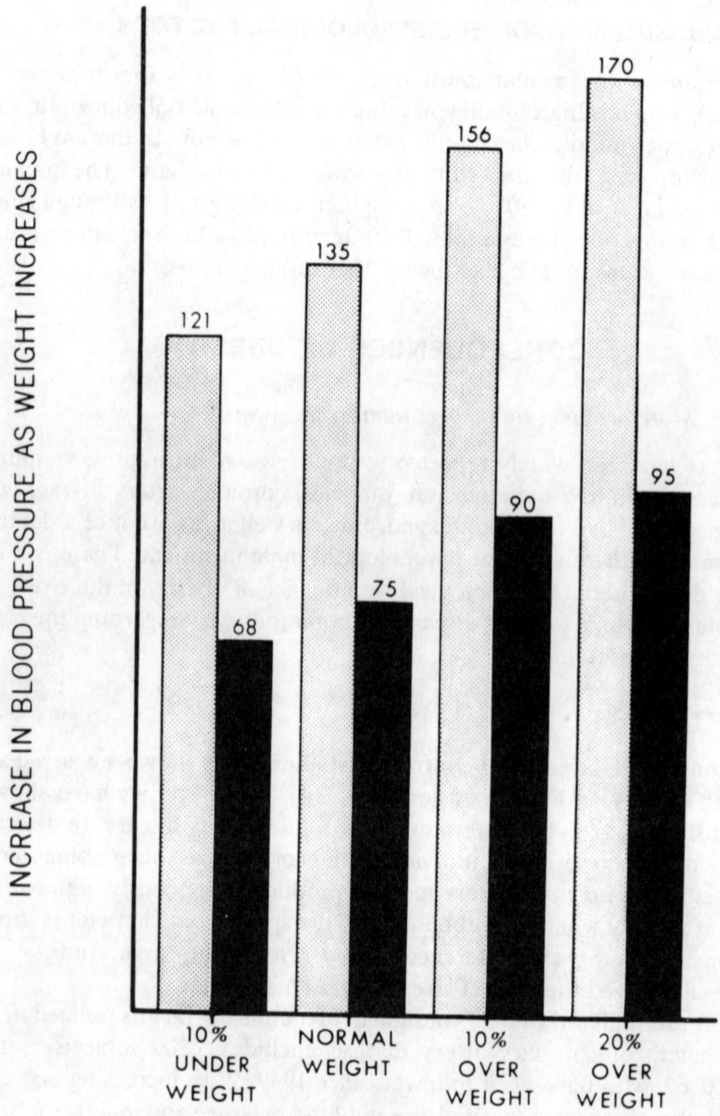

Figure 2.1. Increase in blood pressure as weight increases.

both the Framingham study and the Keys study, obesity did not correlate significantly with risk of developing coronary artery disease when the effect of blood pressure was controlled.

The question of whether obesity in childhood predisposes to hypertension is not settled. The Muscatine study[30] of 4,829 schoolchildren over a 14-month period, found 23% to have weights relative to the group greater than 110% and among this obese group, 20.6% had levels of systolic blood pressure greater than the 90th percentile, and 28.4% had diastolic pressures greater than the 90th percentile. Furthermore, 17.7% and 24.3% had levels of elevated serum cholesterol and elevated triglyceride levels, respectively, above the 90th percentile. This study, therefore, shows a relationship between obesity and hypertension and elevated triglyceride and cholesterol levels in children. Consequently, if obesity in childhood persists and the chance of hypertension developing later increases, this study suggests that the relationship of obesity to blood pressure has its origins in childhood.

The mechanisms through which obesity affects blood pressure are not known. It has been suggested that the obese may consume excess sodium as well as excess calories, resulting in hypertension, or that the excess adipose tissue results in an increased blood flow which results in increased cardiac output due to an increased stroke volume in the presence of the normal heart rate.

In summary, the HEW Committee[31] studying obesity and hypertension, states:

1. More hypertension exists amongst the obese than the non-obese;
2. The obese hypertensive experiences a greater risk of coronary artery disease than the non-obese hypertensive; and
3. Mortality rates for obese hypertensive persons are higher than for persons with obesity alone or hypertension alone.

ATHEROSCLEROSIS

The relationship between obesity and atherosclerosis has been studied in great detail in the Framingham study. No association between overweight and the rate at which atherosclerotic heart disease develops was found when the obese and non-obese were matched for blood pressure and serum cholesterol. However, once atherosclerotic heart disease did develop, angina and sudden death were more likely to occur, particularly in obese men. In discussing this apparently paradoxical finding, Kannel and colleagues[28] conclude that the factors involved in the pathogenesis of atherosclerosis are not necessarily the same as those that precipitate clinical events (for example, angina) and affect mortality, and they propose the following explanation. The obese may require twice the oxygen consumed by non-obese individuals, presumably due to increased blood flow to excessive adipose tissue. Increased oxygen demands of the obese individual and the associated increased cardiac workload require a supple coronary vascular bed capable of dilating to increase the coronary blood flow and the atherosclerotic person, with a narrowed vessel lumen, does not seem able to do this. Therefore, myocardial ischemia and pain may occur when any additional workload is placed on the heart. Furthermore, there are mechanical disturbances in the obese who may have an elevated diaphragm and decreased respiratory excursion and may require increased effort breathing and moving about, and these disturbances may cause a lowered vital capacity, carbon dioxide retention, and increased oxygen debt.

In the Framingham study, the risk of cerebral vascular accidents in men was found not to be related to obesity, when other factors were controlled. Among women, there was a small but definite increased risk in the obese for congestive heart failure and brain infarction.

Another important negative correlation in the Framingham study was found between obesity and intermittent claudication. This atherosclerotic disease was more common in the lean than in the obese. However, there is a potent correlation between intermittent claudication and smoking. Anecdotal reports, as well as a few small studies, suggest that smokers are leaner than non-smokers. Hence, smoking, leanness, and intermittent claudication may be interrelated.

To summarize these findings, obesity may reversibly predispose to elevated serum cholesterol, elevated triglycerides, and hypertension, which are known to be powerful risk factors in the development of atherosclerotic heart disease. Obesity, *per se*, is not clearly associated with the rate of development of coronary artery disease but is associated with an increased incidence of sudden death and angina, once atherosclerotic heart disease develops. Since as much as 50% of the American population may suffer a coronary or stroke, it seems wise to correct obesity even if its only influence is to mediate other risk factors which predispose to atherosclerosis (See Fig. 2.2). Furthermore,

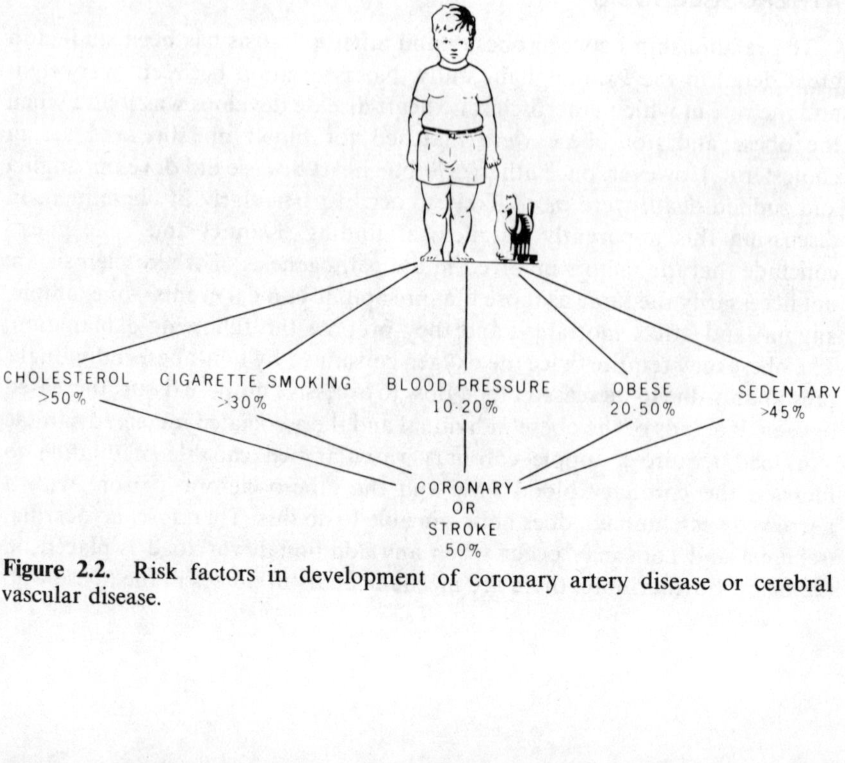

Figure 2.2. Risk factors in development of coronary artery disease or cerebral vascular disease.

insurance companies have long noted that the earlier the onset of overweight in adult life, the more pronounced an effect it has on mortality in later life. Probably, this statement can be extrapolated to childhood, indicating that childhood obesity that persists is associated with a higher mortality rate.

DIABETES

Although there is doubt that obesity predisposes to atherosclerotic heart disease, it is clear that overweight subjects develop diabetes mellitus more often than the lean, and that death from diabetes is nearly 4 times as common among the obese. In the Framingham study,[28] diabetes developed 3 times as often among obese individuals. It is known that adipose tissue in vitro and probably in vivo, is less sensitive to insulin. In the obese the fasting level of immunoreactive insulin is increased, although prior to clinical onset of diabetes true fasting blood sugar is not elevated. The insulin response to oral glucose is greatly elevated in the obese and this may be evidence of peripheral resistance to insulin. It is postulated that an increase in adipose tissue requires an increased production of insulin from the pancreas; this eventually results in failure of the pancreas to produce insulin resulting in diabetes. Furthermore, serum triglycerides are known to be elevated in the obese and this may be secondary to both metabolic and endocrine effects. Obesity may cause a decreased sensitivity to insulin, resulting in increased insulin production, which may stimulate the liver to produce excess endogenous, very low density lipoproteins, presumably by enhancing lipogenesis and lipoprotein packaging and by preventing hepatic triglyceride breakdown. In patients with moderate or severe glucose intolerance, there is impaired lipoprotein lipase synthesis which results, via an entirely different mechanism, in elevated triglycerides. Also, triglycerides may be elevated secondary to excess fat intake in the obese; dietary fat, after hydrolysis to partial glycerides and fatty acids, is absorbed from micelles. Therefore, either excess or insufficient insulin may result in an increase in triglycerides, either by an increase in production or a decrease in breakdown, and excess dietary fat may result in an increase in serum triglycerides from a combination of increased supply and decreased breakdown.

GALLSTONES, GOUT, AND CARCINOMA

Obese adults are also more likely to develop gallstones than non-obese adults. Furthermore, diabetics also have an increased incidence of gallstones. In Horn's study,[32] women below the age of 50 who had gallstones were 25 pounds heavier, on the average, than women without gallstones. Van der Linden[33] found a small but significant correlation between subscapular and triceps skinfold thickness and the incidence of surgically proven cholelithiasis. In 90% of gallstones, cholesterol is the major ingredient. For cholesterol stones to form there must be an excess of cholesterol in the bile; this excess could result from a decreased cholesterol holding capacity or increased cholesterol concentration. It has been shown that both increased cholesterol intake[34] and increased cholesterol production in obese individuals[35, 36] caused increased secretion of biliary cholesterol without markedly affecting bile acid secretion. These factors may promote gallstone formation in the obese.

Gout is also thought to occur more commonly among the obese population. Anecdotal reports, including those from Shakespeare and Benjamin Franklin, have attributed the occurrence of acute gouty arthritis to the ingestion of very rich foods.

Blitzer and colleagues[37] in a retrospective study of 56,111 women who belong to TOPS (Take Off Pounds Sensibly) found that among obese women endometrial carcinoma occurred 1.62 times as often in women who were obese teenagers as compared to those obese women who were not obese as teenagers. This study, although poorly controlled and without laboratory verification of the carcinoma, does sample a large group of obese women and suggests that long-standing obesity may predispose to endometrial carcinoma.

MINOR EFFECTS OF OBESITY

There are less dramatic, but still annoying consequences of obesity. Obese infants are more likely to have genu varum (bowlegs) and the deposition of fat on outer thighs increases this appearance. After age 3–4 children who are obese more commonly have genu valgum (knock-knees). Also, obese youngsters have a decreased exercise tolerance. They are also subject to more frequent and more severe respiratory infections, probably due to a decreased ventilatory function. Adolescent obese boys are more likely to have gynecomastia with an enlarged areola and increased fat pads beneath the areola; this is particularly embarrassing and may limit participation in sports even further, thereby increasing the obese youngster's tendency to be more sedentary. Obese adolescents and adults are more subject to non-specific gastrointestinal symptoms including bloating and vague abdominal distress. Varicose veins are more common among the obese. Various skin diseases are more common (organisms are more likely to multiply in the warm, moist skinfolds of the obese). Amenorrhea and dysmenorrhea are also more common in the obese and may be related to the associated endocrine disturbances seen in obesity. Obesity is also known to worsen osteoarthritis.

BODY IMAGE

A major consequence of obesity, particularly in adolescents, is a defective body image. The body image incorporates one's view of one's self psychologically, physically, and interpersonally. Even the normal weight adolescent must incorporate into his body image radical changes in size, body proportions, and primary and secondary sex characteristics. The obese youngster must incorporate even more radical changes in body size and proportions. There is evidence that childhood obesity may become more pronounced in adolescence, and some cases of juvenile obesity may begin in adolescence. In addition, puberty begins earlier in heavier adolescents, and this may affect their peer relationships. Menarche begins earlier in obese girls. Since obesity is not acceptable in our society and since adolescence is a period of exquisite sensitivity to peer criticism, the obese adolescent is particularly vulnerable. The obese adolescent may be ridiculed and teased, with resulting stunting in social development. It is generally thought that adolescence is the period when one's body image is "imprinted" or fixed; changes in body size and proportion after adolescence are less likely to be incorporated into one's body image. Consequently, the deleterious effects on self-esteem may not be reversible after adolescence, or perhaps even during adolescence.

In evaluating the psychological ramifications of obesity, there are many confounding variables, as well as significant problems in sample selection, and these may bias results. However, it does seem that obese youngsters are more prone to problems with body image.

OVERALL SUMMARY OF CONSEQUENCES

In summary, obesity is associated with a wide variety of diseases, including hypertension, atherosclerosis, gout, cholelithiasis, and psychological disturbances. Mechanical trauma of obesity also accounts for annoying and sometimes serious complications. Although the etiological significance of obesity is not clear in many of these problems, it seems likely that correction or prevention of obesity would result in decreased morbidity and mortality from these diseases.

References

1. Gold DD: Psychological factors associated with obesity. Am Fam Physician 13: 87–91, 1976.
2. Bauer J, cited in Mossberg H: Obesity in children: a clinical prognostical investigation. Acta Paediatr Suppl II: 5–120, 1948.
3. Bruch H: Obesity in childhood. I. Physical growth and development of obese children. Am J Dis Child 58: 457–484, 1939.
4. Asher P: Fat babies and fat children: the prognosis of obesity in the very young. Arch Dis Child 41: 672–673, 1966.
5. Eid EE: Follow-up study of physical growth of children who had excessive weight gain in first six months of life. Br Med J 2: 74–76, 1970.
6. Charney E, Goodman HC, McBride M, et al: Childhood antecedents of adult obesity: do chubby infants become fat adults? N Engl J Med 295: 6–9, 1976.
7. Taitz LS: Infantile overnutrition among artificially fed infants in the Sheffield region. Br Med J 1: 315–316, 1971.
8. Shukla A, Forsyth HA, Anderson CM, Marwah SM: Infantile overnutrition in the first year of life: a field study in Dudley, Worcestershire. Br Med J 4: 507–515, 1972.

9. Jelliffe DB, Jelliffe EF: Fat babies: prevalence, perils and prevention. Environ Child Health Monogr 41: 124–159, 1975.
10. Mullins AG: The prognosis in juvenile obesity. Arch Dis Child 33: 307–314, 1958.
11. Johnson ML, Burke BS, Mayer J: The prevalence and incidence of obesity in a cross-section of elementary and secondary school children. Am J Clin Nutr 4: 231–238, 1956.
12. Hathaway ML, Sargent DW: Overweight in children. J Am Diet Assoc 40: 511–515, 1962.
13. Abraham S, Nordsieck M: Relationship of excess weight in children and adults. Pub Health Rep 75: 263–273, 1960.
14. Garn SM, Clark DC: Trends in fatness and the origins of obesity, Pediatrics 57: 443–456, 1976.
15. Colley JRT: Obesity in school children. Br J Prev Soc Med 28: 221–225, 1974.
16. Lloyd JK, Wolff OH, Whelen WS: Childhood obesity: a long-term study of height and weight. Br Med J 2: 145–148, 1961.
17. Haase KE, Hosenfeld HZ: Zer Fett sucht in kind esalter. Z Kinderheilkd 78: 1, 1956.
18. Mossberg H: Obesity in children: A clinical prognostical investigation. Acta Paediatr Suppl II: 5–120, 1948.
19. Build and blood pressure study. Vol 2. Chicago Society of Actuaries, 1960, pp 230–237.
20. Mayer J: Obesity in childhood and adolescence. Med Clin North Am 48: 1347–1358, 1964.
21. Kriezc A: Relationship between intelligence and relative prevalence of obesity. Hum Biol 46: 109–113, 1974.
22. Stunkard AJ: From explanation to action in psychosomatic medicine: the case of obesity. Psychosom Med 37: 195–236, 1975.
23. Goldblatt PB, Moore ME, Stunkard AJ: Social factors in obesity. JAMA 192: 1039–1044, 1965.
24. Silverstone JT, Gordon RP, Stunkard AJ: Social factors in obesity in London. Practitioner 202: 682–688, 1969.
25. Garn SM, Clark DC, Guire KE: Growth, body composition, and development of obese and lean children. Curr Concepts Nutr 3: 23–46, 1975.
26. Whitelaw GL: The association of social class and sibling number with skinfold thickness in London schoolboys. Hum Biol 43: 414–420, 1971.
27. Orma E, Karvonen MJ, Keys A: "Cuff" hypertension. Lancet 2: 51, 1960.
28. Kannel WB, LeBauer EJ, Dawber TR, McNamara PM: Relation of body weight to development of coronary heart disease: the Framingham study. Circulation 35: 734–744, 1967.
29. Keys A, Aravanis C, Blackburn H, et al: Coronary heart disease: overweight and obesity as risk factors. Ann Intern Med 77: 15–27, 1972.
30. Lauer RM, Conner WE, Leaverton PE, et al: Coronary heart disease risk factors in school children: the Muscatine study. J. Pediatr 86: 697–706, 1975.
31. Obesity and Health: US Dept HEW, US Pub Health Serv Nat Center for Chronic Disease Control, Arlington, Va., pp 23–32.
32. Horn G: Observations on the etiology of cholelithiasis. Br Med J 2: 732–737, 1956.
33. Van der Linden W: Some biological traits in female gallstone disease patients. Acta Chir Scand [Suppl 269]: 74–79, 1961.
34. Quintao E, Grundys M, Ahrens EH: Effects of dietary cholesterol on the regulation of total body cholesterol in man. J Lipid Res 12: 233–247, 1971.
35. Miettinen TA: Cholesterol production in obesity. Circulation 44: 842–850, 1971.
36. Grundy SM, Meltzger AL, Adler RD: Mechanisms of lithogenic bile formation in American Indian women with cholesterol gallstones. J Clin Invest 51: 3026–3043, 1972.
37. Blitzer PH, Blitzer EC, Rimm AA: Association between teenage obesity and cancer in 56,111 women: all cancers and endometrial carcinoma. Prev Med 5: 20–31, 1976.

CHAPTER

3

Natural History of Obesity

The pathogenesis of obesity is difficult to study because multiple factors are involved. Although a grossly obese individual is easy to identify, the determination of the actual lean body mass and fat content is difficult. Fat content in humans is a characteristic that exists on a continuum: that is, a certain percentage of fat is not only normal but necessary, and the optimal fat content at various ages, particularly in infants and children, is not known. Once obesity has been arbitrarily defined, there is a plethora of factors that impinges on the ontogenesis of obesity, including genetics, early learned feeding patterns, and psychological and cultural factors.

GENETICS

The nature-nurture conflict is perhaps nowhere better exemplified than in the study of obesity. It has long been observed that obesity tends to run in families, but a more definitive evaluation of the genetic contribution to obesity has been difficult to obtain because environmental influences on obesity also run in families. There have been six major approaches to the problem: twin studies, adoptive studies, large epidemiological studies, evaluation of somatotypes in families, animal studies, and studies of rare genetic diseases in humans associated with obesity. These methods are all open to criticism. Not one of the studies is without an alternative interpretation, but taken together they clearly indicate a genetic factor in obesity, with an unknown mode of genetic transmission.

CONFOUNDING VARIABLES IN GENETIC STUDIES

Withers[1] has discussed some of the problems in the study of the genetics of human obesity. Most early studies evaluated obesity in terms of an all-or-none condition, whereas in fact, fatness varies continuously throughout the population. In the geneticist's terminology, the phenotype being studied in obesity is the product of a varying multifactorial genetic situation developing in varying situations.

Another factor confounding the findings of genetic studies is assortive mating, which is the non-random selection of a mate. For example, it is known that a husband and wife tend to have similar weights. Although this may be influenced by common eating patterns, it is probably also a consequence of selection of a partner with similar physical characteristics, including weight and somatotype. This is an example of assortive mating.

Laboratory genetic studies ideally study the genetic consequences of random mating; this is technically termed panmixis. The condition of random mating is necessary for operation of the Hardy-Weinberg principle which states that in a large panmixis population in which there is no migration or selection against a particular genotype, and the mutation rate remains constant, the proportions of various genotypes will remain unchanged from one generation to another. Since probably none of these assumptions is correct for human obesity, the study of the genetics of obesity is considerably more difficult than laboratory studies. Various statistical methods have been devised to correct for these environmental influences but all are based on assumptions which may or may not apply to the real situation. For a detailed statistical evaluation of some of the problems, see *Methodology in Medical Genetics* by A. E. Emery.[2] The studies to be described are attempts to solve the dilemma of the relative genetic contribution to the problem of obesity.

POSSIBLE ERRORS IN TWIN STUDIES

Studies of monozygous twins (derived from splitting of a single fertilized ovum at an early stage of development) who have an identical genetic constitution and who are raised in different environmental situations would seem to be an ideal solution to studying the genetic contribution to obesity.

There is a variety of problems in twin studies starting with difficulties in determining whether like-sex twins are actually identical (monozygous) or non-identical (dizygotic, derived from the independent release and subsequent fertilization of two separate ova). Examination of fetal membranes is the time-honored method but is not always unequivocal (e.g. dichorionic twins are more likely to be dizygotic but may be monozygotic), and this information is not always available. The similarity method is often utilized and includes blood group typing, determination of certain phenotypes demonstrable in serum erythrocytes and leukocytes, and dermatoglyphics. Using this method, the probability that a given set of twins is monozygous can be calculated. Some studies do not state how zygosity was determined.

A second problem is that twins may be subjected to a different prenatal environment. For example, one monozygotic twin may suffer an impaired placental circulation. An underlying principle in twin studies is that if variation of a characteristic is entirely genetically determined, the correlation coefficient between monozygotic twins, who have all their genes in common, would be 1.0. Correspondingly, the correlation coefficient observed in dizygotic twins (or siblings) would be expected to be 0.5. Therefore, comparison of monozygotic twins raised together and raised apart, based on the assumption that subsequent postnatal environmental differences account for the difference in correlation from 1.0, may be biased from the outset.

In most twin studies, the following methodological criticism applies. Although the contribution of environment can be studied statistically when the genetics are constant, or vice versa, the contribution of genetics can be studied when the environment is held constant; when both genetics and environment are varying, as in dizygotic twins, these comparisons are probably invalid. Ideally, monozygotic twins raised in a common environment should be compared to monozygotic twins raised in different environments.

Another criticism of twin studies has been made by Edwards[3] who argues that since all diseases have some genetic predisposition, the estimation of such parameters may be a costly way of confirming expectations without providing any useful measure of the intensity of this predisposition. These caveats aside, however, twin studies have yielded interesting, although conflicting, data about the possible heritability of obesity.

RESULTS OF TWIN STUDIES

Von Verschuer[4] compared body weights of 57 pairs of identical twins and found that the deviation in weights was 1.39% for those in the same environment, and 3.60% for those identical twins raised separately. In this study, intra-twin differences in body weight were the greatest of all the parameters measured. However, only four pairs of twins were judged obese and the determination of fatness was in terms of body weight, not skinfold thickness. A second study[5] compared dizygotic twins and found a body weight difference of 10.0 pounds, nearly identical to the 9.9-pound difference this study found between identical twins raised separately. In contrast, Shields'[6] study of intra-twin differences in body weights of identical twins raised together and separately were the same.

Brook and colleagues[7, 8] have recently evaluated the skinfold thicknesses of 222 pairs of like-sex twins of whom 78 were monozygotic and 144 were dizygotic. This study has the advantage of measuring triceps and subscapular skinfold thicknesses, known to be a more reliable method of estimating fat content than body weight. This study evaluates fat content as a continuous characteristic and estimates heritability using correlation coefficients. They conclude that genetic factors are more important in determining trunk fat (estimated by triceps skinfolds). Also, genetic factors appear to play a greater part in determining limb fat in girls than boys. Furthermore, over 10 years of age, heritability was high for both trunk and limb fat in both boys and girls, but for younger children environmental influences appeared to have greater influence over trunk and limb fat.

One problem with this study is that there were only a few sets of twins who were actually obese and these were not investigated separately. Therefore, the study applies strictly only to heritability of skinfold thickness over the normal population and findings in the obese population may be different. Also the youngest set of twins was 3 years old and it is well known that the rate of growth of fat is greater at earlier ages. However, if Brook's findings are applicable to the obese population, one implication is that control of environmental factors in the younger age groups may prevent obesity, but attempts to adjust environmental factors in later age groups may be more difficult because of the strong genetic influence at this time.

THRESHOLD MODEL

A theoretical model of multifactorial inheritance that has been applied to the genetics of obesity is the "threshold model."[9] According to this model there is some underlying graded attribute that is related to the cause of obesity. This attribute is called the individual's liability and it includes the genetic predisposition and environmental circumstances that render an individual more or less vulnerable to obesity. According to this theory, the curve of liability to obesity has a normal distribution in both the normal and obese populations, but in the obese group the curve is shifted to the right because they have a higher mean liability. The point on the curve beyond which all individuals are obese is called the threshold. As shown in Figure 3.1, a small increase in mean body fatness in the population shifts the curve to the right and dramatically increases the number of individuals exceeding the threshold value defined as obesity. Therefore, if the series of assumptions regarding the threshold model apply to obesity, small decrements in the mean body fatness level in the population, which might be achieved by environmental changes, would have a large impact in decreasing the prevalence of obesity.

ADOPTIVE STUDIES

Another approach to the genetic problem is to study adoptive parent-child pairs. Withers[1] studied 142 families with at least one adopted child; 13 of the families also had a natural child. The correlation coefficient for body weight between father/natural child, mother/natural child, father/adoptee, and mother/adoptee were calculated and found not to be statistically significant.

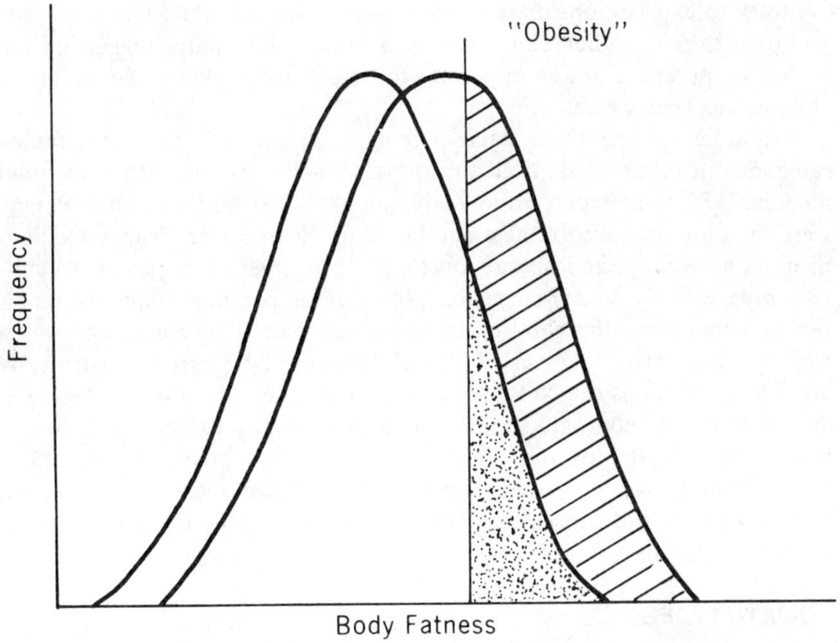

Figure 3.1. Threshold model of multifactorial inheritance. A small shift in body fatness dramatically increases prevalence of obesity. (Reprinted with permission from C. G. D. Brook: Postgrad Med J 53:95, 1977.)

Although this study provides some evidence against a genetic contribution to body weight, the study was via mail questionnaires, the sample size is small, and weight rather than skinfold thickness was evaluated.

More recently, Garn[10] has argued against the genetic explanation of fatness similarities in families citing results from the Ten-State Nutrition Study. Triceps and subscapular skinfold thicknesses were measured in 429 adoptive parent-child pairs and compared to skinfold data on 198 pairs of genetically unrelated siblings. These data were also compared to 6,372 pairs of serologically verified biological parent-child pairs and 3713 biological pairs of siblings. There was no statistically significant difference between the correlations for the biological sibling pairs and the genetically unrelated siblings. This study, which has accurate skinfold data from a large group of subjects, provides strong support for dominance of environmental factors in the determination of level of fatness.

In the Ten-State Nutrition Study, there were highly significant correlations in skinfold measurements between parents and children.[11] Parent-child fatness correlations were approximately 0.25 for various parent-child combinations (father/son, father/daughter, mother/son, mother/daughter).

Contrary to expectation, there were no significant differences in the correlations between mother/child pairs and father/child pairs suggesting that sex of the parent is not as important in determining level of fatness in the child as has been assumed.

In another use of these data, parents were divided into three fatness categories in terms of skinfold thickness: lean (below the 15th percentile), medium (15th to 85th percentile) and obese (85th percentile and up). Parents were then grouped into fatness combinations: lean x lean, lean x medium, medium x medium, and obese x obese, etc. The level of fatness of the child rises progressively with the level of fatness of the parental mating combination. Furthermore, the children of two obese parents become more obese with age. For example, by age 17 the children of obese parents, statistically, are 3 times as fat as the children of lean parents. At first glance, these data appear to overwhelmingly support the genetic theory of obesity. However, in this study, husbands and wives were similar in degree of fatness. Since husbands and wives are usually genetically unrelated, these correlations are probably either the consequence of assortive mating or common environmental conditions.

SOMATOTYPES

As has been noted earlier, measurement of weight is only a rough estimate of body fatness. An important interrelated factor is body build, which also has a genetic component. Somatotyping is a method of quantifying body build into three major categories: endomorphy, ectomorphy, and mesomorphy. Sheldon's[12] technique of determining somatotype utilized three photographs of each subject. The subject is photographed from the front, the back, and the side. Each of the three pictures is analyzed for each trait (endomorphy, ectomorphy, or mesomorphy) and rated on a scale from 1–7 where 1 is the minimum and 7 is the maximum degree of the trait. Endomorphy refers to roundness of the subject and the fact that these subjects gain fat easily. Mesomorphy refers to muscular structure. Ectomorphy refers to linearity or tallness (See Fig. 3.2). Although this technique seems to be a logical method of categorizing body build, it is time consuming and using it requires skill.

Withers[1] evaluated somatotypes of 130 obese and 250 control subjects and their relatives. However, determination of somatotype of the relatives of the obese was from verbal description by the obese subjects and the somatotype of the control subjects and relatives was determined from the subjects' self-report using a questionnaire about body build. This procedure is subject to serious errors. With these limitations in mind, Withers tentatively concludes that the mother contributes endomorphy to the son and the father contributes mesomorphy to the daughter. The important aspect of this study is that it considers the factor of body build which is complicated genetically. That the

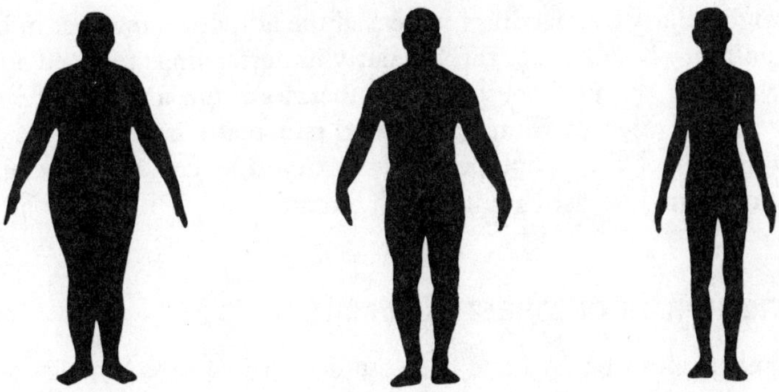

Figure 3.2. Somatotypes. (Reprinted with permission from F. Stare: Obesity Data and Directions for the 70s. New York, Medcom Publ, 1973.)

genetic inheritance of body build is multifactorial seems apparent. For example, in Shields'[6] study of monozygotic twins, stature, which in part determines ectomorphy, has a higher intra-twin correlation than body weight. Withers[1] (p. 88) summarizes the problem succinctly: "In somatotype terminology, the clinician is interested in obesity as in endomorphy, whereas overweight may be the result of a high degree of mesomorphy."

ANIMAL STUDIES

Although results from animal studies cannot be directly extrapolated to the obese patient, an experimental animal model might facilitate planning for clinical investigations. In a number of strains of rats and mice, obesity or the susceptibility to obesity is genetically transmitted. Mayer[13] initially noted that genetically obese mice differ in a number of metabolic ways from mice who were obese following destruction of the hypothalamus with gold thioglucose. He cited the genetically obese mice as an example of "metabolic" obesity. The animals treated with gold thioglucose developed hypothalamic obesity and Mayer considered this an example of "regulatory" obesity.

The Zucker[14] fatty rat (genetic symbol: *fa/fa*) inherits obesity as an autosomal recessive Mendelian trait. Johnson and colleagues[15] have studied the metabolically obese Zucker rat in a series of experiments designed to evaluate the relationship between development, nutrition, and genotype. During the 1st month of life, nutrition and genotype influenced the rat's growth. At 3 months of age, genotype became the major determinant of body weight. Early overfeedings increased the adipocyte number in both the obese and non-obese Zucker rat, but early underfeedings reduced adipocyte number *only* in the non-obese rat. Furthermore, the amount of immunoreactive insulin released from the isolated pancreatic islets of these animals was a function of the genotype and was uninfluenced by early nutrition. These studies are interesting but may or may not be applicable to the human situation.

GENETIC FORMS OF OBESITY IN MAN

The genetics of obesity have been studied in five rare genetic conditions known to be associated with obesity. These diseases are: Laurence-Moon-Bardet-Biedl (LMBB) syndrome, the Alström-Hallgren syndrome, the Prader-Willi syndrome, the Morgagni-Stewart-Morel syndrome (the syndrome of hyperostosis frontalis interna), and triglyceride storage disease. These conditions are discussed in detail in Chapter 4.

PRENATAL INFLUENCES

Pre-pregnancy weight and maternal weight gain during pregnancy are highly correlated with birth weight. There is some evidence that higher birth weight is correlated with later obesity. Therefore, prenatal influences which are associated with an increased birth weight may predispose a child to adult obesity. Furthermore, one of the most interesting theories about obesity is that there are three critical periods in the development of adipose tissue cellularity: the last part of gestation, the 1st year of life, and early adolescence. If this theory has validity, maternal nutrition, particularly in the last trimester, may dramatically influence the potential for later obesity.

PRE-PREGNANCY WEIGHT

Several studies have documented the relationship between pre-pregnancy weight and birth weight of the infant. In one study[16] of 3,939 Caucasian women divided in three groups by weight, light, medium, and heavy, the incidence of low birth weight infants (2,500 g and under) decreased with increasing pre-pregnancy weight of the mother. Conversely, the incidence of excessive-size infants (4,000 g or over) increased with increasing pre-pregnancy weight of the mother. This study evaluates a large group of women whose weights, heights, and obstetric courses are known.

PATTERN OF WEIGHT GAIN IN PREGNANCY

Evaluation of the prenatal influences requires an understanding of the normal pattern of weight gain and its relationship to growth of fetal and maternal tissue. In studies ranging over the last 30 years,[17, 18] weight gain during pregnancy has been shown to be approximately 24 pounds (11 kg). This may be an optimal as well as average weight gain since the best overall reproduction performance (i.e. the lowest combined incidence of obstetric complications) also apparently occurs at about 24 pounds. However, probably the pattern of weight gain is more important than the total weight gain. The usual pattern is a minimal weight gain in the first trimester (1–2 kg) and then a progressive accumulation of approximately 0.35–0.4 kg/week to term. Most of the weight accumulation during the second trimester is related to the maternal compartment and most of the gain during the third trimester is related to the fetal compartment[19] (See Fig. 3.3). At term, the mother accounts for slightly more than half the weight gain and the fetus slightly less than half the total weight gain. Approximately 10% (1–2 kg) of the average weight gain of 11 kg is fat.

Numerous large studies have documented a possible correlation between weight gain during pregnancy and birth weight of the infant. Niswander and Jackson[20] studied several thousand black and white patients and found that smaller weight gains were associated with a higher risk of a low-birth-weight infant which is known to be associated with a higher perinatal morbidity and mortality. On the other side of the coin, with massive weight gain, there was an associated increase in weight of the infant, hence an increased risk of an excessive-sized infant.

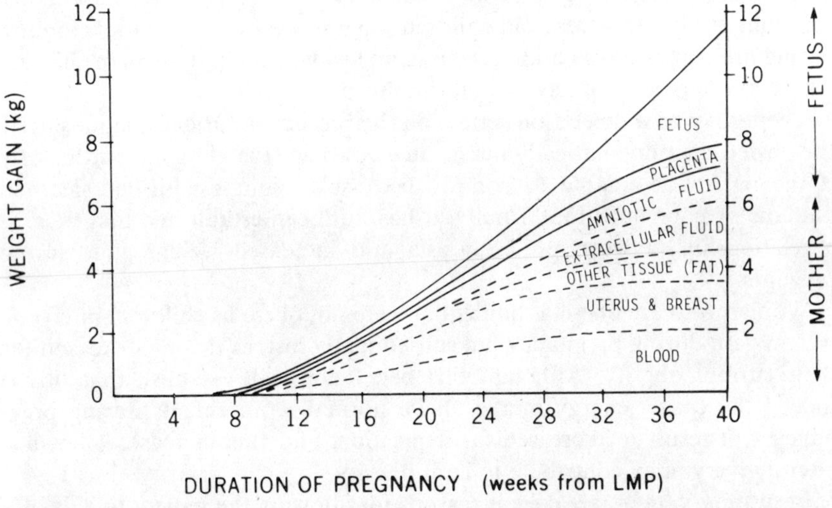

Figure 3.3. Pattern and components of average maternal weight gain. (Reprinted with permission from R. M. Pitkin: Clin Obstet Gynecol 19:489, 1976.)

In an interesting retrospective study,[21] 300,000 19-year-old Dutch inductees whose mothers were exposed to famine during World War II were studied. The inductees were divided into two groups: the mothers of the first group were exposed to famine in the first or second trimester and the second group was exposed to famine in the third trimester or early postnatal life. In the first group there were significantly higher obesity rates among the inductees; in the group exposed to famine late in pregnancy and early postnatal life, there were significantly lower obesity rates. Although this study is subject to the same defects found in any retrospective study, it does provide some evidence for the theory that the third trimester and early postnatal periods are critical for increase in cellularity of adipose tissue.

The dilemma is whether to restrict weight gain to prevent toxemia and possibly later obesity or to allow free weight gain to prevent low birth weight infants and decrease perinatal mortality. The current consensus is that restriction of weight gain to less than the probably optimal 24 pounds is hazardous in a number of ways. First, there is the increased risk of perinatal mortality. Second, severe dietary restriction to limit calories may result in displacement of other nutrients in the diet. Optimal protein utilization in pregnancy requires a minimum of approximately 30 Kcal/kg/day.[22]

During the last decade, a popular practice was to place an obese woman entering pregnancy on a severely limited diet even encouraging these patients to conclude pregnancy with a net loss in the hope of preventing some of the complications known to be more common in obese pregnant women, such as hypertension and diabetes mellitus. This is dangerous not only for the reasons noted above but because severe dietary restriction results in catabolism of fat stores, which in turn produces ketonemia. This is of importance since one study[23] of 4-year-old children suggests that women with ketonuria during pregnancy have children who score less well on IQ tests than children whose mothers did not have ketonuria during pregnancy.

There may be a deleterious effect on the physician-patient relationship if the obstetrician dogmatically insists on a restricted weight gain, particularly if the patient is unable to comply because of long-established, learned patterns of poor nutrition. Finally, it has not been established that there is a relationship between pre-eclampsia and increased weight gain during pregnancy.[18]

Women who are obese as adults but were not obese as children, often cite weight gain during pregnancy not subsequently lost, as the major reason for their current obesity. Although this belief does not establish that this is indeed the cause, energy intake above normal requirements during pregnancy will result in increased fat deposition, and this increase, if not lost after delivery, may contribute to later obesity.

In summary, there are cogent reasons for allowing the patient to gain 10–12 kg during pregnancy whether obese or not. A gain in excess of this may be appropriate for a woman who is initially underweight. However, weight gain in excess of energy requirements, particularly in the last trimester, may predispose both infant and mother to later obesity.

BREAST-FEEDING TO PREVENT OBESITY

REASONS FOR SHIFT TO FORMULAS

Infant feeding practices have changed dramatically in the last 50 years. Formulas were available in the late 1800's, but the first simulated human milk was developed in 1919.[24] Since then, food technology has developed proprietary milk formulas that more closely resemble human milk. In the United States mothers have enthusiastically accepted commercial formulas for infant feeding and it is now the exception, rather than the rule, to breast-feed. Formula feeding rose from 50% to 80% from 1950 to 1970.[25] The reasons for this dramatic increase are complex and involve cultural and commercial pressures. Culturally, the availability of artificial formulas has sometimes been viewed as a scientific triumph. Also, working mothers have found bottle formulas more convenient. Then, the breast as a sexual symbol has been epitomized in newspapers, magazines, and television and its practical usefulness as a source of infant nutrition has not been nationally lauded.

The infant food industry has promoted artificial formulas emphasizing the convenience of formulas and prepared infant foods. This industry is "big business." In 1975, Jelliffe and Jelliffe[26] estimated annual sales at about $400,000,000.00 in the United States alone. It comes as no surprise, therefore, that the baby food industry has a definite financial stake in encouraging formula feeding whether or not this is really advantageous to the infant or mother.

The medical profession has been surprisingly ignorant about breast-feeding and infant nutrition. Most medical schools do not have courses in nutrition nor are the practical aspects of breast-feeding taught to students so that they might later assist their patients who choose to breast-feed. In fact, what has been the prevalent attitude until very recently among pediatricians was summarized by Robert Hutchinson of London (quoted by Jelliffe and Jelliffe,[26] p. 143): "What you need to know about infant feeding can be written on the back of a postage stamp." That this laissez-faire attitude about infant nutrition is incorrect has been established in a variety of studies. First, recent information about the mother-child relationship has had a significant impact on our views. "Bonding," the immediate postnatal attachment between mother and child, may well be different between the breast-fed and bottle-fed child. The development of trust in the infant and the response of the mother may be enhanced during the intimacy of breast-feeding. Later childhood and adult development is, at least in part, influenced by the quality of this mother-child dyad with important implications for later eating behavior. To encourage bottle-feeding which is, after all, only an experiment of the last 50 years, may be to encourage a change in the mother-child relationship that is deleterious to both.

COMPOSITION OF BREAST MILK VS. COMMERCIAL FORMULAS

There have been numerous studies documenting differences between cow's milk and human milk.[27] Figure 3.4 illustrates some of the differences. Cow's milk has more protein than human milk. Human milk has large amounts of lactoferrin whereas cow's milk has miniscule amounts. Alpha-lactalbumin occurs in a larger percentage in breast milk. Also the immunoglobulins in human milk are species-specific and therefore differ from those in cow's milk. Lysozyme occurs in much higher concentrations in breast milk. There is less casein in breast milk than in cow's milk and it has a different physiochemical composition in the two species.

Fat content is greater in breast milk than in cow's milk, providing about 50% of the total calories. In breast milk the long-chain unsaturated fatty acids predominate whereas saturated fatty acids predominate in cow's milk. Furthermore, the fat content of breast milk has a diurnal variation, with a higher fat content in the mornings. The composition of breast milk is influenced by maternal diet—an increased carbohydrate intake by the mother results in an increase in fat content in breast milk.

In order to prepare formulas which more closely resemble breast milk, manufacturers start with non-fat cow's milk and add carbohydrates, vegetable oils, vitamins, or minerals. However, what has been added to "humanize" a commercial formula often does not do so; for example, coconut oil, which contains primarily saturated fatty acids, has been added to some proprietary formulas, but this does not "humanize" the formula. In addition, many of the protein components of breast milk are species-specific and a modified cow's milk does not substitute.

It has been known for years that the composition of breast milk changes during nursing from foremilk which is "watery" to white thick milk which has a higher fat content. Hall[28] theorizes that a change in texture, taste, or smell of the milk triggers an appetite control mechanism from within the infant resulting in appropriate milk intake for the baby. In contrast, commercial formulas have a uniform concentration, flavor, and smell, and thus may fail to trigger the infant's internal regulatory system. According to this theory, overfeeding could easily result with an excessive weight gain and this might predispose to later obesity.

One supposed advantage of proprietary milk has been its lower cholesterol content. This is based on the observation that lower cholesterol values in the adult are associated with diminished risk of atherosclerosis. Fomon[25] has

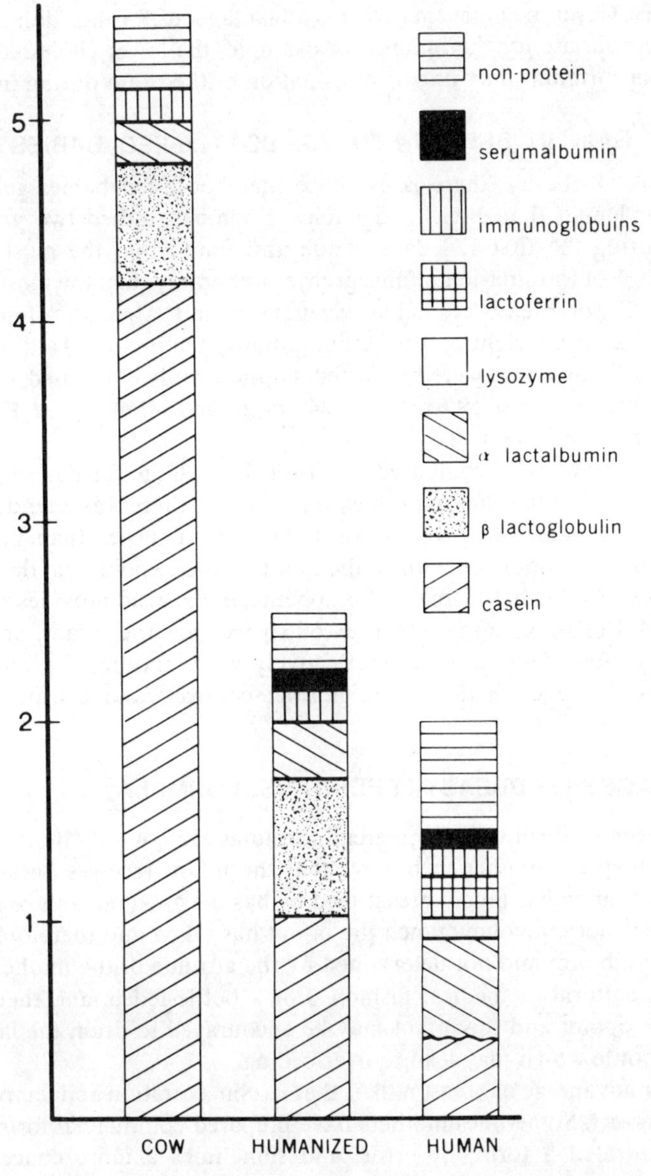

Figure 3.4. Differences between cow's milk and human milk. (Reprinted with permission from L. Hambraeus, E. Forsum, and B. Lönnerdal: Nutritional aspects of breast milk versus cow's milk formula. In L. Hambraeus, L.-Å. Hansson, and H. McFarlane (eds.) Food and Immunology. Symposia of the Swedish Nutrition Foundation XIII. Stockholm, Almgvist and Wiksell, 1977.)

documented a higher cholesterol level in breast-fed infants, particularly females. However, he notes that what is advantageous for the adult may well not be appropriate for the infant. For example, the lower cholesterol levels in artificial formulas may impair myelination of the brain during infancy.

WEIGHT GAIN IN BREAST-FED VS. BOTTLE-FED BABIES

In terms of obesity, there is evidence that bottle-fed babies gain more weight for length than breast-fed babies. Fomon[25] studied two groups of infants during the first 120 days of life and found that the most rapidly growing 10% of formula-fed infants grew more rapidly than the most rapidly growing 10% of breast-fed babies. Neumann and Alpaugh[29] found that doubling the birth weight occurs earlier in bottle-fed infants. Taitz[30] studied 261 infants, 21 of whom were breast-fed. Of these, only 4% gained above the 90th percentile whereas 59.6% of the 240 bottle-fed infants were above the 90th percentile in weight.

Ounsted and Sleigh[31] compared small-for-dates, large-for-dates, and normal infants and found that in both extreme groups there was a tendency for the breast-fed babies to revert toward the median faster than bottle-fed babies. This study does not confirm the traditional viewpoint that the smaller the baby's size at birth, the smaller his appetite, but instead provides evidence for powerful self-regulating appetite controls within the infant, and these controls apparently operate more effectively when the baby is breast-fed. This study, however, had only 36 normal controls, and confirmation is needed.

ADVANTAGES OF BREAST-FEEDING VS. FORMULA

It has been claimed that commercial formulas are not only more convenient but allow the mother to be sure that the infant receives an adequate intake. As Fomon has noted, breast-feeding has the great advantage that the mother does not know how much the infant has taken and therefore intake really is ad libitum and not determined by the attitude of the mother or the prevailing cultural or medical fashion. For a bottle-fed infant, there is an artificial endpoint and the infant may be encouraged to drain the last drop from the bottle which may lead to overfeeding.

Another advantage of breast milk is that its concentration and temperature are also correct. Sometimes mothers have prepared commercial formulas in too concentrated a form, by error, and sometimes a more concentrated formula has been prepared to increase weight gain in the mistaken belief that greater weight *per se* is advantageous. A number of investigators have implicated over-concentrated feeds in the etiology of some cases of the sudden infant death syndrome ("crib deaths"). Taitz[30] suggests that some formulas and semi-solids may be in fact hyperosmolar. The resulting solute load and demand on the infant kidney to excrete the excess electrolytes and urea may lead to greatly increased water requirements. In this situation, a mother may erroneously think that the child is hungry, when in fact he is thirsty, and she may give him more of a hyperosmolar formula, thereby worsening the situation. It has been postulated, but not proven, that this hyperosmolar state may predispose the infant to the sudden infant death syndrome.

Some evidence[32] suggests that there is an association between widely spaced meals and an increased risk of obesity, hypercholesterolemia, impaired glucose tolerance, and atherosclerosis. Frequent suckling, perhaps more likely in the breast-fed infant, may have important metabolic advantages.

DEFICIENCIES OF FORMULAS

In the course of development of various commercial formulas, a number of serious deficiencies has been discovered. For example, one formula on the market several years ago resulted in convulsions, subsequently shown to be due to a lack of vitamin B_6, a nutrient known to be present in human milk, but not recognized as essential. Another potentially fatal syndrome which occurs more frequently in bottle-fed infants is acrodermatitis enteropathica; a deficit in absorption is probably the etiological factor in this syndrome. These examples are but two of the many hazards of various formulas, and they illustrate our ignorance about the complex composition of breast milk and the importance of each constituent. The reader is referred to Jelliffe[33] for a more complete listing of various syndromes that may be due to deficiencies in commercial formulas.

PHYSICIANS' ROLE IN BREAST-FEEDING

Perhaps one of the most difficult aspects of mothering at present is that on all sides the mother has advice from "experts" including relatives, the baby food industry, and the medical profession, with the consequence that nearly all mothers feel guilty about some aspect of their child rearing. As one very caring mother observed, "Guilt goes with the job."[34] Certainly the infant food industry has used overt and covert methods to induce mothers to utilize more of their products, often inducing guilt in the process. The medical profession might help the situation by remembering the first rule of medicine, "First do no harm," and evaluate substitutes for breast milk critically before endorsing their use. It has been wryly noted by Jelliffe and Jelliffe (p. 150)[26]

> " . . . If human milk (or more exactly, the process of breast feeding) were "discovered" the scientist responsible would undoubtedly receive the Nobel Prize. "Mammalac"—or whatever the discovery might be termed—would be hailed for its "cost-effectiveness," for its nutritional value and for its anti-infective contracep-

tive properties, as well as for its easy delivery in even the most remote home in all weathers!"

Breast-feeding alone from a well nourished mother provides adequate nutrients for the first 4–6 months of life. Commercial formulas may be necessary for an infant whose mother cannot breast-feed, or for an infant who is separated from the mother for long periods. There may be a reversal in the trend to bottle-feeding as more parents become aware of the advantages of breast-feeding. La Leche League Organization[35] has done much to encourage breast-feeding and to disseminate information about the more practical aspects of nursing. The support and knowledge of the medical profession could substantially influence this avant-garde trend toward breast-feeding. Skulka et al.[36] report that of a group of mothers who were bottle-feeding, 81% said no doctor or nurse advised them to breast feed, and 16% said this was mentioned only casually. More informed input from physicians is necessary.

EARLY FEEDING PATTERNS

EFFECT OF SOLID FOODS ON OBESITY

There has been a dramatic rise in the early introduction of solid foods with some infants receiving solids in the 1st week of life. Skulka and associates[36] studied 300 infants and found that 1.7% received solid food in the 1st week, 20% had received solid food by the 3rd week, almost 40% had solids by the 4th weeks, and 93% had solids by the 13th week. Ounsted and Sleigh[31] found that 138 of 191 infants were receiving cereals by 8 weeks. The addition of solids to the diet results in a change of nutrients with very little evidence that this is helpful or even safe.

The diet of an infant totally breast fed contains approximately 6% of calories from protein, 56% from fat, and 38% from carbohydrate (principally lactose). Anderson[37] estimates that in the "typical" baby diet in the United States combining both milk and solid food, 8% of the calories are from protein, 12% from fat, and 80% from carbohydrates. Skulka et al.[36] found that the average daily protein intake was 32.7 g, markedly higher than the 20 g/day recommended by Britain's Department of Health.[38] Fat intake in this study was 5.7 g/kg/day in boys, and 6.5 g/kg in girls, higher than the 3–4 g/kg/day recommended.[39] Carbohydrate intake was 1–3 g/kg/day higher in all age groups than the recommended 12 g/kg/day.

The consequences of these changes in nutritional content have yet to be determined, but a number of dangers can be easily hypothesized. For example, although little is known about the early imprinting of taste preferences in human infants, in animals these preferences are known to be established early and are remarkably persistent.

If this is the case for humans, an early introduction to sweet foods might well establish a preference for sugar with important implications for later dieting. Another potential hazard relates to the neonate's gastrointestinal tract known to be more permeable to macromolecules; foreign substances in the cow's milk and solid foods are readily absorbed and may become antigenic.

Also, "weaning" has taken on a new meaning. Whereas it once meant a gradual addition of solid foods associated with a decrease in milk intake, it now often means addition of solids without a decrease in milk intake. Therefore there is often a sharp increase in caloric intake when solids are added.

Jelliffe and Jelliffe (p. 136)[26] have traced some of the changes in infant feeding practices by quoting various pediatric textbooks written over the last 80 years. A few examples are:

> "Eggs, meats and vegetables should not be given until the second year." (1896)
>
> "Cereal may be given at the end of the first year." (1912)
>
> "About the sixth or seventh month, it is advised to begin feeding cooked, strained cereals." (1927)
>
> "Cereal, or pureed fruit or vegetable may be started late in the second or third month." (1962)
>
> "It has become fashionable to introduce cereals from the age of 2–3 months or even younger. . . . The majority of infants thrive on milk alone until 4–5 months." (1970)

REASONS FOR EARLY INTRODUCTION OF SOLID FOODS

Emotional, Social and Economic Pressures

First, fear of underweight is certainly legitimate in a society with scant food supplies: a thin, puny baby in such circumstances *is* likely to die. Only in the last century have any parts of the world had more than enough food for a large segment of the population, and therefore it is only recently that overnutrition, particularly in infants, has been recognized as a problem.

Second, overfeeding may represent guilt on the part of the caretaker. Many women are seeking roles other than wife and/or mother, and this change may exact an emotional cost in the form of guilt. In this context it is interesting to note that Skulka and co-workers[36] found a general tendency among mothers of bottle-fed babies to give solids even earlier than 4 weeks in contrast to mothers of breast-fed babies.

Another interpersonal factor involved in the early introduction of solid foods is competition. Some parents may compete with each other to introduce solids as early as possible in order to demonstrate superiority.

Commercial Pressures

A factor that may well be the most important is the influence of the baby food industry. Mothers are bombarded with advice on how to feed their youngsters. This advice is based on marketing and cost considerations rather than scientific evidence as has been documented by Anderson[37] who describes some changes made in solid baby foods since 1969. These changes (adapted from Anderson (pp. 42–43)[37]) have included:

1. *Sodium:* All manufacturers have recently discontinued the use of added salts.
2. *Sucrose:* There has been decreased use of sugar. Corn sweeteners have been substituted for sucrose in some products.
3. *Discontinued ingredients:* Monosodium glutamate, sodium nitrate, and nitrite are no longer added to baby foods.
4. *Fat:* One manufacturer has increased the amount of fat in strained meats 23.0% with a resultant increase in caloric density and reduction in protein calories.

That these changes are not predicated on scientific nutritional data seems obvious.

Probably many mothers are bewildered by the various claims of baby-food manufacturers and would welcome sound nutritional counseling by their pediatrician or family physician. Despite our relatively sketchy information about infant nutrition, two major recommendations can be given to mothers:

1. Breast-feeding for the first 4–6 months not only provides all the nutrients the baby needs, but probably decreases the likelihood of later obesity.
2. Adding solid foods only *after* 4 months of age also may decrease the potential for obesity.

DECELERATION OF GROWTH IN EARLY CHILDHOOD

NORMAL PATTERN OF WEIGHT GAIN

Determining which children may be predisposed to later obesity is difficult but is facilitated by an understanding of what is known about normal growth and development. Infancy can be described as the era of rapid growth, childhood as the period of stable growth, and adolescence as the era of shifting growth influenced by sex hormones.

Most full-term infants regain their birth weight by 10 days and weight gain after this averages 20 g/day for the first 5 months and then 15 g/day until near the end of the 1st year. The average infant will usually double his birth weight by 5 months and triple it by 1 year. During the 2nd year the average child will gain about 5–6 pounds (2.5 kg) and about 5 inches (12

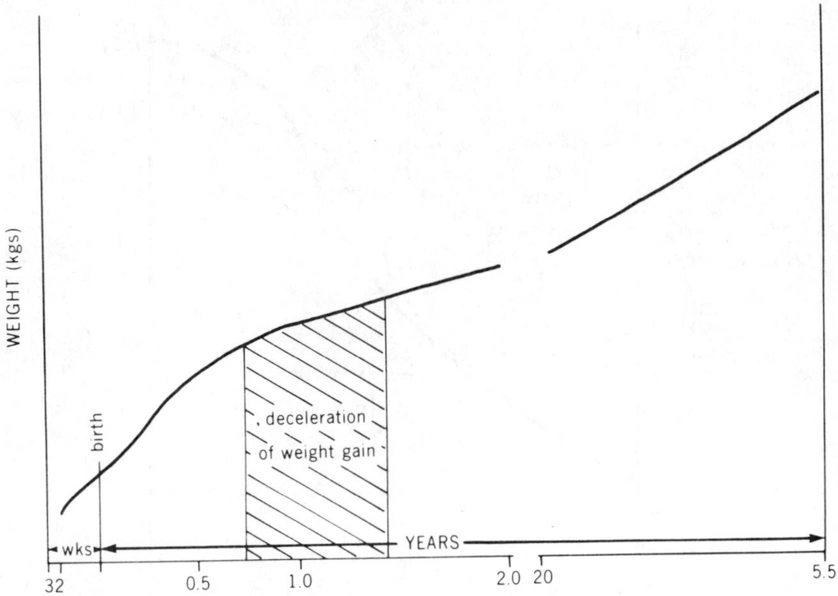

Figure 3.5. Weight gain in late fetal life and first 5 years. Note rapid rate of weight gain in last trimester and first 6–8 months of life. Weight gain decelerates at approximately 10 months.

cm) in length. Near the end of the 1st year and during the 2nd year there is a deceleration in this very rapid rate of growth.

Figure 3.5 shows the average course of weight gain of boys and girls from late fetal and postnatal growth through 5 years of age. As shown on the graph the slope is sharpest in late fetal life and during the first 6–8 months (indicating a more rapid rate of growth). After about age 2 in both boys and girls there is a gradual increase in rate of weight gain until adolescence (Fig. 3.6) when there is again a sharp increase in weight gain beginning at the average age of 11 in girls and 12–13 in boys.

DECREASE IN GROWTH RATE AT 10 MONTHS

There is normally a decrease in rate of growth at about 10 months of age, with an associated decrease in the infant's appetite, which may extend well into the 2nd year. This decrease in appetite is frequently misinterpreted by the mother as illness, or more often as a failure in the mother-child relationship. She may try to correct for what is a normal phenomenon by encouraging the infant to eat more, with consequent overnutrition. Well-meaning relatives and friends may worsen the situation. The physician is

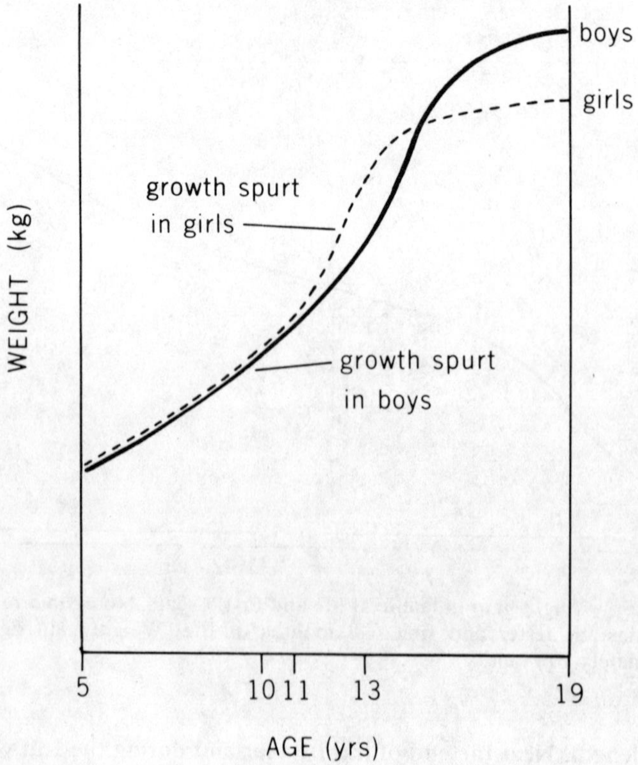

Figure 3.6. Growth patterns in childhood and adolescence. Note stable growth during childhood. The onset of the growth spurt is approximately age 11 in girls and age 13 in boys.

often the last one consulted but he can often obviate the problem by telling the mother in advance that the infant is likely to have a decrease in appetite and that intake should decrease accordingly.

GROWTH PATTERN OF ADIPOSE TISSUE

The pattern of growth of different tissues varies. For example, growth of more than 50% of the brain occurs in fetal life. By the end of the 1st year the brain has attained two-thirds of its mature size and by the end of the second year four-fifths of its adult size. The growth of adipose tissue, however, has a markedly different, probably biphasic, pattern. At birth, the female infant has slightly more adipose tissue and is slightly less muscular than a newborn male infant.[40] Testosterone produced by the fetal testis may account for this slight increase in muscularity of the male newborn. In both sexes there are probably critical periods of marked increase in adipose cell number. The first is in late fetal life, extending into the 1st year of life. Although adipose cell number probably continues to increase throughout childhood, it is at a much lower rate until just before or during adolescence when there is apparently another critical period of rapidly increasing adipose cell number. Evidence for the first critical period of rapid growth is convincing (See Chapter 7), but the details of the postulated second critical period are less clear. Figure 3.7 compares the critical periods of increasing cell number for brain, skeleton, muscle, and adipose tissue.[41]

MIDDLE AND LATE CHILDHOOD

STRESS AND OBESITY

As a youngster leaves infancy and enters childhood there are an increasing number of social and interpersonal factors that affect growth and weight. Although childhood is normally a period of stable growth, obesity may start in childhood. The clinical impression of several authors[42, 43] is that a precipitating event can often be noted in this age group. For example, obesity may follow tonsillectomy, other surgery, or an enforced period of bedrest. A move to a new neighborhood, a mother starting work, or a bout of encephalitis have all been identified[44] as precipitating factors in childhood obesity. The children so identified may not have any earlier history of weight or feeding problems.

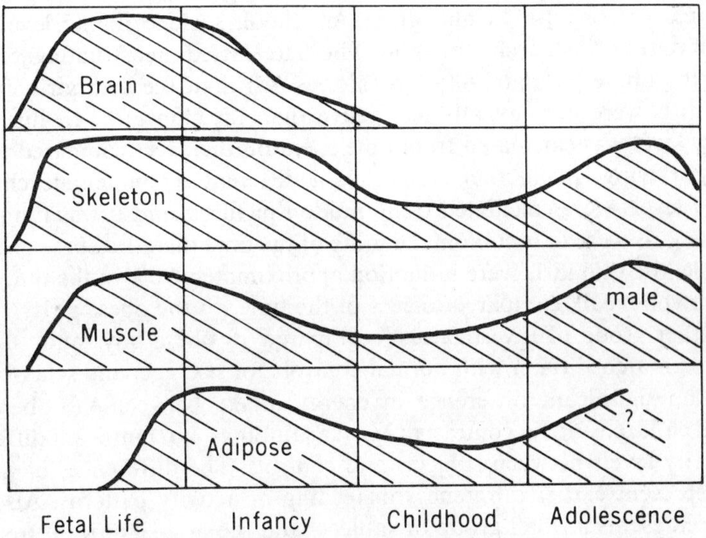

Figure 3.7. Critical periods of increasing cell number for brain, muscle, skeleton and adipose tissue. (Reprinted with permission from D. W. Smith: Major Problems in Clinical Pediatrics, Vol. 15. Philadelphia, W. B. Saunders Co., 1977, p. 2.)

Although feeding is one of the primary forms of nurturance in infancy, it is only with dawning awareness of interpersonal relationships that a child may begin to use food intake to control or please important people in his environment. Refusing to eat is common and probably normal at times, particularly in toddlers who may say no to any request, but refusing to eat or agreeing to eat may become a weapon in families who use food to bribe or withhold food to punish. In families where food substitutes for affection, a pattern of eating when starved for affection may result in obesity. Also in childhood, the youngster begins to be exposed to a wide variety of cultural influences which influence eating patterns.

ACTIVITY LEVELS IN OBESE CHILDREN

Differences in activity levels between normal and obese children become clearer in childhood. In babyhood, placid infants are more likely to gain excessive weight than very active babies, although in "demand" feeding, as epitomized by breast-feeding, probably less active infants adjust their intake to suit energy expenditure. That this may not be a correct theory, however, is suggested by Mayer's study[45] of 31 infants from 0–15 months: no correlation between food intake and weight gain was found, but it was noted that the fatter babies were quiet and placid with a moderate intake, and the thinner babies were active with a larger intake.

Differences in activity levels in childhood have been studied intensively by Mayer and associates. In one study,[46] 28 thin girls and 28 obese girls were compared, pairing for height, grade in school, socioeconomic levels, and time of onset of menarche for those who had started menstruating. Surprisingly, the obese girls ate 300–400 calories *less* than the thin girls, but the obese girls were dramatically less active than the thin girls. In this study, activity level was calculated from time spent on their feet compared to time sitting or lying. In another study[47] of a different set of female children, activity levels were calculated using motion pictures, and it was found that the thin girls were in motion much more of the time than the obese girls. For example, the thin girls were in motion approximately 90% of the time when playing volleyball, compared to 50% of the time for the obese girls.

Another group of investigators[48] compared 10 obese boys and 10 obese girls and matched them with normal controls for sex, age, and school. They found no significant difference in energy intake between the obese and normal children and, in contrast to Mayer's findings, no significant difference in activity levels between subjects and controls. The differences in weights may represent earlier differences in feeding or activity patterns. Also, this study represents a small group of subjects and the non-significant trend for obese boys to exercise less might be significant in a larger study.

Griffiths and Payne[49] compared two groups of normal weight 4- and 5-year-olds divided into two groups on the basis of whether their parents were obese or non-obese. They found that food intake in the group with obese parents was less than in the group with normal weight parents. Energy expenditure at rest was less for the obese group than the normal group. The children with normal weight parents had significantly more energy available for activity than the children with obese parents. Although only 20 children were evaluated, this study raises a number of questions. Do these differences result from environmental or metabolic factors? Are these factors acquired or genetic? Most importantly, could children at risk be relatively easily identified *before* the onset of obesity so that preventive measures might be initiated?

CULTURAL TRENDS AND PHYSICAL ACTIVITY

Over the last century in the United States and other developed countries, there has been a dramatic shift to less and less physical activity as a consequence of a variety of important sociocultural changes including industrialization, automobiles, and television. The number of hours the average child spends watching television is not known with certainty, but the time is significant and during this time the child is usually not exercising and may be overeating. There are more obese girls than boys, and this may be related in part to the decreased emphasis on sports and physical activities for girls compared to boys.

Mayer has led the way in identifying lack of adequate activity as a significant factor in the pathogenesis of obesity. In a successful experiment involving several hundred schoolchildren, Mayer[50] found that adding an hour of exercise to the children's school regimen resulted in a weight reduction in about 60% of these youngsters. Furthermore, this plan obviated the numerous complications inherent in limiting food intake in growing children. Unfortunately, after the experiment, the school returned to its previous routine and a recent survey of the same children found that the effect which lasted during the 4 years of the study was obliterated 3 years after the program was eliminated. Mayer[50] concludes, bitterly, that obesity in children can be treated but "it seems to have very little permanent value in a society that is geared to prevent any child from moving a muscle unless he absolutely insists upon it."

CLASSIFICATION OF CHILDHOOD OBESITY

A variety of classification systems of childhood obesity has been proposed. These classification schemes are described in detail in Chapter 1, but briefly the three main types of childhood obesity are as follows. The first type has been named "constitutional obesity"; it has its onset in infancy and is thereafter characterized by growth of fat that develops at a steady physiological rate.

The second category of obese children has been variously termed "symptomatic," or "malignant" or "progressive" and refers to a group of youngsters whose obesity has its onset in childhood between the ages of 2 and 12. These obese children are often relatively inactive, often fail in school, and are emotionally unstable. Furthermore, their growth pattern deviates progressively from normal with incremental weight gains. A third group of obese children are those with inappropriate eating habits. Infants and adolescents are at greatest risk for this problem.

RARE CAUSES OF OBESITY IN CHILDHOOD

Hypothroidism and Cushing's syndrome may have their onset in childhood, although this is rare. Youngsters with gonadal dysgenesis (XO chromosome state) or with growth hormone deficiency may be obese. However, usually these patients can be easily identified by other stigmata of their disease. A youngster of short stature whose height has not increased since the onset of his obesity should have an endocrinologic evaluation.

OBESITY SECONDARY TO CHRONIC DISEASE

Obesity may occur in children with chronic diseases who are required to be inactive or it may occur in those who receive steroids for lengthy periods. A dramatic example of the mechanical problems that can occur with obesity is seen in youngsters with myelomeningocele. Not only are these patients inactive due to muscle weakness or paralysis of their lower extremeties, but often they receive excessive caloric intake through overprotective feeding or by eating from frustration.

As Ruckard and associates[51] have noted, youngsters who cannot straighten their legs out completely due to paresis are at a mechanical disadvantage requiring a muscular force equivalent to 3½ times the child's body weight to walk reasonably well. Under these conditions the negative effect of excessive body weight on ambulation is magnified 3½ times and obesity itself may literally confine these patients to wheelchairs for life. A multidisciplinary approach to treatment of these children should include early family nutritional counseling as well as the more traditional medical, psychological, and socioeconomic aspects of treatment.

EVALUATION OF CHILDHOOD OBESITY

In summary, the rare youngster with an endocrine or chromosome disorder or known familial disorder should be identified and treated if possible. The child who is inactive due to chronic illness will require extensive multidisciplinary treatment. Finally, the vast majority of obese children will not have these conditions and to devise an adequate treatment program, the following information (adapted from Neumann (p. 119)[42]) is needed:

1. Birth weight—onset of obesity and precipitating events, if any.
2. Early feeding history—breast vs. bottle feeding.
3. Age of starting solids.
4. Mother's or family's perception of what quantity their child should eat.
5. Record of weights and heights—particularly in the 1st year of life.
6. Family history of obesity—and any disease aggravated or induced by obesity, particularly diabetes and hypertension.
7. Twenty-four hour recall for activity and food intake for a typical weekday and weekend day.
8. Assessment of family relationships—particularly mother-child relationship.
9. Degree of dependency, maturity, motivation.
10. Somatotype.
11. Triceps fat measurement.
12. Figure drawings to evaluate body image.

ADOLESCENCE

The specific biologic event of the adolescent years is pubescence: i.e., the maturing of the sex organs and the development of secondary sex characteristics. In addition to these dramatic changes, it is also the time when an individual attains his mature size and stature.

ADOLESCENT GROWTH SPURT

On the average, girls enter puberty earlier and their mid-adolescent growth spurt is approximately 2 years earlier than boys. There is a marked difference in the amount and distribution of adipose tissue between the sexes.

Although both boys and girls increase their body fat in early adolescence, by mid-adolescence girls normally accelerate the deposition of fat whereas boys may even lose body fat in absolute amounts during the last part of the adolescent growth spurt. As a consequence of these sharp sex-related differences, girls have almost twice as much body fat by the end of adolescence.

After 6 months of age there is normally a decline in adiposity in both sexes, more pronounced in boys than girls. In mid-childhood, girls have a gradual increase in adiposity, and by mid-adolescence girls have a rate of increase of deposition of fat that is at its greatest velocity since infancy. In boys, the amount of adipose tissue does not normally increase until early adolescence when there may be a small increment in total fat. Although both boys and girls have an increase in adipose tissue in mid-adolescence, the growth spurt in boys commences with an increase in lean body mass. There is an absolute increase in total body fat during adolescence but there is a decrease in the percentage of adipose tissue, more marked in boys than girls.

In both sexes, there is an increase in muscle mass, more marked in boys than girls. Muscle mass (as calculated from creatinine clearance) doubles in boys from ages 10 to 17. There is also an increase in muscle mass in girls but by approximately age 13 height-years girls have attained their mature complement of muscle mass whereas boys continue to increase their muscle mass until height-age 17. Although boys have reached 80–85% of their mature height by the time they enter puberty, their body mass is normally doubled between 10 and 18.

Boys and girls complete their dramatic differences in distribution of fat, muscle, and bone during adolescence. The adolescent growth spurt is greater in the male in all measurements except for hip width. In shoulder width the difference in velocity of growth is still greater than in most other measurements.

HORMONAL CONTROL OF PUBERTY

The adolescent sex-related differences in body fat, muscle mass, and body contours are under hormonal control as is the development of the sex organs. The nature of this hormonal control is not known with certainty, but much research is underway. Several hormones are known to influence the amount of adipose tissue. Insulin excess, hydrocortisone excess, and pituitary growth hormone deficiency result in an excess of adipose tissue. Estrogen increases adiposity and testosterone reduces the amount of adipose tissue. Thyroxine deficiency results in a small increase in adiposity.

Cheek,[52] theorizes that sex differences between growth hormone and insulin secretion are responsible for the sex differences in body fat and muscle mass. Growth hormone is known to influence nuclear replication and insulin influences cytoplasmic growth. This investigator determined which hormone was dominant by inspecting nuclear number in the muscle vs. the ratio of protein/DNA. The theory is that just prior to the onset of puberty in boys, the male becomes more responsive to growth hormone at the tissue level with rapid cell multiplication in muscle. There is growth of the lean body mass with a corresponding increase in protein and calorie intake. Increased androgen secretion augments cytoplasmic growth in muscle. Fat deposition increases in the male, but less than muscle, probably because both growth hormone and testosterone tend to decrease the amount of adipose tissue. In the female, follicle stimulating hormone (FSH) escalates just prior to puberty with resultant estrogen increase which restricts the action of growth hormone at the tissue level. Insulin is postulated to predominate in influence, resulting in a greater growth of adipose tissue in girls.

PUBESCENCE

In boys, adolescence begins at about age 12 and ends at age 18. In *early adolescence* (average ages 12 to 13), there is an increase in the size of testes and scrotum. In *middle adolescence* (average ages 13 to 16) there is first development of pubic hair, then axillary hair, and a continued increase in size of scrotum and testes and growth in size of the penis. There is a marked growth spurt with a maximum rate of increase at about the time pubic hair begins to grow. Prostate and seminal vesicles mature and spontaneous or induced emissions follow but the sperm are inadequate in number and fertility for fertilization. Voice changes begin as the larynx enlarges. In *late adolescence* (average ages 16 to 18) there is development of facial and body hair, pubic and axillary hair become more dense, the voice deepens, the testes and penis continue to grow, and sperm are adequate in number and motility for fertilization. Growth in height decelerates. By 17¾ years, 98% of boys have reached mature stature.

In girls, development begins earlier and lasts approximately from ages 10 to 16. In *early adolescence* (average ages 10 to 11) there is rounding of hips, and breasts are elevated and in the "bud stage." In *middle adolescence* (average ages 11 to 14) pubic hair begins to develop followed by development of axillary hair. There is a marked growth spurt with maximum rate of height increase 18 months before menarche. Menarche (first menstrual period) occurs and there is associated labia enlargement and a change in vaginal secretions (more acidic). Breasts form early glands. In *late adolescence* (average ages 14 to 16) axillary and pubic hair continues to develop, breasts fill out forming the adult configuration, menstruation is well established, and growth in height decelerates and ceases at the average age of 16¾ years.

The above descriptions of changes that occur in puberty are average ages at which these biological events occur and vary considerably among individuals. For example, in some normal boys the penis growth has finished before it has even started in others. Furthermore, the relationship between the various series of events in puberty is not fixed. For example, certain stages of breast development do not necessarily precede, accompany, or follow certain fixed stages of pubic hair development. Therefore, the ages at which various series of changes start and finish vary as well as the relationship between the different series of events (See Figure 3.8). Furthermore, as Tanner[53] has noted, giving average ages for various pubertal events provides less information than noting the sequence and tempo of pubescent changes in relationship to the peak height velocity.

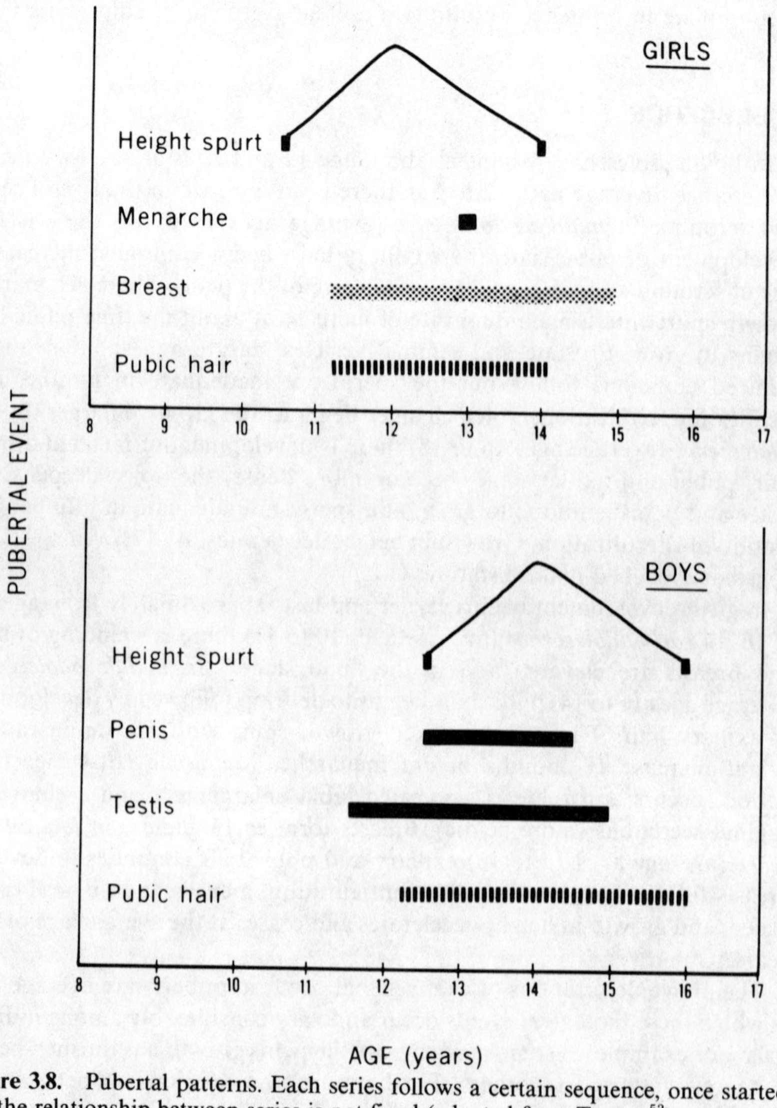

Figure 3.8. Pubertal patterns. Each series follows a certain sequence, once started, but the relationship between series is not fixed (adapted from Tanner[53]).

INFLUENCE ON BODY IMAGE

The maturation of the sex organs and the changes in size, stature, and proportions result in a profound change in body image. Body image is a rather nebulous concept that incorporates one's view of himself, physically, emotionally, and interpersonally (See Chapter 8 for details). Adolescence is characterized by an intense awareness of one's own body and often a painful sensitivity to even the slightest criticism from peers. Although the sequence and tempo of pubertal changes may be irrelevant in terms of eventual physical development, any deviation from one's peers may have catastrophic and perhaps permanent effects on body image and self-esteem. The nature and quality of interpersonal relationships in adolescence, particularly with peers, are likely to influence one's body image. Although results are still tentative, body image appears to stabilize during adolescence. For example, a 30-year-old slender woman may still perceive herself as fat if she was obese in adolescence, particularly if she was teased or criticized by family or peers. An obese teenager may develop an accurate view of himself physically and may have good self-esteem with consequent accurate body image, but this requires support from his family and positive understanding relationships with his peers. More often, the obese teenager is ridiculed and develops negative subjective feelings about his or her body. These negative subjective self-evaluations and misperceptions about body size (many obese teenagers overestimate actual body size) may interact with other factors that tend to promote obesity. For example, the obese teenager who probably already exercises less than his age mates, may refuse to exercise in school or elsewhere, fearing ridicule, and this in consequence results in decreased expenditure of calories.

CRITICAL WEIGHT MAY TRIGGER MENARCHE

Although changes in hormone secretion may account for the differences in muscle and fat content, the trigger for the changes in hormone secretion or the changes in sensitivity to certain hormones remains obscure. Frisch[54] has proposed that there is a direct relationship between critical body weight and crucial events of puberty, particularly menarche. The changing growth patterns in the last two centuries in the developed countries, termed the "secular trend," have resulted in a great change in the rate of maturation and to a lesser extent the ultimate size of individuals. During the last century menarche has started 3 to 4 months earlier each decade[55] and final height has been attained earlier at approximately age 18 compared to age 23 a century ago. Parenthetically, many comparisons of stature compare 18-year-olds from a century ago to 18-year-olds of today and erroneously conclude that there are greater increases in height than there actually are: an 18-year-old in 1850 was still growing in height and an accurate comparison would be between contemporary 18-year-olds and 23-year-olds in 1850. During the last century, nutrition has improved greatly, children increase their weight sooner, and Frisch concludes that this earlier attainment of a critical weight accounts for earlier menarche, as well as for the other less easily documented events of puberty. That is, today children are bigger sooner and girls therefore reach the mean critical weight sooner. She predicts that this secular trend toward earlier menarche will end when successive generations are a constant weight at puberty.

Obese girls tend to have an earlier menarche[56] and consequently advanced sexual and skeletal maturity for their age. Frisch and others have documented a relationship between various events of puberty in both boys and girls that are associated with certain weights. Early and late maturing girls gain the same amounts of weight from initiation of the spurt to menarche (approximately 17 kg), although late maturers grow more slowly than early maturers. In a large study of 201 girls and 209 boys, Frisch found that in girls, initiation of the growth spurt occurs at the mean weight of 31 kg, the peak velocity of growth at a mean weight of 39 kg, and menarche at a mean weight of 47 kg. Age and height at which these events occurred differed greatly as well as the pace at which they occurred. In boys, the initiation of the growth spurt was at the mean weight of 37 kg, and the peak velocity was at 47 kg. Again, age and height at which these events occurred differed, but the mean weights for the crucial events were the same.

On the other hand, menarche is delayed by malnutrition, perhaps because the critical weight is reached later. In undernourished girls, menarche occurred at the same mean weight although 2 years later and at a significantly taller height than in the control group.[54]

Frisch concludes that weight *per se* is the trigger for puberty. Although the mechanism by which weight might trigger the onset of puberty is not known, there are several possibilities. For example, the attainment of the critical weight may cause a change in metabolic rate affecting the hypothalamic-ovarian feedback by decreasing the sensitivity of the hypothalamus to estrogen which might in turn affect growth hormone output. Alternatively, a change in metabolic rate might influence the hypothalamus to stimulate the pituitary to increase output of growth hormone. Although Frisch's theory accounts for some of the known data, her work has yet to be replicated and has not been widely accepted.

There are implications of these findings. First, since it is known that menarche is likely to occur between 43 and 51 kg for 50% of girls, girls nearing 43 kg should receive counseling from their mothers about the management of a menstrual period and its meaning. We could advise parents to discuss sex, reproduction, and menses with their young daughters when they weigh approximately 90 pounds and, therefore, we could correctly time receipt of this information. A second implication of Frisch's work relates to the increase in prevalence of obese teenagers in our overnourished society. These children are likely to enter puberty earlier because they reach the critical weights sooner and therefore may be prone to a variety of psychological problems.

PSYCHOLOGICAL PROBLEMS OF EARLY MENARCHE

The principal psychological problem of an early menarche is that physical changes may start before a child is emotionally ready to incorporate these changes into her body image. Also a youngster who has matured early may be expected by her elders to accomplish more or to be more psychologically sophisticated than she is. A girl may become exquisitely sensitive about breast development or gain in height, at a time when her age mates are relatively insensitive. The resultant teasing may not only be painful at the time, but can have a permanent deleterious effect on the girl's subjective feelings about her appearance. Not only is an obese teenager likely to be teased about her size, but also, she must deal too early with the tremendous changes of adolescence. The following case illustrates some of the problems that can occur even when pubertal events are only slightly early.

> Debra is a 15-year-old attractive girl who appears 18. At age 8 when she weighed 65 pounds, she noticed a lump in her left breast and her mother phoned her physician fearing Debra had breast cancer. Physical examination revealed that her left breast was beginning normal pubertal growth. During the next 2 years, Debra began to grow in height and was taller than her peers, and she began to develop feminine contours. She felt embarrassed about her developing breasts, and she was teased by both her peers and relatives. Her menstrual periods began at age 11, before any of her girlfriends, when she weighed 95 pounds. In the course of her development she had a trusting relationship with her mother and was able to discuss some of these matters openly with her. Debra was easily embarrassed and sensitive about how her body looked. By age 13 she was no longer the tallest girl in her peer group, and by age 15 she was 5′6″ and was shorter than many of her contemporaries. However, at 15, she still felt "out of place" and "older" than her age mates. She dressed in stylish clothes rather than jeans and thought girls her age considered her "snooty." She said she liked her body now but wished she was going to be taller, because she wanted to be a model. She thought that boys her age or a year older were immature and uninteresting, but she was frightened by directly aggressive approaches of 18-year-olds saying she was not ready for sexual involvement. She was doing well in school, was looking forward to driving and a part time job at age 16, and was planning to go to college. She complained that she was expected to make wise decisions when she often felt she needed more guidance. She decided to come for a psychiatric consultation, scheduled her own appointment, arranged her own transportation, and wanted advice as to whether she should pretend not to care for a certain boy her age or tell him that she liked him.

Debra is an example of a teenager who has had many of the typical adjustment problems of adolesence, but slightly out of step with her peers. Her early development has resulted in a mild sense of alienation from her peers, but she will probably be able to cope with her problems effectively because she has a strong sense of identity and mature, flexible ego-defense mechanisms. She will probably develop into a competent mature adult. However, for many youngsters with less ego strength, an early onset of puberty can be markedly more difficult, often devastating.

ADULT-ONSET OBESITY

INCREASING FAT CONTENT DURING ADULTHOOD

There are a number of factors that influence the development of adult onset obesity. Several investigators[57–59] have studied changing body composition in adult life. Fat content continues to change throughout adult life, although the rate of change is less than during puberty. At the beginning of puberty, body fat represents approximately 20% of total body weight. By the end of puberty in males there has been a relative and absolute decrease in body fat to approximately 15% total body weight and in females the percentage of fat has increased to 25% total body weight. After about age 18, however, there is a continuing rise in percentage of body fat in both sexes.

Associated with this steady increase in body fat there is a reciprocal decrease in lean body mass. Concomitant with the rise in fat content, there is a decline in body water and a gradual decrease in body density.[60]

DECLINE IN PHYSICAL ACTIVITY

Physical activity normally declines during adult life, resulting in decreased energy expenditure. If caloric intake remains unchanged, there will be a gain in weight. Furthermore, Nelson and colleagues[61] found a decrease in basal metabolic rate with age and conclude that obesity can develop even if exercise remains constant and food intake is decreased. They estimate that a man weighing 70 kg (154 pounds) eating 2400 kcal and expending 2400 kcal at the age of 30 would weigh 91 kg (201 pounds) at age 62 if no changes were made in food intake or activity levels. Probably exercise influences the percentage of fat content. Several studies of normal subjects during exercise[60, 62, 63] have demonstrated a decrease in total fat content and increase in muscle mass with or without a change in weight. With regular continued exercise, body composition can remain constant over many years,[57, 64] although the amount of exercise may have to increase.

One animal study[65] shows that restriction of physical activity may lead to a paradoxical increase in food intake. Rats were exercised up to 8 hours per day. In the rats exercised between 1 and 5.5 hours per day, food intake was proportional to energy expenditure. Below 1 hour per day food intake increased inappropriately, and above 5.5 hours per day, food intake did not match expenditure and the rats lost weight. If humans paradoxically increase food intake after exercise falls below certain levels, our sedentary society is in double jeopardy for obesity.

In a sedentary society where foods rich in fat and carbohydrate are readily available, it is not surprising that weight regularly increases with age and that a large proportion of the population has "middle aged spread." Although there is cultural pressure to remain slim, very few practical measures are readily available. There are gymnasiums and playing fields, but these are often at a distance from home or work that precludes their use. Convenience foods are more and more a part of the daily food intake and although these foods could be nutritionally sound, usually they are high in sugar and fat content.

CIGARETTE SMOKING AND OBESITY

Several other factors are thought to affect weight gain in adult life. For example, cigarette smokers often gain weight when they stop smoking. Khosla and Lowe[66] reported on body weights of 17,836 miners and found that the men who had never smoked were, on the average, 12 pounds heavier than smokers, over age 40. In men who had previously smoked, weights approached those of the non-smokers. Another study[67] of 224 ex-smokers (154 and 70 women) found that 68% gained weight.

MEAL FREQUENCY

In our culture, there is a tendency toward a decreased frequency of meals in adulthood, and this practice may promote obesity. It has been noted by Fábry and colleagues[68] that the intake of a small number of large meals tends to increase the deposition of fat and overweight in adults. Skinfold thickness measurements were used to estimate fat deposition. A decrease in meal frequency was also associated with hypercholesterolemia and reduced glucose tolerance.

PSYCHOLOGICAL FACTORS

The relationship between obesity and psychological factors in adult onset obesity is unclear. Many obese patients state that they eat to relieve depression or anxiety, but so do many normal weight individuals. Perhaps the pattern of overeating in response to stress is more consistent in those prone to obesity or perhaps in certain individuals there is a change in their biological "set-point" to a higher level in response to stress (See Chapter 5). Stunkard[69] has identified two groups of obese adult patients who appear to eat consistently in response to stress. One group is described as having "night eating syndrome" which occurs in approximately 5% of the adult obese population. These patients, usually women, eat almost exclusively at night and are often nauseous in the morning. This abnormal pattern is intensified by stress. The other relatively uncommon eating pattern associated with stress is the "binge eating syndrome." These patients, typically women, will eat huge amounts of food voraciously and indiscriminately and a precipitating stress can often be clearly identified. Usually the patient feels remorseful after eating. The patient may be able to maintain a normal weight by stringent dieting between episodes, but often she is mildly obese. This syndrome has also been called bulimia, bulimarexia, and the binging-purging syndrome. There has been much recent interest in the condition because of its possible relationship to anorexia nervosa.

EFFECT OF CRUCIAL LIFE EVENTS

It seems likely that emotional factors can contribute significantly to many types of adult obesity but the nature and extent of that contribution are not clear. Anecdotal observation and epidemiological studies have found that some critical events in life, particularly in women, seem to be associated with weight gain.

In one study,[70] married women without children were heavier than single women, at the same ages. Although the weight gain associated with the use of oral contraceptives has been shown in various studies to be due to fluid retention, many women state that they cannot lose the weight gained even after stopping the medication.

Pregnancy is associated with weight gain. McKeown and Record[71] found that, on the average, a woman would be 4 pounds heavier 2 years after her first pregnancy than if she had not become pregnant; after the second pregnancy the weight gain would be 5.9 pounds, and after the third or more 6.2 pounds. Furthermore, women who are obese before pregnancy tend to gain more weight than lean women.

Although Kannel and Gordon[72] (Framingham study) found no correlation between menopause and weight gain, many obese women cite menopause as a factor in their obesity. Marriage, pregnancy, and menopause are all highly significant emotional events in the life of a woman and psychological influences are doubtless part of the complex multi-factorial etiology of adult-onset obesity.

Although critical life events have not been associated with obesity in men, the decade from 20 to 30 appears to be the one with the greatest change in weight. This is a time when most men marry and begin to raise families, and it is also a time when their careers start. The psychological impact of these significant life events on eating and exercise patterns of men has yet to be determined.

In summary, there is a multiplicity of factors that can affect weight and predispose to obesity in adult life. These include a tendency to a more sedentary life, possibly in association with an increased intake of high calorie foods spaced at less frequent intervals than in childhood or puberty. Stress and significant life events may also be associated with the onset of obesity. The interplay of these factors is probably unique for each individual.

References

1. Withers RFJ: Problems in the genetics of human obesity. Eugenic Rev 56: 81–90, 1964.
2. Emery AE: Methodology in Medical Genetics: An Introduction to Statistical Methods. Edinburgh, Churchill Livingstone, 1975.
3. Edwards JH: The value of twins in genetic studies. Proc Soc Med 61: 227–229, 1968.
4. Von Verschuer O: Die vererbungsbiologische Zwillingsforschung. Ergeb Inn Med Kinderheilkd 31: 35–120, 1927, cited by Bray GA: The Obese Patient. Philadelphia, WB Saunders Co, 1976.
5. Newman HH, Freeman FN, Holzinger KJ: Twins: A Study of Heredity and Environment. Chicago, Univ of Chicago Press, 1937.
6. Shields J: Monozygotic Twins Brought Up Apart and Brought Up Together. London, Oxford Univ Press, 1962.
7. Brook CGD, Huntley RMC, Slack J: Influence of heredity and environment in determination of skinfold thickness in children. Br Med J 2: 719–721, 1975.
8. Brook CGD: Genetic aspects of obesity. Postgrad Med J 53(Suppl 2): 93–97, 1977.
9. Falconer DS: The inheritance of liability to certain diseases estimated from the incidence among relatives. Ann Hum Genet 29: 51–76, 1965.
10. Garn SM, Bailey SM: Fatness similarities in adopted pairs (letter). Am J Clin Nutr 29: 1067–1068, 1976.
11. Garn SM, Clark DC: Trends in fatness and the origins of obesity. Pediatrics 57: 443–455, 1976.
12. Sheldon WH: Atlas of Men. New York, Harper and Bros, 1954.
13. Mayer J: The obese hyperglycemic syndrome of mice as an example of metabolic obesity. Am J Clin Nutr 8: 712–718, 1960.
14. Zucker LM, Zucker TF: Fatty, a new mutation in the rat. J Hered 52: 275–278, 1961.
15. Johnson PR, Stern JS, Greenwood MRC, Zucker LM, Hirsch J: Effect of early nutrition on adipose cellularity and pancreatic insulin release in the Zucker rat. J Nutr 103: 738–743, 1973.
16. Peckham CH, Christianson RE: The relationship between pre-pregnancy weight and certain obstetric factors. Am J Obstet Gynecol 111: 1–7, 1971.
17. Chesley LC: Weight changes and water balance in normal and toxic pregnancy. Am J Obstet Gynecol 48: 565, 1944.
18. Maternal Nutrition and the Course of Pregnancy: Summary Report: Committee on Maternal Nutrition, Food and Nutrition Board, National Academy of Sciences. Washington DC, US Government Printing Office, 1970.
19. Pitkin RM: Nutritional support in obstetrics and gynecology. Clin Obstet Gynecol 19: 489–513, 1976.
20. Niswander K, Jackson EC: Physical characteristics of the gravida and their association with birth weight and perinatal death. Am J Obstet Gynecol 119: 306–313, 1974.
21. Ravelli GP, Stein ZA, Susser MW: Obesity in young men after famine exposure in utero and early infancy. N Engl J Med 295: 349–353, 1976.
22. Oldham H, Sheft BB: Effect of calorie intake on nitrogen utilization during pregnancy. J Am Diet Assoc 27: 847–854, 1951.
23. Churchill JA, Berendes HW: Intelligence of children whose mother had acetonuria during pregnancy. In: Perinatal Factors Affecting Human Development. Pan American Organization Committee on Medical Research, Pan American Sanitary Bureau, Washington, DC, Sci Pub No 185: 30–35, 1969.
24. Gerstenberger HJ, Ruh HO: Studies in the adaptation of an artificial food to human milk. Am J Dis Child 17: 1–37, 1919.
25. Fomon SJ: A pediatrician looks at early nutrition. Bull NY Acad Med 47: 569–578, 1971.
26. Jelliffe DB, Jelliffe EF: Fat babies, prevalence, perils and prevention. Environmental Child Health Monograph 41: 123–159, 1975.
27. Hambraeus L: Proprietary milk versus human breast milk in infant feeding. In Nutrition in Pediatrics. Ped Clin North Am 24: 17–36, 1977.
28. Hall B: Changing composition of human milk and early development of an appetite control. Lancet 1: 779–781, 1965.

29. Neumann C, Alpaugh M: Birthweight doubling time: a fresh look. Pediatrics 57: 469–473, 1976.
30. Taitz LS: Infantile overnutrition among artifically fed infants in the Sheffield region. Br Med J 1: 315–316, 1971.
31. Ounsted M, Sleigh G: The infant's self regulation of food intake and weight gain. Lancet 2: 1393–1397, 1975.
32. Fabry P, Tepperman J: Meal frequ•ncy—a possible factor in human pathology. Am J Clin Nutr 23: 1059–1068, 1970.
33. Jelliffe EFP: Infant feeding practices: associated iatrogenic and commerciogenic diseases. In Nutrition in Pediatrics. Ped Clin North Am 24: 49–62, 1977.
34. Baram L, personal communication.
35. Address: La Leche League International: 9616 Minneapolis Ave, Franklin Park, Illinois 60131.
36. Skulka A, Forsyth HA, Anderson CM, Marwah SM: Infantile overnutrition in the first year of life: a field study in Dudley, Worchestershire. Br Med J 4: 507–515, 1972.
37. Anderson TA: Commercial infant foods: content and composition. In Nutrition in Pediatrics. Ped Clin North Am 24: 37–47, 1977.
38. Department of Health and Social Security (1970) Reports on Public Health and Medical Subjects, No 120. London, HMSO.
39. MacKeith R, Wood G: Infant Feeding and Feeding Difficulties. Ed 4. London, Churchill, 1971.
40. Tanner JM: Variability of growth and maturity in newborn infants. In: Origins of Behavior: The Effect of the Infant on Its Caregiver. Lewis M, Rosenblum LA (eds). New York, John Wiley & Sons, Inc., 1974.
41. Smith DW: Growth and Its Disorders. In: Major Problems in Clinical Pediatrics. Vol 15, Philadelphia, WB Saunders, 1977, p 2.
42. Neumann CG: Obesity in pediatric practice: obesity in the pre-school and school-age child. In Nutrition in Pediatrics. Ped Clin North Am 24: 117–122, 1977.
43. Court JM: Obesity in childhood. Med J Aust 1: 888–891, 1977.
44. Forbes GB: Obesity in Ambulatory Pediatrics. Green M, Haggart YE (eds). Philadelphia, WB Saunders Co, 1968.
45. Mayer J: The fat baby. Postgrad Med 44: 277–288, 1968.
46. Johnson ML, Burke BS, Mayer J: The prevalence and incidence of obesity in a cross-section of elementary and secondary schoolchildren. Am J Clin Nutr 4: 231–238, 1956.
47. Bullen BA, Reed RB, Mayer J: Physical activity of obese and non-obese adolescent girls appraised by motion picture sampling. Am J Clin Nutr 14: 211–223, 1964.
48. Wilkinson PW, Parkin JM, Pearlson G, et al: Energy intake and physical activity in obese children. Br Med J 1: 756, 1977.
49. Griffiths M, Payne P: Energy expenditure in small children of obese and non-obese parents. Nature 260: 698–700, 1976.
50. Mayer J: The role of exercise and activity in weight control. In: Weight Control. Eppright ES, Swanson P, Iverson CA, (eds). Ames, Iowa, Iowa State Univ Press, 1955.
51. Ruckard K, Brady MS, Gresham EL: Nutritional management of the chronically ill child. In Nutrition in Pediatrics. Ped Clin North Am 24: 157–174, 1977.
52. Cheek DB: Body composition, hormones, nutrition, and adolescent growth. In: Control of the Onset of Puberty. Grumbach MM, Grave GD, Mayer FE (eds). New York, John Wiley & Sons, 1974, pp 424–447.
53. Tanner JM: Sequence and tempo in the somatic changes in puberty. In: Control of the Onset of Puberty. Grumbach MM, Grave GD, Mayer FE (eds). New York, John Wiley & Sons, 1974, pp 448–470.
54. Frisch RE: Critical weight at menarche, initiation of the adolescent growth spurt, and control of puberty. In: Control of the Onset of Puberty. Grumbach MM, Grave GD, Mayer FE (eds). New York, John Wiley & Sons, 1974, pp 403–423.
55. Tanner M: Secular trend toward earlier physical maturation. Tijdschr Geneesk 44: 524–539, 1966.
56. Zacharias L, Wurtman R, Schatzoff M: Sexual maturation in contemporary American girls. Am J Obstet Gynecol 108: 833–846, 1970.

57. Forbes RM, Reina JC: Adult lean body mass declines with age: some longitudinal observations. Metabolism 19: 653–663, 1970.
58. Behnke AR: Anthropometric evaluation of body composition throughout life. Ann NY Acad Sci 110: 450–464, 1963.
59. Young CM, Blondin J, Tensuan R, Fryer JH: Body composition studies of "older" women, thirty to seventy years of age. Ann NY Acad Sci 110: 589–607, 1963.
60. Friis-Hansen: Hydrometry of growth and aging. In Human Body Composition. Brozek J (ed). Oxford, Pergamon Press, 1965, pp 191–209.
61. Nelson RA, Anderson LF, Gastineau CF, et al: Physiology and natural history of obesity. JAMA 223: 627–630, 1973.
62. Bjorntörp P: Effect of physical conditioning in obesity. In: Obesity in Perspective. Bray GA (ed). Fogarty International Center Series on Preventive Medicine, Vol II, Part 2. Washington DC, US Government Printing Office, 1976.
63. Keys A, Brozek J: Body fat in adult man. Physiol Rev 33: 245–325, 1953.
64. Keys A, Taylor HL, Grande F: Basal metabolism and age of adult man. Metabolism 22: 579–587, 1973.
65. Mayer J, Marshall NB, Vitale JJ, et al: Exercise, food intake and body weight in normal rats and genetically obese adult mice. Am J Physiol 177: 544–548, 1954.
66. Khosla T, Lowe CR: Obesity and smoking habits by social class. Br J Prev Soc Med 26: 249–256, 1972.
67. Wynder EL, Kaufman PL, Lesser RL: A short-term follow-up study on ex-cigarette smokers. Am Rev Resp Dis 96: 645–655, 1967.
68. Fábry P, Fodor J, Hejl Z, et al: The frequency of meals: its relation to overweight, hypercholesterolaemia and decreased glucose tolerance. Lancet 2: 614–615, 1964.
69. Stunkard AJ: The Pain of Obesity. Palo Alto, Bull Publ Co, 1976.
70. Lowe CR, Gibson JR: Changes in body weight associated with age and marital status. Br Med J 2: 1006–1008, 1955.
71. McKeown T, Record RG: The influence of weight and height on weight associated with pregnancy in women. J Endocrinol 15: 423–429, 1957.
72. Kannel WB, Gordon T: 3. Obesity and cardiovascular disease: the Framingham study. In: Obesity Symposium, Dec 4–15, 1973. Burland WL, Yudkin J, Samuel P (eds). London, Servier Research Institute, 1971.

CHAPTER

4

Endocrinological and Other Uncommon Causes of Obesity

T. Scott Douglass, M.D.*

Despite their frequent concern regarding a "glandular problem," patients with obesity seldom have an underlying disease process causing their problem. The more significant the obesity the less likely it is that endocrinologic dysfunction is responsible. Essential obesity is common. Endocrinological diseases associated with obesity are uncommon and none give rise to massive obesity. While hypothalamic lesions may cause obesity, they are usually associated with other neurological findings, or in association with obvious systemic diseases. Nonetheless, the obese patient should be specifically evaluated for possible underlying organic disease. Those individuals who require special testing can usually be readily identified by history and physical examination.

THYROID DISEASE

Thyroid deficiency, contrary to popular misconception, is not a cause of obesity. Certainly obesity occurs in patients with myxedema, but when it occurs, it is an independent process. Plummer,[1] in 1940 at the Mayo Clinic, studied 100 consecutive patients with well established hypothyroidism; he found no evidence of increased obesity in this group of individuals, either before or after treatment with thyroid replacement. Hypothyroidism from either primary or secondary causes can produce fluid accumulation and

* Associate Consultant, Internal and Preventive Medicine, Mayo Clinic and Mayo Foundation; Instructor, Mayo Medical School.

consequent weight gain. Simple unexplained weight gain, however, is rarely the only clue to this diagnosis. Hypothyroidism should not be difficult to recognize if thought about at this point, as typical associated symptoms and physical features of hypothyroidism will usually be present when fluid accumulation is significant. The typical features of hypothyroidism are well known; these include cold intolerance, dry skin, dry hair, brittle nails, constipation, fatigue, menorrhagia, hoarse voice, and muscle cramps. Fluid accumulation in myxedematous tissue explains the finding of myoedema and the delayed relaxation phase of deep tendon reflexes in hypothyroidism. Soft tissue swelling in the wrist gives rise to a medically treatable cause of the carpal tunnel syndrome. If the patient has a goiter or the typical appearance of myxedema the diagnosis may be obvious at once (Fig. 4.1). On the other hand, subtle hypothyroidism or sometimes even advanced thyroid deficiency, may not be readily apparent. For this reason a total serum thyroxin or other appropriate screening test should be performed if there is any doubt concerning the patient's thyroid status. From a clinical standpoint patients being evaluated for obesity expect their thyroid function to be tested, and since even the best clinical diagnosticians have sometimes been fooled by hypothyroidism it is usually wise to document thyroid status chemically.

The biochemical establishment of hypothyroidism is usually straightforward and should be used to confirm the clinical diagnosis before instituting replacement therapy. When appropriate thyroid replacement is begun, negative water balance is produced, and the tissues rid themselves of the excess fluid that has accumulated. This initial fluid weight loss through diuresis occurs within the first 2 weeks of treatment, and may be as much as 5 to 8 pounds, but is seldom greater![1] This figure is probably generous since it is based on data from the treatment of a population of myxedema patients whose myxedema was probably more severe than is commonly encountered today.

Scientific studies have failed to substantiate any benefit from the routine administration of thyroid hormone in the treatment of obesity. There is no place for thyroid hormone supplements in the treatment of obesity in the clinically or chemically euthyroid individual. Careful clinical and chemical assessment of patients receiving thyroid replacement therapy is indicated and the goal should be the establishment of a euthyroid state.

Some patients may be tempted to use thyroid replacement because of a placebo effect or because of a mild euphoria which sometimes accompanies exogenous hyperthyroidism. While hyperthyroidism can produce weight loss it is achieved at the expense of lean body mass out of proportion to the loss of adipose tissue.[2] The use of thyrotoxic doses of thyroid hormone is therefore metabolically unsound as well as dangerous.

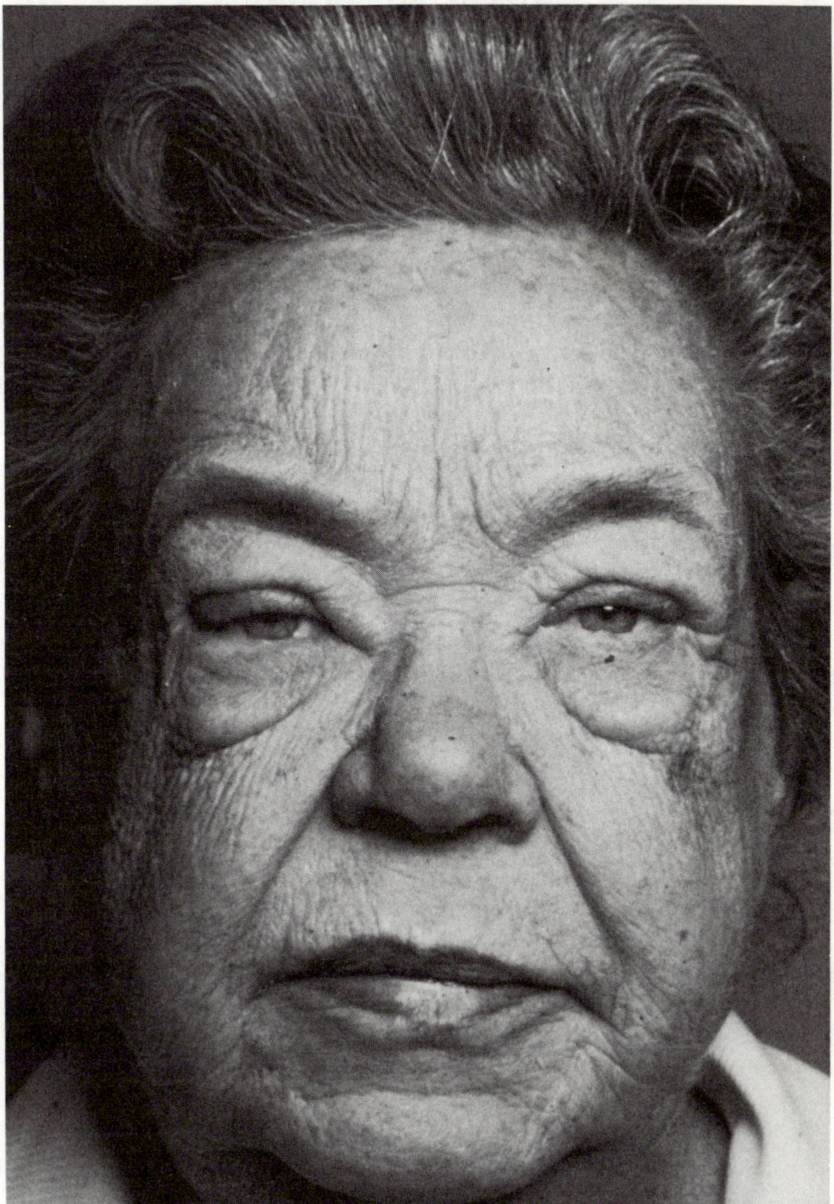

Figure 4.1. Hypothyroidism.

HYPERCORTISOLISM

Hypercortisolism (Cushing's syndrome), whether endogenous or exogenous, may lead to obesity. Cortisol is an appetite stimulant and this is a main contributor to the obesity of hypercortisolism. As with thyroid deficiency it is usually easily recognized when the constellation of characteristic clinical features are present. These include hypertension, osteoporosis, carbohydrate intolerance, thin skin, pink striae, and a peculiar pattern of fat distribution which helps to distinguish it from simple obesity (Fig. 4.2). Fattening appears to take place in a centripetal or truncal distribution. Actually, this truncal distribution of fat, seen in hypercortisolism, is more apparent than real. Obviously it is not possible for cortisol to exert a selective effect on centrally located fat storage depots. What happens appears to be a

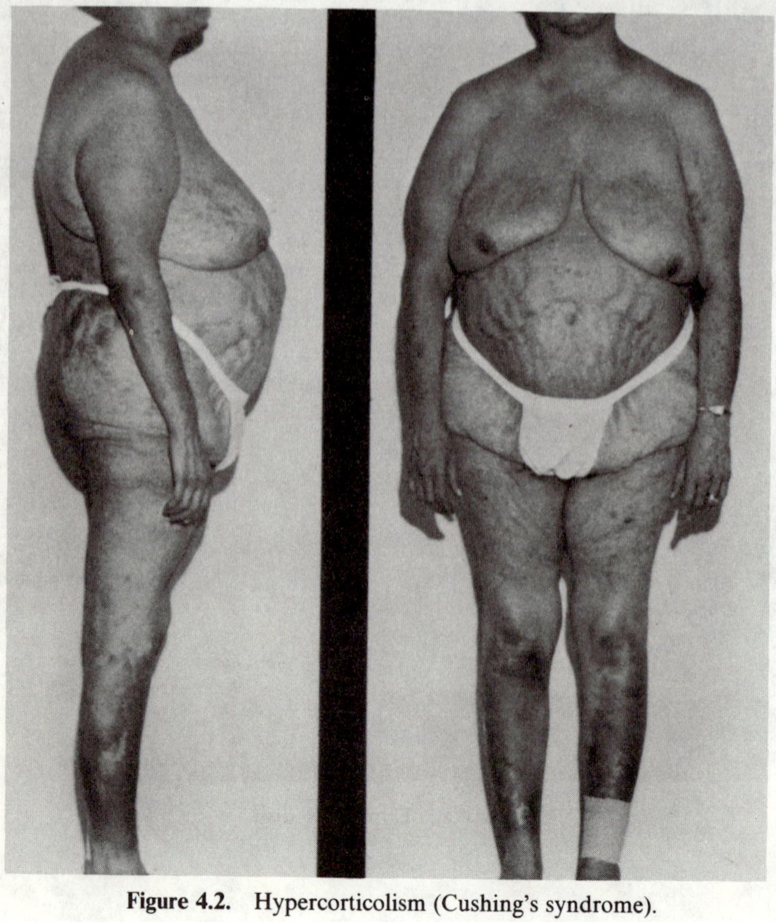

Figure 4.2. Hypercorticolism (Cushing's syndrome).

combination of two factors. First, fat storage takes place in all fatty tissues throughout the body, but more fat seems to occur about the trunk because more fat cells are located here. Simultaneously, cortisol exerts a catabolic effect on lean body mass and since more muscle tissue is located peripherally in the extremities, more wasting occurs there. It is the combination of these two effects that produces the characteristic pattern of the distribution of fat seen in hypercortisolism. Essential obesity may be associated with elevated urinary 11-hydroxycorticosteroid and 17-ketogenic steroid excretion; however serum cortisol levels are usually normal, and their diurnal variation is unaffected by uncomplicated simple obesity.[3] If serum or urinary determinations of cortisol secretion are elevated, the diagnosis of hypercortisolism is excluded by the demonstration of suppressability with dexamethasone.

INSULINOMA

Insulinoma is another unusual endocrinological disorder which has been considered and can be a cause of obesity. The diagnostic problem is compounded by the elevation of serum insulin levels which occurs with essential obesity. An insulinoma is a functioning insulin-producing islet cell tumor of the pancreas; an insulinoma may be single or multiple. The problem is one of hypoglycemia. If the individual does not eat frequently enough, he develops typical symptoms of hypoglycemia, including symptoms related to epinephrine excess (tremors; diaphoresis, tachycardia) and those of neuroglycopenia (drowsiness, incoordination, restlessness, syncope, and/or seizures).

The diagnosis of insulinoma is established by demonstrating inappropriately elevated endogenous plasma insulin levels, relative to low plasma glucose levels. This can usually be accomplished by fasting under controlled conditions in a hospital setting and obtaining simultaneous plasma insulin and glucose levels when symptoms of hypoglycemia occur or at the end of 72 hours. The tolbutamide test may also be used. Arteriography is usually performed in an attempt to localize the tumor and determine its extent before surgical exploration is undertaken to remove the tumor. Very rarely, non-pancreatic tumors may secrete insulin. Diazoxide and streptozotocin are additional therapeutic modalities.

Hyperinsulinism has been suggested as a possible mechanism leading to simple obesity, but while it is interesting that some individuals with insulinoma tend to be obese, the relationship between insulinomas and obesity is not as great as might be expected. In 60 consecutive cases of insulinoma seen at the Mayo Clinic, only 11 patients were found to be obese at the time of diagnosis.[4]

It has been observed that a number of obese people with insulinomas apparently did not begin to gain weight until they had made the conscious association between eating and avoiding their spells. In other words, increased feeding behavior and consequent obesity, at least in some cases, appears to be the result of learned behavior, rather than increased hunger or hypothalamic stimulus.

The situation is analogous to the insulin-taking diabetic who, on a fixed dose of insulin, begins having insulin reactions, increases his caloric intake to prevent symptoms, and subsequently gains weight. It has been demonstrated experimentally in animals that exogenous insulin administration results in the development of obesity.[5] Both situations, however, are different from the mild, chronic hyperinsulinism present in simple obesity in which more complex factors are involved in regulating feeding behavior.

GONADAL DISEASES

HYPOGONADISM

Hypogonadism has been associated with obesity. Testosterone is an anabolic steroid and alters metabolism by increasing the proportion of lean body mass relative to fat. Animal producers have been aware of this for a long time and have used castration on a commercial basis to increase feed efficiency and produce animals with a higher fat-to-muscle ratio. It is interesting to note that castration less reliably produces obesity in humans than in other animals. This may also be related to more complex factors involved in human eating behavior. In women there appears to be no consistant effect of castration related to obesity. No abrupt increase in obesity occurs in women at menopause. Weight gain occurring in the 50's in women is consistent with the trend established in their 20's, 30's, and 40's.

The tendencies toward altered fat/muscle ratios in humans as a result of gonadal failure is independent of whether it is primarily in nature due to trauma, testicular infection, congenital syndromes such as Klinefelter's (seminiferous tubule dysgenesis), or idiopathic causes. Secondary gonadal failure may be due to pituitary insufficiency with failure to synthesize the gonadotropin-luteinizing hormone (LH) and follicle-stimulating hormone (FSH) or it may be due to hypothalamic failure to elaborate appropriate releasing factors. Gonadal hormone replacement is indicated only when specific deficiencies exist and is otherwise not useful in the treatment of obesity.

POLYCYSTIC OVARY SYNDROME

There is an increased prevalence of obesity associated with polycystic ovary (PCO) syndrome. It is not, however, a homogenous entity. The Stein-Leventhal[6] syndrome (Fig. 4.3) classically is characterized by obesity, hirsutism, oligomenorrhea, and infertility in association with polycystic ovaries. It represents one end of the spectrum of PCO disease. At the other end of

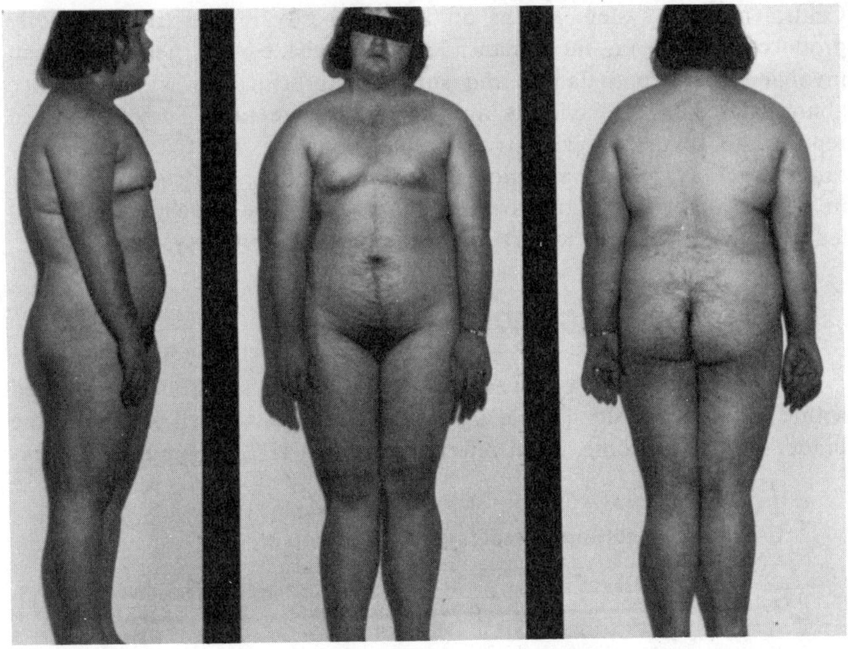

Figure 4.3. Stein-Leventhal syndrome.

this spectrum are women with polycystic ovaries who do not appear to develop any of the other classically associated clinical features. Most, however, do tend to have some features of the Stein-Leventhal syndrome, and these women tend to be a little heavier, a little more hairy, and have more menstrual irregularities. The syndrome most frequently must be differentiated from Cushing's syndrome.

The etiology of the PCO syndrome is not completely understood. Hypothalamic, ovarian, adrenal, and peripheral hormone metabolism all appear to be involved. While the endocrinological abnormalities present in PCO syndrome have been extensively studied, no direct hormonal basis for the increased prevalence of obesity has been demonstrated. The onset of obesity frequently tends to occur about the time of puberty and usually appears to be related to increased caloric consumption beginning about this time. The basal metabolic rates in women with the PCO syndrome are normal and they can lose weight with caloric restriction. Beyond this not much is known regarding obesity in the PCO syndrome.

HYPOTHALAMIC SYNDROMES

The hypothalamus, limbic system, and other related central nervous system structures play an important role in regulating feeding behavior.

Central nervous system lesions producing obesity in rats can be readily produced.[7] However, in humans, lesions of the central nervous system involving the hypothalamus and surrounding structures which produce abnormal feeding behavior leading to obesity are rare. They have been reported to occur following trauma, infections, or from compression by tumors such as craniopharyngiomas or Hans-Schüller-Christian disease, or in association with obvious systemic disease processes such as childhood leukemia with leukemic infiltration of the central nervous system.

CHILDHOOD OBESITY

Pediatricians have long recognized characteristic syndromes associated with childhood obesity (Table 4.1). One of the most well known is the Prader-Willi[8] syndrome, often referred to as the HHHO syndrome of hy-

Table 4.1
Childhood syndromes associated with obesity.

Disease	Characteristic Features
1. Laurence-Moon-Bardet-Biedl (LMBB) Syndrome	• obesity • retinal degeneration • mental retardation • polydactyly • hypogenitalism
2. Alstrom-Hallgren Syndrome	• obesity • childhood blindness • nerve paralysis • diabetes mellitus
3. Prader-Willi Syndrome	• obesity • short stature • mental retardation • hypogonadism
4. Morgagni-Stewart-Morel Syndrome	• obesity • virilism • hyperostosis

potonia, hypomentation, hypogonadotrophic hypogonadism, and obesity. Obesity usually becomes evident during the first decade of life and is frequently a most difficult problem since the child's voracious appetite, if unchecked, can lead to profound obesity (Fig. 4.4).

Another syndrome associated with obesity presenting in childhood is the Laurence-Moon-Bardet-Biedl[9] syndrome (Fig. 4.5). These children have decreased intellectual functioning, hypogonadism, retinitis pigmentosa, polydactyly, and a tendency to obesity that begins in childhood, but usually is not as striking as is seen in the Prader-Willi syndrome.

Other rare syndromes of obesity are the Alström-Hallgren syndrome, characterized by obesity, blindness in childhood, nerve paralysis, and diabetes mellitus, and the Morgagni-Stuart-Morel[10] syndrome which occurs in older women and is characterized by virilism, obesity, and hyperostosis.

METABOLIC VARIATIONS IN OBESITY

Medical science has sought in vain for some pathophysiological abnormality or humoral factor responsible for essential obesity. While a number of biochemical variations have been described in association with the condition, none has been proven to be the cause. A partial list of metabolic variations found in obesity are presented in Table 4.2.

INSULIN ABNORMALITIES

The observation of pancreatic islet cell hypertrophy in obesity suggested the possibility of altered insulin metabolism.[11] This was subsequently also observed in hypothalamic-induced obesity in rats.[12] Elevated fasting and postabsorptive insulin levels in non-diabetic obese subjects have been found by a number of other investigators[13, 14] (Fig. 4.6).

An interesting phenomenon noted in hypothalamic-induced obesity in rats is that lesions of the ventromedial nucleus (VMN) produce a rise in plasma-insulin levels in a few days even before obesity occurs, and this appears to be independent of the overfeeding as overfed sham-operated rats don't develop hyperinsulinism.[15]

In essential obesity, while some yet-to-be-clarified hypothalamic and other associated central nervous system structures may be playing some role in producing hyperinsulinism,[5] other mechanisms also appear to be involved. Peripheral tissues, specifically fat and muscle, have been shown to be relatively resistant to the effects of insulin in the obese state,[16–19] and the size of the fat cells appears to correlate directly with the degree of insulin resistance.[20] Physical training has been found to decrease hyperinsulinism in obesity, independent of weight loss, and suggests that muscle metabolism plays an important role in the hyperinsulinism of obesity.[21]

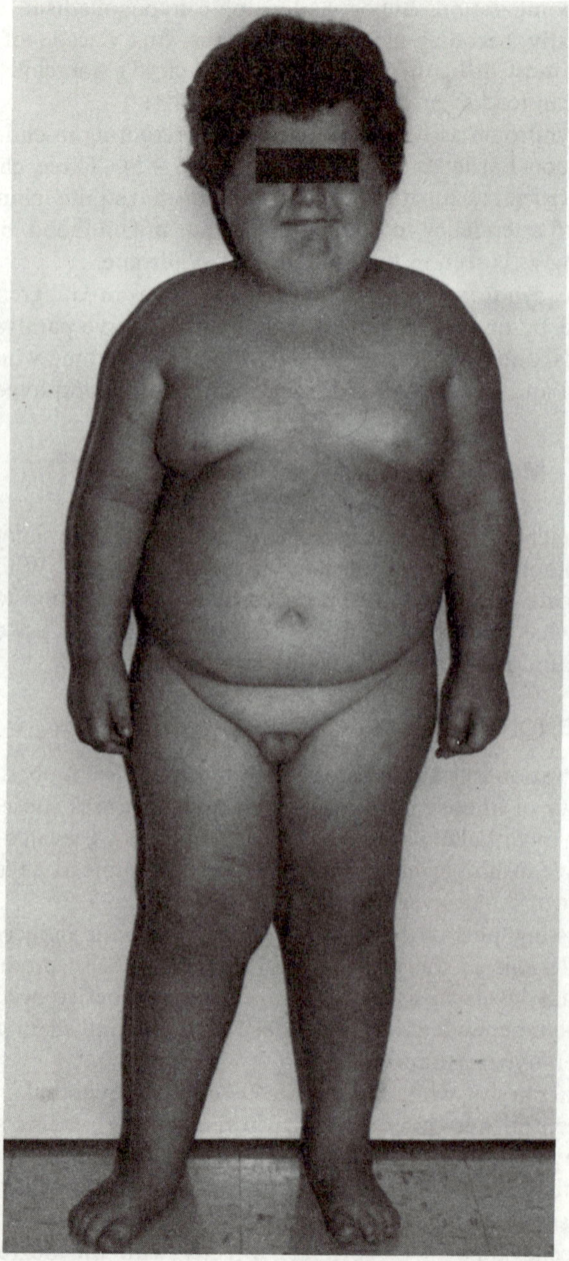

Figure 4.4. Prader-Willi syndrome. Note hypogonadism marked obesity, and short stature.

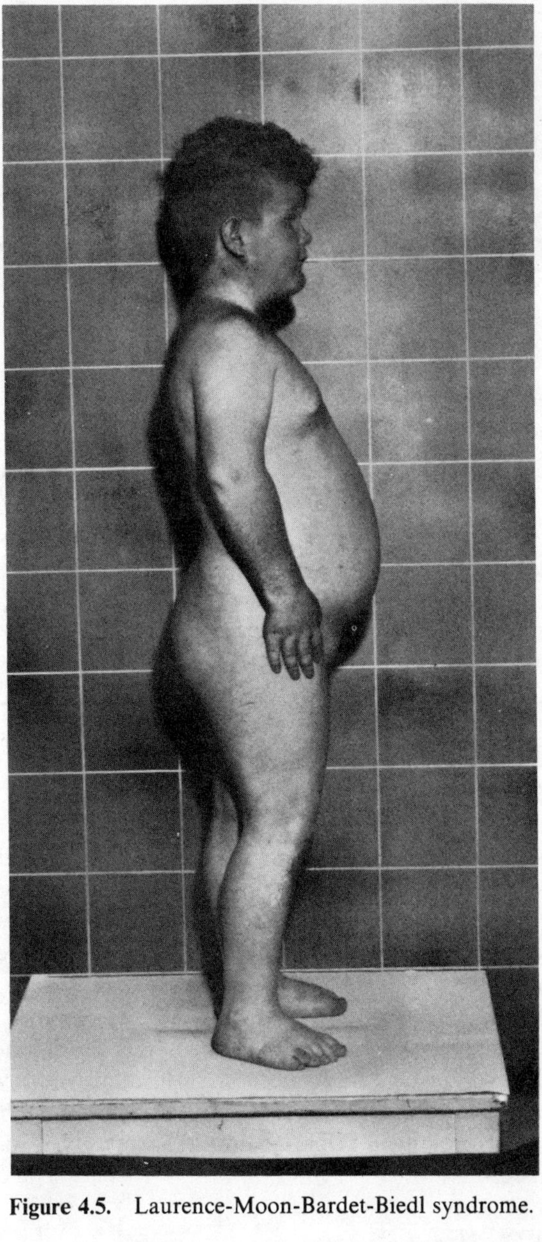

Figure 4.5. Laurence-Moon-Bardet-Biedl syndrome.

Table 4.2
Metabolic variations in obesity.

METABOLIC VARIATIONS IN OBESITY
• Hyperinsulinism
• Resistance to ketosis
• Carbohydrate intolerance
• Blunted growth hormone responsiveness
• Hyperlipidemia
• Hyperaminoacidemia

Obese individuals seem to be relatively resistant to the development of ketosis. In the thin individual ketosis develops relatively quickly following only several hours of fasting.[22] However, in the obese person it may be a matter of days before ketosis develops. It has been suggested that hyperinsulinism in obesity plays a part here by facilitating the use of free fatty acids by non-ketogenic metabolic pathways.[23] However, it may also reflect to some extent the increased hepatic and muscle-glycogen stores present in the overfed individual.

Obesity is strongly correlated with carbohydrate intolerance. It has been long observed that obesity frequently precedes the development of adult onset diabetes, and that weight reduction can bring about improvement and/or normalcy of carbohydrate metabolism. At the present time, however, it is still unproven that prolonged hyperinsulinism in obesity leads to insulin-dependent diabetes.[24, 25]

GROWTH HORMONE

Growth hormone, in addition to its essential role in facilitating growth in pre-pubertal individuals, is also involved in metabolic adaptive adjustments

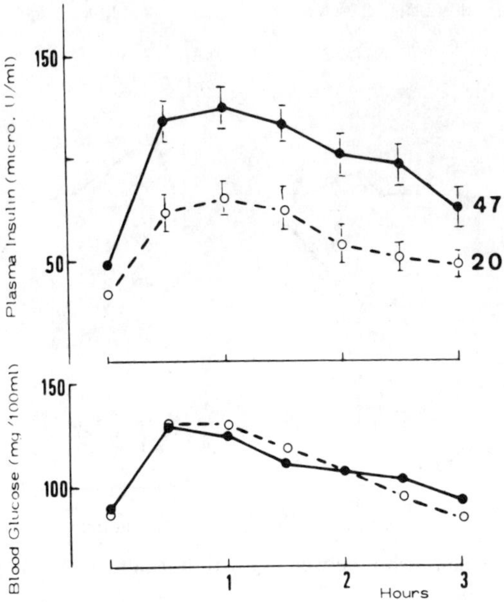

Figure 4.6. Fasting and Post-absorptive insulin levels in non-diabetic obese subjects.

to food deprivation by promoting nitrogen retention, carbohydrate sparing, and fat mobilization. The secretion of growth hormone is under hypothalamic control. In the non-obese individual following a glucose load, there is normally an initial suppression of growth hormone secretion followed later by a rise in growth hormone to above basal levels. However, in the obese individual, while initial post-absorptive suppression of growth hormone occurs normally, late secretion of growth hormone is subnormal. Similarly, the response of growth hormone secretion to hypoglycemia, arginine infusion, and fasting is blunted by obesity[26] (Fig. 4.7). Growth hormone responsiveness to these various stimuli is restored by weight reduction to ideal weight.

Insulin normally facilitates protein synthesis and tends to lower serum amino acid levels; however, certain amino acids (valine, leucine, isoleucine, tyrosine, and phenylalanine) have been found to be elevated in the serum of obese individuals. It has been suggested that this represents another manifestation of insulin resistance at the tissue level.[27, 28]

LIPIDS

Hyperlipidemia is frequently associated with obesity. It is predominantly a problem of hypertriglyceridemia rather than hypercholesterolemia.[29, 30]

The Frederickson-Levy Type IV lipoprotein pattern is the type most commonly seen in association with obesity.[30, 31] The association of other

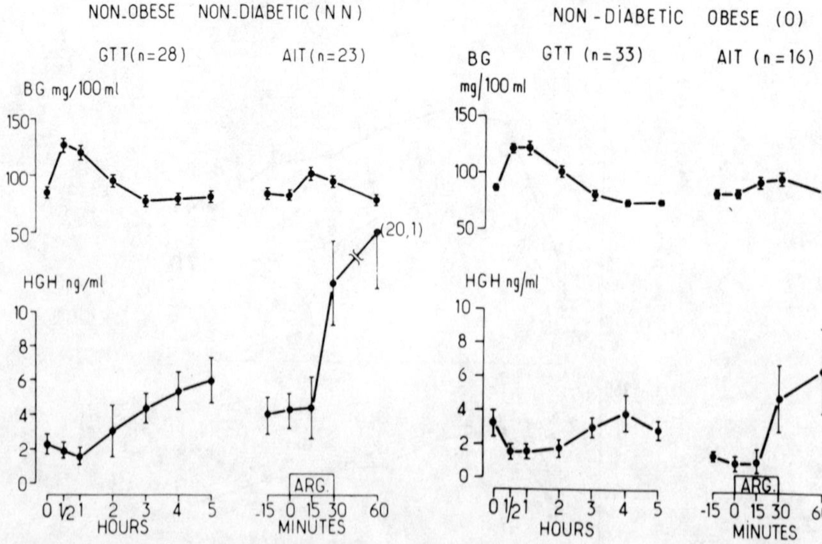

Figure 4.7. Relationship between growth hormone and hypoglycemia.

lipoprotein patterns with obesity is less clear. Hypertriglyceridemia associated with obesity will frequently be corrected by caloric restriction seen before significant weight loss occurs. Decreasing the proportion of carbohydrates in the diet, especially concentrated sugars and alcohols, is also helpful in modifying hypertriglyceridemia.

Hyperlipidemia in obesity results from endogenous overproduction[32] and/or impaired plasma clearance of lipids.[33] Hyperinsulinism probably plays a role in producing hypertriglyceridemia by facilitating hepatic very low density lipoprotein (VLDL) synthesis.[34] Hypertriglyceridemia has been shown to be associated with hyperinsulinism in both non-obese as well as obese individuals.[35]

Free fatty acid (FFA) metabolism is altered in obesity. Basal plasma levels are elevated and the normal rise usually seen with fasting is blunted in obesity.[36] Insulin administration decreases plasma FFA levels by suppressing lipolysis, but less efficiently in obesity due to insulin resistance.[37]

Free fatty acids have consistently been found to be elevated in obesity. This is probably explained by two factors: (1) increased lipolysis occurs as a consequence of increased adipocytes and (2) altered lipolysis and esterification occur in obesity.

ENERGY EXPENDITURE

Despite the metabolic variations that occur with obesity, physiological studies show that obese persons are not any more efficient in their use of calories for energy production than their leaner counterparts. When body surface area, a measure of body size, is taken into consideration in interpreting the metabolic rate under basal conditions, it appears that obese individuals have no difficulty in mobilizing fat stores as a source of energy, in fact they tend to burn fat more rapidly than normal weight individuals in order to satisfy their greater energy requirements.[38]

Obviously a number of complex factors are related to the metabolic variations found in what some have called "simple" obesity. It appears that these variations represent not the cause but only a consequence of obesity and the calories needed to maintain it.

References

1. Plummer WA: Body weight in spontaneous myxedema. Tr Am A Study: Goiter, pp 88–98, 1940.
2. Kyle JH, Ball MF, Doolan PD: Effect of thyroid hormone on body composition in myxedema and obesity. N Engl J Med 275: 12–17, 1966.
3. Schteingart DE, Conn JW: Characteristics of the increased adrenocortical function observed in many obese patients. Ann Ny Acad Sci 131: 388–403, 1965.
4. Service JF: Insulinoma: clinical and diagnostic features of 60 consecutive cases. Mayo Clin Proc 51: 417–429, 1976.
5. Strickler EM: Hyperphagia. N Engl J Med 298: 1010–1013, 1978.
6. Stein JF, Leventhal ML: Amenorrhea associated with bilateral polycystic ovaries. Am J Obstet Gynecol 29: 181–191, 1935.
7. Schacter SJ: Some extraordinary facts about obese humans and rats. In: The Psychology in Obesity, Dynamics in Treatment. Kiell N (ed). Springfield, Ill, Charles C Thomas, 1973, pp 15–38.
8. Dunn HG: The Prader-Labhart-Willi syndrome: review of the literature and report of nine cases. Acta Pediatr Scand (Suppl) 186: 1–38, 1968.
9. Laurence HE: Obesity, mental retardation, polydactyly, retinal pigmentation and hypogenitalism (Laurence-Moon-Biedl syndrome): case report. Bull N Engl MC 6: 285–290, 1944.
10. Grollman A, Rousseau PJ: Metabolic craniopathy: a clinical and roentgenologic study of so-called hyperostosis frontalis interna. JAMA 126: 213–217, 1944.
11. Ogilvie RF: Sugar tolerance in obese subjects: a review of 65 cases. Q J Med 4: 345, 1935.
12. Kennedy GC, Parker RA: The islets of Langerhans in rats with hypothalmic obesity. Lancet 2: 981–982, 1963.
13. Karam JH, Grodsky GM, Forsham PH: Excessive insulin response to glucose in obese subjects as measured by immunochemical assay. Diabetes 12: 197–204, 1963.
14. Vague PH, Boeuf G, Depieds R, Vague R: Plasma insulin levels in human obesity. In: Pathology of Adipose Tissue. Vague J (ed). New York, Excerpta Medica, 1969, pp 203–225.
15. Slaunwhite RW, Goldman JL, Bernardis LL: Sequential changes in glucose metabolism by adipose tissue liver of rats after destruction of the ventromedial hypothalamic nuclei; effect of three dietary regimens. Metabolism 21: 619–631, 1972.
16. Rabinowitz D, Zierler K: Forearm metabolism in obesity and its response to intra-arterial insulin: characterization of insulin resistence endurance for adaptive hyperinsulinism. J Clin Invest 41: 2173–2181, 1962.
17. Bagdade JD, Bierman EL, Porte D: Significance of basal insulin levels in the evaluation of the insulin response to glucose in diabetic and non-diabetic subjects. J Clin Invest 46: 1549–1557, 1967.
18. Perley MJ, Kipnis DM: Plasma insulin responses to oral and intravenous glucose: studies in normal and diabetic subjects. J Clin Invest 46: 1954–1962, 1967.
19. Butterfield WJH, Abrams ME, St John DJB, Whichelow MJ: The intravenous glucose tolerance test: peripheral disposal of the glucose load in controls and diabetics. Metabolism 16: 19–34, 1967.

20. Salans LB, Knittle JL, Hirsch J: The role of adipose cell size and adipose tissue insulin sensitivity in the carbohydrate intolerance of human obesity. J Clin Invest 47: 153–165, 1968.
21. Bjorntörp P, DeJounge K, Sjöström L, Sullivan L: The effect of physical training on insulin production in obesity. Metabolism 19: 631–638, 1970.
22. Bagdade JD, Bierman EL, Porte D: Counter regulation of basal insulin secretion during alcohol hypoglycemia in diabetic and normal subjects. Diabetes 21: 65–70, 1972.
23. McGarry JD, Foster DW: Regulation of ketogenesis and clinical aspects of the ketotic state. Metabolism 21: 471–489, 1972.
24. Sims EAH, Goldman RF, Gluck CM, et al: Experimental obesity in man. Trans Assoc Am Phys 81: 153–170, 1968.
25. Sims EAH, Horton ES, Salans LB: Inducible metabolic abnormalities during development of obesity. Annu Rev Med 22: 235–250, 1971.
26. Tchobroutsky G, Rosselin G, et al: Growth hormone secretion in obese subjects with and without diabetes. In: Pathophysiology of Adipose Tissue. Vague J (ed). New York, Excerpta Medica, 1969, pp 269–288.
27. Felig P, Marliss E, Cahill GF: Plasma amino acid levels and insulin secretion in obesity. N Engl J Med 281: 811–816, 1969.
28. Pozefsky T, Felig P, Tobin JD, et al: Amino acid balance across tissues of the forearm in postabsorptive man: Affects of insulin at two-dose levels. J Clin Invest 48: 2273–2282, 1969.
29. Montoye HJ, Epstein FH, Kjelsberg MD: Relationship between serum cholesterol and body fatness: an epidemiologic study. Am J Clin Nutr 18: 397–406, 1966.
30. Nestel PJ, Goldrick B: Obesity: changes in lipid metabolism and the role of insulin. Clin Endocrinol Metab 5: 313–335, 1976.
31. Blacket RB, Woodhill JN, Leelarthaepin B, Palmer AJ: Type IV hyperlipidemia and weight-gain after maturity. Lancet 2: 517–520, 1975.
32. Schoenfeld G, Pfleger B: Utilization of exogenous-free fatty acids for the production of very low density lipoprotein triglyceride by livers of carbohydrate fed rats. J Lipid Res 12: 614–621, 1971.
33. Nestel PJ, Austin W, Foxman C: Lipoprotein lipase content triglyceride uptake in adipose tissue of rats of differing body weights. Lipid Res 10: 383–387, 1969.
34. Reaven GM, Lerner RL, Stein MP, Farquhar JW: Role of insulin in endogenous hypertriglyceridemia. J Clin Invest 46: 1756–1767, 1967.
35. Bagdade JD, Bierman EL, Porte D: Influence of obesity on the relationship of insulin and triglyceride levels in endogenous hypertriglyceridemia. Diabetes 20: 664–672, 1971.
36. Gordon ES. Metabolic aspects of obesity. Adv Metab Disord 4: 229–296, 1970.
37. Nestel PJ, Matark: Relationship between resistance to insulin and body weight. Aust Ann Med 15: 301–304, 1966.
38. Nelson RA, Anderson LF, Gastineau CF, et al: Physiology and natural history of obesity. JAMA 223: 627–630, 1973.

CHAPTER 5

Etiology and Pathogenesis of Obesity: Food Intake

The literature reporting research on the etiology of obesity is voluminous and contradictory. In large part this reflects our ignorance of the basic mechanisms controlling hunger and eating behavior in the normal weight individual. Many of the theories of the regulation of body weight have been derived from animal studies and the relationship to clinical forms of human obesity is tenuous. Although the search for one theory to account for the regulation of hunger, eating, and body weight in the non-obese population is certainly necessary, it is probably fruitless to search for one theory that can account for the various forms of clinical obesity. In animal studies various different types of obesity have been identified and it would be surprising if human obesities were less complex.

In reviewing the experimental work and theoretical constructs on obesity, it is helpful to remember that etiology refers to initial causes of the condition and pathogenesis is the mechanism of development of the disease state. Most of the experimental studies have focused on the pathogenesis of obesity whereas psychodynamic theories have usually posited both an etiology and pathogenesis for obesity, albeit with relatively few well controlled experimental data.

REGULATION OF ENERGY BALANCE

That energy balance is normally maintained within rather precise limits is often overlooked. What is surprising is not that a percentage of the population is obese, but that generally there is a relatively narrow range of body weight for any individual adult. The outside limits of possible weights that can support life are not known with certainty, but probably range from approximately 50 pounds (one anorexia nervosa patient who was 5′4″) to over 1,000 pounds. The fact that most people are at weights well within these outside physiological boundaries suggests some type of regulatory mechanism. When actual food intake is calculated over a period of years, it is apparent that some type of energy balance mechanism must exist. For example, Passmore[1] noted that an average woman actually gains 11 kg between the ages of 25 and 65; during this period she eats roughly 20 tons of food; her weight increase corresponds to an average daily error of only 350 mg of food, as compared with the exact amount required for energy balance.

EARLY THEORIES OF REGULATION OF ENERGY

Historically, philosophers initially speculated that feelings of hunger, assumed to control food intake, originated in the abdominal cavity. Galen (138–201 AD) said that the gnawing sensations and pangs which accompany prolonged food deprivation were due to contractions of the stomach which he identified as the primary seat of hunger. Then "central" theories of the control of hunger became popular. For example, Magendie, Tidewald, and Milne-Edwards[2] postulated a "hunger center" in the brain sensitive to depletion of nutrients. Claude Bernard, in the 19th century, was the first to recognize that the composition of the fluids bathing the cells of multi-cellular organisms must be controlled. He proposed that the stability of this internal environment which he named the "milieu organique intérieur" gave the body a degree of functional freedom from the variability of the external environment. André Mayer,[3] in 1939, applied this theory to the regulation of energy balance. He determined food intake, energy expenditure, and body reserves, and demonstrated that food intake was regulated to maintain homeostasis of the body. He postulated a short-term daily regulation of food intake influenced by temperature, energy expenditure, and composition of diet and a long-term regulation which corrects errors of the short-term mechanism.

HOMEOSTATIC REGULATION OF ENERGY BALANCE

The homeostatic regulation of energy balance can be summarized by the following formula:

$$\text{Energy in} - \text{energy out} = \text{difference in energy reserves}$$

Excess energy in the body is stored primarily in adipose tissue. Therefore, if food intake exceeds energy expenditure there will be an increase in adipose tissue stores, resulting, if incorrected, in obesity. Conversely if energy expenditure exceeds food intake, adipose stores will be catabolized and depleted, as in anorexia nervosa. In the great majority of the population, however, energy reserves remain relatively constant with only a slight increase with age, indicating a long-term precise regulation of balance between energy in and energy out.

Much of the work to be described represents a search for the mechanism of this energy regulation. It is conceivable, of course, that either food intake or energy expenditure might be regulated either separately or conjointly but most of the work has focused on the regulation of food intake. This is partly because some animal experiments have demonstrated that the degree of corpulence following experimental manipulation is primarily due to an increase in food intake.

However, part of the reason that regulation of energy expenditure has not been as closely studied as food intake is because it is much more difficult to monitor than food intake. There are three major determinants of energy expenditure and all are difficult to calculate. The first, basal metabolism, is the sum total of the minimal activity of all tissues under steady state conditions and provides energy for protein synthesis, brain metabolism, maintenance of ionic balance across cells, and the contraction of the myocardium, gastrointestinal, and other continuously functioning muscle groups. Basal metabolism cannot be directly measured and its calculation rests on a number of assumptions that may not be operative in a given experimental situation. The second major determinant of energy expenditure is physical activity. Here again, calculation of calories expended relies on the measurement of indirect parameters. The specific dynamic action of food ((SDA) also known as the thermic effect of food) is the third major determinant of energy utilization. This effect refers to the increase in energy consumption following ingestion of food. Relatively little work has been done in this area and calculation of the SDA rests on the difference between oxygen consumption at rest and following a meal; a number of confounding variables might alter this calculation.

Direct calorimetry can be used to determine the sum total of all three effects but is very time consuming and often impossible to use in the clinical or experimental situation, and, furthermore, does not provide specific information about any of the three major determinants of energy expenditure. Therefore, much experimental work has evaluated food intake which can be calculated easily by using food of known composition and predetermined caloric content.

Recently there has been much exciting work studying changes in adipose tissue stores (energy stores), the third variable in the energy balance equation. This research will be discussed in detail in Chapter 7.

"HUNGER" AND "SATIETY" ARE SUBJECTIVE TERMS

In considering various theories of the regulation of energy consumed, hunger and eating (food intake) are ubiquitous terms. Hunger is a subjective state which is not well understood. Eating or food intake is a behavior and is more easily measured in the laboratory; eating may or may not mean that the animal or human is hungry. Likewise, satiety is a subjective state whereas termination of eating is a behavior.

It may well be that the subjective states of hunger and satiety are in fact the crucial factors determining food intake, but this has not been clearly demonstrated. Even describing what is meant by hunger and satiety is difficult. For example, Monello and Mayer[4] examined the individual's subjective experience of hunger and satiety by a self-report questionnaire. They defined extreme hunger as "the hungriest you can ever remember being," and ordinary hunger was defined as occurring between 2 hours and ½ hour before a typical weekday meal. They then asked subjects to evaluate the subjective sensations at the beginning of eating and at the end of a meal. They found that the number of reported physical sensations were greater during extreme hunger than during ordinary hunger: gastric sensations were reported most frequently, and mouth, throat, and head sensations slightly more often than overall body sensations. Furthermore, there was a marked sex difference of subjective experience of hunger. More women reported negative moods of irritability and tenseness than men when experiencing ordinary hunger. This sex difference was more marked among adults than among adolescents. At the end of a meal, most subjects described sensations of gastric bulk, feelings of satisfaction, warmth, and relaxation. This study highlights the fact that hunger and satiety are subjective terms and vary in meaning between individuals.

SEARCH FOR PHYSIOLOGICAL CORRELATE OF HUNGER

For centuries, scientists have attempted to define a physiological correlate of the subjective state of hunger. In the 18th century, Haller (cited in Mayer and Thomas[2]) ascribed the desire to eat to "intolerable pain" due to rubbing against one another of the folds of the empty stomach. Cannon and Washburn in 1912[5] reported that contractions of the stomach, which when empty except for a gastric balloon, were associated with abdominal sensations similar to those reported by some people when they said they were hungry. Carlson[6] concluded that these "gastric hunger contractions" regulated food intake by converting changes in the internal milieu into an experience which motivated food-seeking behavior. However, dramatic evidence against the theory of regulation of hunger by gastric contractions is that individuals who have had their stomachs removed continue to report hunger sensations and maintain their food intake.[7]

More recently Stunkard and Koch[8] have investigated the relationship between hunger and gastric motility in obese and normal subjects. There was little correlation between the perceptual experience of hunger and gastric motility in obese subjects whereas normal subjects more often reported hunger during gastric contractions. However, later studies clouded this finding. Both obese subjects (at least those judged not to be neurotic) and normal weight subjects had weak and inconsistent relationships between the experience of hunger and gastric motility.[9] Furthermore in this study they were able to teach obese subjects to detect gastric contractions but this did not improve the association between hunger and gastric motility nor the subjects' ability to control their weight.

EXPERIMENTAL EVIDENCE FOR REGULATION OF ENERGY BALANCE

ANIMAL STUDIES

Evidence from experimental work with both animals and humans favors the hypothesis that energy reserves are regulated. When experimental animals are underfed to reduce weight[10] or force fed to gain weight,[11] they spontaneously readjust their food intake when free feeding is allowed.

Another line of data favoring internal regulation of body fat is from experiments with transplantation or removal of adipose tissue. One study[12] found that the percentage of successful transplant of adipose tissue in mice rose from 10% when no fat was removed prior to the transplant in the recipient to 80% when both gonadal fat organs had been removed from the recipient mouse prior to the transplant. Another experiment[13] removed intra-abdominal fat from mice that had a form of genetically transmitted obesity. Following the operations, body weight increased in the operated mice to the same level as in the unoperated controls. Both experiments provide evidence for an internal regulatory mechanism.

EXPERIMENTAL HUMAN OBESITY

In a novel experimental approach to the problem of human obesity, Sims and colleagues[14, 15] induced short-term obesity in normal adult volunteers. Fifteen subjects entered the experiment and most came close to the goal of a 25% increase in weight by consuming high calorie meals. Only four of the subjects gained weight easily and two of these had a family history of obesity or diabetes. During the course of the weight gain, the subjects were, in general, more emotional and less physically active. At the end of the experiment all of the subjects except two who had initially gained weight easily, lost weight promptly by restricting food intake and increasing physical activity. The marked difficulty in gaining weight experienced by most subjects and prompt loss to control levels within a few weeks, suggest a powerful regulating mechanism.

There were important similarities and differences between experimental short-term human obesity and spontaneous obesity. In both, weight gain is mainly central. Studies of lipid content from adipose tissue biopsies showed a high correlation between lipid content per cell and the percentage of body fat (as estimated from body density measurements). Thus, the subjects' fat cells got larger but not more numerous. In contrast, most patients with spontaneous juvenile onset obesity, have an increased number of fat cells.

Endocrine and metabolic trends in the experimental obese group were similar to those reported in the literature for spontaneous obese humans. One major difference was that plasma free fatty acids were decreased in the experimental group whereas in spontaneous obesity levels may be elevated. Serum cholesterol and serum triglycerides are elevated in both groups. In both groups fasting serum insulin and the insulin glucose ratio are increased. In spontaneous obesity there is a decrease in glucose tolerance, and there was a trend to a reduced glucose tolerance in the experimental group. In both types of obesity,[16] in contrast to diabetes, there is a greater secretion of insulin in response to a comparable stimulus than in the normal. In other words, in both spontaneous and experimental human obesity, secretion of insulin is greater than normal in response to a given stimulus and in diabetes, secretion of insulin is less than normal in response to a given stimulus. Growth hormone response to oral glucose is reduced in both types of obesity. Cortisol production is elevated on an absolute basis in both groups but not when related to increase in body size. These findings are summarized in Table 5.1.

REGULATION OF ENERGY INTAKE

Extensive studies of animals with lesions in the ventromedial nucleus (VMN) and lateral nucleus (LN) of the hypothalamus have promoted the search for a regulatory mechanism that controls some factor that ultimately regulates body weight. Animals with lesions in the ventromedial nucleus become obese, lazy, and finicky in their choice of food. Historically, this was thought to indicate damage to a postulated "satiety" center in the ventromedial nucleus of the hypothalamus. There is a vast amount of literature on this topic which is important because any theory that purports to account for the etiology or pathogenesis of obesity must incorporate or explain the findings of this research.

Clearly, regulation of body weight in the rat or goldfish is likely to be strikingly different from the regulation of weight in humans, but a successful animal model of a disease state is often the first step in understanding the human condition. Animal models may well provide an initial understanding of basic biochemical and organic factors in human obesity, but elucidation of critical emotional, cognitive, and social factors which influence the onset and maintenance of obesity will require carefully designed studies of man.

TABLE 5.1
Comparison of spontaneous and experimental obesity (adapted from Sims et al[14]).

	Spontaneous Obesity	Experimental Obesity
Adipose Cell Number	↑	no increase
Blood Lipids		
Serum Cholesterol	↑	↑
Serum Triglycerides	↑	↑ trend only
Plasma Free Fatty Acids	↑	↓
Fasting Serum Insulin and Insulin Glucose Ratio	↑	↑
Intravenous Glucose Tolerance		
k value	↓	↓ trend only
insulin response	↑	↑
Growth Hormone Release Following Oral Glucose	↓	↓
Cortisol	↑	↑

Furthermore, in a number of animal studies "motivation" has been evaluated by defining certain behaviors as indicative of motivation. Whether these behavioral approaches apply to motivation in humans is debatable. With these limitations in mind, the following discussion focuses on the historically important dual center hypothesis and the current tenable theories of the regulation of weight.

DUAL CENTER HYPOTHESIS IMPORTANT HISTORICALLY

Bilateral electrolytic destruction of the VMN in rats is followed by obesity.[17] Brobeck[18] concluded that the obesity was almost entirely due to increased food intake and termed the syndrome "hypothalamic hyperphagia." Other investigators[19] produced the syndrome in other species, including mice, cats, dogs, and monkeys. There is a "dynamic" phase during which there is an increase in food intake and rapid weight gain, and there is a "static" phase during which the lesioned animal reduces the amount eaten but maintains the obese weight. Damage to the area just lateral to the ventromedial nucleus also produces obesity.[17]

Bilateral destruction of an even more lateral hypothalamic area caused animals to become aphagic and die.[20] Furthermore, animals made hyperphagic by ventromedial lesions became aphagic following destruction of the more lateral area. More recent studies[21] have demonstrated that with good nursing care and forced feeding, animals with bilateral lateral hypothalamic lesions will eventually begin eating and gain weight to a stable but lower weight than prior to the lesion.

The "dual center" hypothesis for the regulation of body weight was postulated by Anand and Brobeck.[20] According to this hypothesis, the ventromedial nucleus serves as a "satiety" center and acts as an inhibitor of the "feeding center" located in the lateral hypothalamus. This theory has provided the impetus for two decades of research into the nature of the central brain regulation of body weight. Although current neurotransmitter theories are more elaborate and provide a more tenable explanation of various brain lesions on the regulation of body weight, the importance of the dual center hypothesis historically cannot be overestimated.

EVIDENCE THAT FAVORED THE DUAL CENTER HYPOTHESIS

Support for the theory came from several sources. First, a variety of experimental manipulations in animals have produced the results predicted by the theory. For example, electrical stimulation of the lateral area results in an increase in food intake and electrical stimulation of the ventromedial area does not. When the ventromedial area is anesthetized with procaine, there is an increase in food intake, and injection of procaine into the lateral hypothalamic area results in a decrease in food intake. The supportive experimental data for the theory have been summarized by Bray.[22]

A second major line of support for the theory was electrophysiological studies.[23,24] The electrical firing rate of neurons in the ventromedial nucleus of starved animals is less than the firing rate of the neurons in their lateral hypothalamic areas. Furthermore intravenous glucose feedings result in an increased firing rate of the neurons in the ventromedial nucleus. In rats there is reciprocal electrical activity between the ventromedial and lateral hypothalamic area.[24]

A third area of experimental studies lending support to the theory was anatomic studies[25] showing that in the fasted rat the nucleoli of the ventromedial area are smaller than the nucleoli of the lateral area, implying decreased anabolic activity in the ventromedial area.

One problem with the theory was that it was difficult to demonstrate nerve fibers connecting the ventromedial and lateral areas of the hypothalamus although there is some inconclusive evidence for the existence of these nerve fibers.[26]

TABLE 5.2
Characteristics of lesioned animals.

VMH ANIMALS	LH ANIMALS
• HYPERPHAGIA ("DYNAMIC" PHASE)	• APHAGIA
• LAZINESS	• SENSORY NEGLECT
• FINICKINESSS	
• HYPERINSULINISM	
• INCREASE IN FAT CONTENT	

CHARACTERISTICS OF LESIONED ANIMALS

HYPERINSULINISM IN VMH LESIONED ANIMALS

Recent studies have delineated a number of characteristics of the "hyperphagic hypothalamic" animal that have figured prominently in current theories (see Table 5.2). For example, ventromedial lesions result in hyperinsulinism and an increase in fat stores, even if body weight is maintained at pre-lesion levels by controlling the amount of food available and thereby preventing hyperphagia. There are elevated immunoreactive insulin levels after ventromedial hypothalamic destruction in adult rats when hyperphagia is prevented.[27] When these lesioned animals were permitted to eat ad libitum, the elevation of immunoreactive insulin was positively correlated with subsequent body weight. As noted earlier, short-term experimental human obesity and spontaneous obesity are also correlated with elevated insulin levels. Two possible explanations have been advanced to account for the hyperinsulinism even in the absence of obesity: VMN lesions may cause a direct humoral or nervous effect on the pancreas stimulating insulin release, or, perhaps the lesions result in an endocrine abnormality which results in insulin resistance of peripheral tissue and a consequent rise in insulin level.

Ventromedial hypothalamic rats become fatter even if no increase in weight is permitted by restricting food supplies;[27, 28] that is, there is an increase in percentage of fat. These two findings—hyperinsulinemia and increased percentage of fat even in the absence of weight gain—have provided support for the lipostatic theory of weight regulation initially proposed by Kennedy.[29] The core concept of this theory, to be discussed more fully later, is that the hypothalamus monitors fat content via some metabolite released from fat stores and that adjustments in food intake are made in response to the level of this metabolite.

"FINICKINESS" AND "LAZINESS" OF VMH ANIMALS

Classically, a triad of findings has been considered characteristic of the VMH lesioned animal: increased food intake (resulting in obesity), laziness, and, paradoxically, finickiness in the choice of food. Teitelbaum[30] demonstrated that in the "dynamic" phase of increased food intake, VMN lesioned animals, like normal animals, maintain appreciable food intake despite adulteration of their diet with cellulose or quinine which makes it less palatable. However, in the "static" phase, the obese lesioned animals reject such adulterated foods. Another study found a similar finickiness in VMN lesioned rats, but not in generally obese rats of the same strain.[31]

Lesioned animals were judged "lazy" because they were less likely to strive to obtain food. For example, VMN lesioned rats are less likely to cross an electrical field to obtain food than lean rats.[32]

Both finickiness and laziness have figured prominently in theories of human obesity. Obese human subjects have been observed to be more responsive to the sensory qualities of food[33] and less physically active.[34] Therefore, the VMN lesioned animal that is obese, finicky in food selection, and physically inactive might be an ideal experimental model of human obesity. However, more recent studies have cast some doubt on the conclusion that such animals are finicky or lazy. For example, if rats that have VMN lesions are maintained at their pre-operative weight, they will work as hard for food as non-lesioned lean control rats.[35]

DECREASED "MOTIVATION" IN LH LESIONED ANIMALS

Lateral hypothalamic lesioned animals have been studied more extensively in recent years and it appears that the major behavioral symptom following lateral hypothalamic destruction is a general motivational inertia and decrease in vigilance. Marshall and colleagues[36] found complex sensorimotor deficits in animals with unilateral lateral hypothalamic damage; there were deficits in orientation to contralateral visual, olfactory, and somato-sensory stimuli which the authors termed "sensory neglect." Panskeep[37] concludes that destruction of the lateral hypothalamus decreases "interaction with all biologically relevant stimuli—food, water, temperature" and postulates an impaired capacity to judge biological relevance. Perhaps, behaviorally speaking, LH lesioned animals are analogous to "unmotivated" humans.

AMINE THEORY OF REGULATION OF FOOD INTAKE

NEUROANATOMY

Recent studies of VMH and LH lesioned animals have implicated the biogenic amines in the control of food intake. An understanding of the theory requires knowledge of the neuroanatomy of the amine neurofiber tracts. The *dorsal noradrenergic* pathway originates in the locus coeruleus, ascends lateral and ventral to the periaqueductal gray, and descends to pass over the interpeduncular nucleus, enters the medial forebrain bundle, and is widely distributed to the neocortex and hippocampus. The *ventral noradrenergic* pathway also originates in the lower brain stem (but not from the locus coeruleus) and projects to the hypothalamus, forebrain, and amygdaloid complex. *Serotonergic fibers* arise from the anterior raphe nuclei and project rostrally and medially to gather in the interpeduncular nucleus; the fibers then course through the medial forebrain bundle and terminate in the diencephalon and telencephalon. The *nigrostriatal dopaminergic* system originates in the substantia nigra and terminates in the neostriatum. The *mesolimbic dopamine* system arises near the interpeduncular nucleus and terminates in several forebrain structures, including the amygdaloid complex (See Table 5.3).

Current theories[37] postulate that lesions in the ventromedial and ventrolateral hypothalamus cause the observed effects by interrupting amine pathways, rather than by a local effect on the ventromedial nucleus or lateral hypothalamus. Specifically, disruption of the ventral noradrenergic bundle, which has terminals in the ventromedial nucleus, rather than destruction of the ventromedial nucleus itself, may modulate satiety. Similarly, destruction of the nigrostriatal dopamine pathway may produce a syndrome similar to that seen in the LH lesioned animals, namely a loss of a wide variety of behavioral systems which influence motivation, including food-seeking behavior. In its simplest form, the amine theory states that satiety is controlled by the *ventral noradrenergic* system and motivational aspects of food-seeking behavior are modulated by the *nigrostriatal dopaminergic* system. This theory

TABLE 5.3
Major biogenic amine pathways.

Pathway	Origin	Termination
Doral Noradrenergic Pathway	Locus Coeruleus	Neocortex Hippocampus
Ventral Noradrenergic Pathway	lower brainstem	hypothalamus forebrain amygdaloid complex
Serotonergic Pathway	anterior raphe nuclei	diencephalon telencephalon
Nigrostriatal dopaminergic system	substantia nigra	neostriatum
Mesolimbic dopaminergic system	near interpeduncular nucleus	amygdaloid complex

accounts for some, but not all, of the experimental data. For example, in cats, stimulation of the basal lateral part of the amygdaloid complex inhibits food intake[38] and destruction of the amygdala increases food intake.[39] Since the ventral noradrenergic pathway has terminals in the amygdala, these data provide some evidence for the amine theory of the regulation of weight.

The characteristic lateral hypothalamic syndrome can also be produced by damage to the nigrostriatal dopaminergic pathway at its origin in the substantia nigra.[37] This gives credence to the idea that there is no "feeding center" and that the aphagia resulting from lesions in the lateral hypothalamus is due to interruption of fibers of passage.

VARIANT OF AMINE THEORY

However, an attempt[40] to reproduce the hyperphagia typically seen in the VMH lesioned animals by injecting 6-hydroxydopamine into the mesencephalic portion of the ventral noradrenergic pathway, resulted in only modest weight gains. Thus, hypothalamic hyperphagia may not be a product of primary damage to the ventral noradrenergic pathway. Instead, interruption of the ventral pathway by VMH lesions probably only contributes to the classic syndrome. A mild form of a lateral hypothalamic syndrome can be produced by destruction of the mediolateral serotonergic systems by depletion of brain serotonin with para-chlorophenylalanine.[41] Furthermore, damage to the dorsal noradrenergic system may participate in the lateral hypothalamic syndrome by reducing the reinforcing properties of environmental stimuli.[42] Thus, the classic lateral hypothalamic aphagia of rats may be due to interruption of three amine pathways: the *nigrostriatal dopamine pathway*, the *serotonergic pathway*, and the *dorsal norepinephrine pathway*. Panskepp postulates a more complex role for the ventromedial nucleus and theorizes that it is responsible for the long-term control of feeding by elaborating both excitatory and inhibitory control by an unknown mechanism over the lateral hypothalamic centers. The evidence Panskepp adduces for this theory is based primarily on a reinterpretation of some of the classic experimental findings and some recent work[43, 44] indicating that electrical stimulation of the medial hypothalamus can increase feeding and potentiate lateral hypothalamic cellular activity. Therefore, although the support of Panskepp's variant of the amine theory is thus far scanty, it is very likely that if the biogenic amines are involved in the regulation of body weight, it is in a complex way.

SHORT TERM REGULATION OF ENERGY INTAKE

HUMANS INEFFECTIVE IN SHORT-TERM REGULATION

Since André Mayer's[45] work on the regulation of food intake, both long-term and short-term regulation of body weight have been postulated. A major argument for some short-term mechanism is the observation that satiety, however it may be expressed behaviorally or emotionally in any given individual, occurs rapidly, long before nutrients could be absorbed and directly affect a central regulatory system.

A short-term regulatory system may result in satiety, but there has long been fairly clear evidence that energy balance in man is not regulated during 24 hours.

One study[46] evaluated young soldiers for 7 weeks. They were weighed daily and there was a 0.5-kg change in weight from day to day in more than 30% of the subjects, but there was no relationship between these changes and daily food intake or energy expenditure. Edholm and associates[47] measured the intake and expenditure of 12 military cadets over 14 days and found no correlation between intake and output for the same day, but did find a correlation between the energy expenditure on 1 day and intake 2 days later. (These same investigators were not able to replicate this latter correlation in a later survey in 1970.[48]) The mean intake of all the cadets during the 14-day period was 3,432 kcal/day and the mean expenditure was 3,416 kcal/day; therefore as a *group*, energy intake and energy expenditure were closely balanced. However, this does not mean that individual cadets regulated intake and expenditure closely.[49] The mean intake for each cadet over 14 days plotted against the mean expenditure for each cadet over 14 days reveals no significant correlation. In only two of the cadets did mean intake and expenditure agree within 150 kcal. Therefore, it is invalid to conclude that the study of Edholm et al documents balance of energy over a 2-week period in *individual* subjects.

One difficulty in studying short-term energy balance in animals is that rats, which have certainly been the most popular experimental animals, do regulate energy balance within a 24-hour period, whereas humans do not. However, the common observation that satiety occurs rapidly, at least in normal subjects, is really the cornerstone for the theory that some short-term regulatory system must exist. It seems likely that some short-term mechanism operates to induce satiety but that it is relatively inefficient in maintaining energy balance over a 24-hour period. A long-term regulatory system is thought to correct these errors in energy balance, presumably by altering food intake.

NEUROENDOCRINE EXPLANATIONS OF SATIETY

The usual explanation for short-term satiety is increased vagal afferent activity produced by gastric stimulation.[50] Gastric pre-loading of rats and dogs does reduce subsequent oral intake but not by equivalent amounts.[51,52] In rats, vagotomy decreases the size of the individual meal but frequency increases and caloric intake continues unchanged.[53] These studies indicate that gastric distention probably plays a role in short-term satiety, but it is clearly not the only operative factor.

Short-term satiety may be modulated by hormonal factors in concert with vagal effects. Gastrointestinal hormones are released by the contact of ingested food with the mucosa of the stomach and small intestine. This release is quick enough to account for the short-term satiety which begins within minutes after eating begins. Cholecystokinin (CCK) may be one of these hormonal factors.[54] In rats, CCK was injected into the peritoneum and feeding decreased in a dose-related manner. Endogenous CCK is produced in the upper two-thirds of the small intestine. Although it has yet to be determined whether endogenous CCK reduces food intake in either the rat or man, it may interact with other gut hormones to mediate short-term satiety. These endocrine and vagal factors may affect central brain mechanisms that regulate eating.

PALATABILITY

Another possibility is that palatability or taste in some way controls short-term food intake. Individuals may have different palatability slopes.[55] That is, some individuals may consume more before there is a decrease in palatability. Figure 5.1 illustrates this concept graphically. If more calories were consumed before the taste of a given food was less pleasurable, or even aversive, this might account for obesity in some subjects. Very obese human

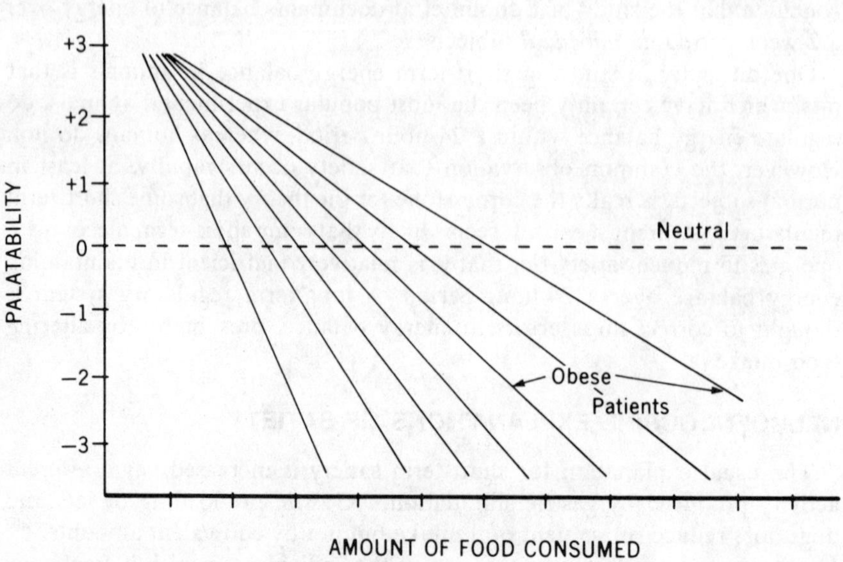

Figure 5.1. Satiety slopes. Obese individuals may consume more food before there is a decrease in palatability. (Reprinted with permission from Hagan[55]).

subjects continue to rate a sucrose solution as pleasant even after gastric pre-loads.[56] Non-obese subjects, however, report a decrease in rate of pleasantness for the sucrose solution after gastric pre-loads. Wooley and Wooley[57] found that caloric ingestion sufficient to inhibit salivation in the non-obese does not do so in the obese. Whether increased salivation reflects increased hunger is a moot point, but this study does provide some evidence for a different gustatory experience in the obese in comparison with normal subjects. A change in taste or palatability, therefore, may determine the amount of food consumed at one sitting, but how this is accomplished is unclear and why long-term regulatory mechanisms do not compensate for short-term errors secondary to prolonged palatability, forms the basis for the set-point theory of Nesbitt.[58]

AMINOSTATIC THEORY

An aminostatic theory of the short-term regulation of energy balance has been recently re-emphasized by Panskepp.[37] An inverse relationship between the levels of amino acids and food intake was noted in one study.[59] Rogers and Leung[60] noted that if an animal were deficient in an amino acid, the usual decrease in food intake could be prevented by injection of that amino acid into the carotid artery, whereas injection of the amino acid into the jugular vein did not prevent a decline in food intake. Therefore, the receptor system for detecting deficiency of the amino acids appeared to be in the brain. Furthermore, feeding can be rapidly suppressed in hungry animals by injecting amino acids (particularly glycine, alanine, and perhaps glutamic acid) into either the medial or lateral hypothalamic areas. Panskepp notes that amino acids are good candidates for short-term control because amino acid information channels could be easily interfaced with the regulation of carbohydrates: for example, a substantial part of the glucose carbon ultimately appears in the amino acid pool in the rat brain.

In summary, energy balance during a 24-hour period is probably regulated, but relatively imprecisely, in humans. Gastric distention resulting in afferent vagal discharge, release of various endocrine factors, and palatability have all been implicated in the regulation of short-term satiety.

LONG-TERM REGULATION OF ENERGY INTAKE

There are several theories that attempt to account for the long-term regulation of energy balance by focusing on control of food intake in normal and obese humans and experimental animals. These theories are based on various feedback control concepts. It is analogous to the regulation of temperature in the house. The thermostat measures the temperature; if the temperature is too high, the furnace shuts off. When the temperature in the house falls below the level set on the thermostat, the furnace turns on and heat increases. Many investigators think that the "thermostat" that controls food intake is in or passes through the hypothalamus; the lipostatic, glucostatic, aminostatic, and thermostatic theories postulate different peripheral signals that are detected by the "thermostat." Any of a variety of errors in the hypothalamus or in the periphery may account for an increase in fat stores. On the other hand, the set point, or "ponderostat," theory states that the "thermostat" itself may be incorrectly set at a high or low value and therefore the behavioral response to the peripheral signal, whatever it may be (lipid, glucose, temperature, or amino acid), is correct in terms of the set point, but may result in obesity or underweight if set too high or too low. Therefore each of these theories is based on feedback control concepts but differs in what metabolite is thought to emanate from the periphery and be sensed by the hypothalamus.

In each of the theories to be discussed, the pathogenesis of obesity, but not the etiology, is stressed. That is, although these are elegant theories, which taken together or separately may account for the development of obesity in some individuals, the initial events that set these mechanisms into operation are not elucidated. For example, although VMH lesioned rats may have many similarities to obese humans, there are only a few reports[62] of obese humans with damage to the hypothalamus from tumor, trauma, or congenital defects. Or, phrased somewhat differently, what causes the "ponderostat" to be set too high or too low?

In contrast, the psychosomatic theorists have made plausible, but for the most part unproven, suggestions about the etiology of disorders of food intake. Bruch,[63] for example, postulates that faulty emotional transactions between the parent and child may cause subsequent eating disorders. Freudian schools maintain that there is an arrest of ego development at the oral phase which is the major etiological factor in the development of later obesity. Both theories have some support, but little proof. Their advantage lies in the attempt to postulate an etiology and pathogenesis for human, rather than rat, obesity. Nonetheless, the following theories of the pathogenesis of obesity have the great advantage of testability, sometimes in humans.

GLUCOSTATIC HYPOTHESIS

The glucostatic hypothesis was initially proposed by Mayer in 1953[64] and provided a unifying theory of the regulation of weight that stimulated research for two decades. According to this theory, there are receptors in the ventromedial hypothalamus that have a special affinity for glucose. An increase in the rate of utilization of glucose by these receptors in the VMN activates mechanisms that terminate eating. Similarly, a fall in the rate of glucose utilization by these receptors results in an increase in feeding. This theory was based on several observations. First, carbohydrate reserves are proportionately much more depleted between meals than are reserves of fat or protein. Second, glucose metabolism, which is regulated by complex endocrine machinery, is itself a regulator of fat and protein metabolism. Third, the central nervous system is known to depend largely on glucose for its needs, yet the CNS has little capacity to store glucose and is dependent on a continuing blood supply of glucose.

The major evidence supporting the glucostatic theory rests on animal experiments in which injections of gold thioglucose sufficient to produce obesity were shown by Mayer and co-workers to destroy selectively cells in the region of the VMN. Furthermore, injection of compounds in which the gold thio-moiety is linked to metabolites other than glucose (for example gold thiomalate or gold thiogalactose) does not produce ventromedial hypothalamic damage or obesity.

The major evidence against the glucostatic theory is that injection of glucose into the ventromedial hypothalamus in animals does not immediately decrease intake.[65] Injections of glucose into the medial but not the lateral hypothalamus in rats does decrease food intake the day *after* treatment although there is no immediate effect.[37] Therefore, although initially proposed as a short-term regulator of food intake by Mayer, it is more likely that, if operant at all in humans, the glucostatic component serves as a long-term regulatory mechanism.

THERMOSTATIC HYPOTHESIS

According to the thermostatic hypothesis,[66] heat production as reflected by changes of body temperature, regulates food intake. Homeothermic animals (those that regulate temperature within narrow limits) eat more in cold than in hot environments. The anterior hypothalamus is thought to modulate body temperature. In one study,[67] the pre-optic region of the anterior hypothalamus in rats was destroyed and these animals had inappropriate feeding responses: they overate in hot environments and underate in cold environments. A study[68] of thermic responses of anorexia nervosa patients also provides some support for this theory. These emaciated young women in whom food intake is clearly inappropriate to their needs, also have abnormal responses to heat and cold: a functional or anatomic lesion in the anterior hypothalamus might account for these findings. Although environmental temperature does influence food intake, it probably acts in concert with other factors that regulate intake.

THE LIPOSTATIC THEORY

The lipostatic theory,[69] states that the body somehow senses the amount of fat reserves and that eating behavior is aligned with the sensed amount of fat. A variety of substances have been candidates for the peripheral signal which is sensed by the hypothalamus. According to one variant of the theory a metabolite from fat stores is present in greater or lesser amounts depending on whether lipolysis or lipogenesis occurs peripherally. This metabolite is "sensed" by the ventromedial hypothalamus which results in an increase or decrease in feeding. That is, if food intake has been less than the energy expenditure, energy stores will decrease (lipolysis will occur) and some peripheral metabolite from lipolysis will increase and then be "sensed" by the ventromedial hypothalamus which will in turn result in an increase in food intake. Similarly, a decrease in the metabolite resulting from an increase in lipogenesis (and thereby increasing adipose tissue stores) will be sensed by the hypothalamus which will effect a decrease in food intake.

The three major metabolites released from adipose tissue are free fatty acids, glycerol, and prostaglandins. Glycerol is the likely candidate for the peripheral metabolite because it is released into the circulation in proportion to the rate of hydrolysis of triglycerides. The hypothalamus metabolizes glycerol more rapidly than do other parts of the brain, although the blood brain barrier does not have any special permeability to glycerol.[69] Glycerol may act as an indirect messenger. Perhaps glycerol is converted to glucose in the liver and then sensed by hepatic glucoreceptors which relay the change in glucose levels to the hypothalamus via the vagus nerve. See Figure 5.2 for schematic representation of this variant of the lipostatic theory. Free fatty acids, the second major metabolite of adipose tissue fluctuate rapidly during the day and therefore are unlikely to serve as a messenger for the long-term

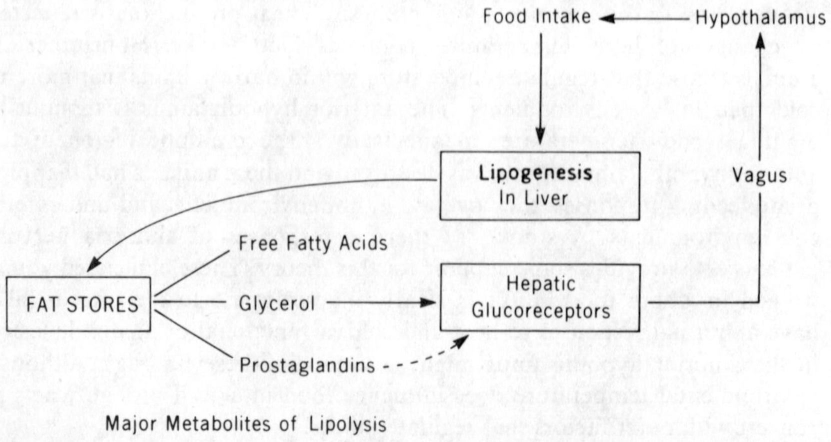

Figure 5.2. Lipostatic theory: Glycerol as the signal. The three major metabolites of lipolysis are free fatty acids, glycerol, and prostaglandins. Glycerol can be readily converted to glucose which may be a signal to the hepatic glucoreceptors. Information may be relayed to the brain via the vagus nerve.

regulation of food intake. Prostaglandins also are possible messengers but there is little evidence substantiating this idea.

ENDOCRINE VARIANT OF LIPOSTATIC THEORY

An endocrine modus operandi has been proposed for the lipostatic theory. Woods and colleagues[70] propose that insulin and growth hormone occur in a certain ratio that determines body weight. Specifically, when the insulin/growth hormone ratio increases, adipose tissue stores increase and when the insulin/growth hormone ratio decreases adipose tissue stores decrease. The insulin/growth hormone ratio may determine the amount of body fat stores by influencing the rate of formation of fat (lipogenesis) and the rate of breakdown of fat (lipolysis). This mechanism is presumed to account for the long-term regulation of fat stores rather than day-to-day fluctuations.

The evidence for this theory is plausible and is based, in part, on well accepted data for humans. For example the known actions of insulin include the following. Insulin enables most tissues to take up glucose and use it as fuel or store it as glycogen; it causes fatty acids to be taken up by the liver and converts them to triglycerides which are stored in adipose tissue (lipogenesis); insulin increases the uptake of amino acids by muscle, liver, and other tissues; and with growth hormone, insulin promotes the conversion of amino acids to stored proteins. Growth hormone promotes the growth of bone, connective tissue, and other tissues. It also has a protein sparing action: during a fast it suppresses the breakdown of stored protein but promotes the breakdown of stored triglycerides to free fatty acids within adipose tissue (lipolysis). Thus, growth hormone and insulin have opposite effects on adipose tissue: growth hormone promotes lipolysis and insulin promotes lipogenesis. Therefore the amount of stored fat (energy reserves) is at least partially determined by the relative amounts of insulin and growth hormone present.

Thus, the endocrine variant of the lipostatic theory is that the ratio of insulin to growth hormone is what is sensed by the ventromedial hypothalamus which in turn modulates feeding. That is, short-term factors (for example social pressures to diet, or emotional factors) might result in decreased food intake. This would result in a decrease in insulin and increased growth hormone levels which would be "sensed" by the lateral hypothalamus, either directly or relayed from the ventral medial hypothalamus to the lateral hypothalamus by neural or humoral means. Increased activity of the lateral hypothalamus would result in an increase in feeding and consequent lipogenesis with an increase in fat stores. Conversely, short-term influences might result in overeating and an increased insulin/growth hormone ratio which would be "sensed" by the ventral medial hypothalamus, resulting in increased activity of the VMN resulting in decreased insulin and increased growth hormone. Feeding would decrease and lipolysis occur. (See Fig. 5.3)

Although the actions of growth hormone and insulin as enumerated by Woods and colleagues[70] are well accepted for humans, most of the proof for this endocrine theory is from animal studies. For example, animals that cannot secrete insulin do not gain weight even when the ventral medial hypothalamus is destroyed.[71] Furthermore, animals made obese prior to subsequent bilateral ventromedial hypothalamic lesions do not become more obese after this destruction.[72] Conversely, animals rendered underweight do not become more underweight following lateral hypothalamic destruction.[73]

Some evidence from human studies also fits well with the endocrine variant of the lipostatic theory. For example, growth hormone levels are elevated in marasmus, Kwashiorkor, and anorexia nervosa which should stimulate feeding according to this theory, and would be biologically adaptive in all three conditions. However, although it is well documented that at least some obese subjects have elevated insulin levels and decreased growth hormone levels, it is not clear why this does not result in a subsequent decrease in feeding, as predicted by the theory. In order to account for spontaneous obesity with this theory, an abnormality in the hypothalamus

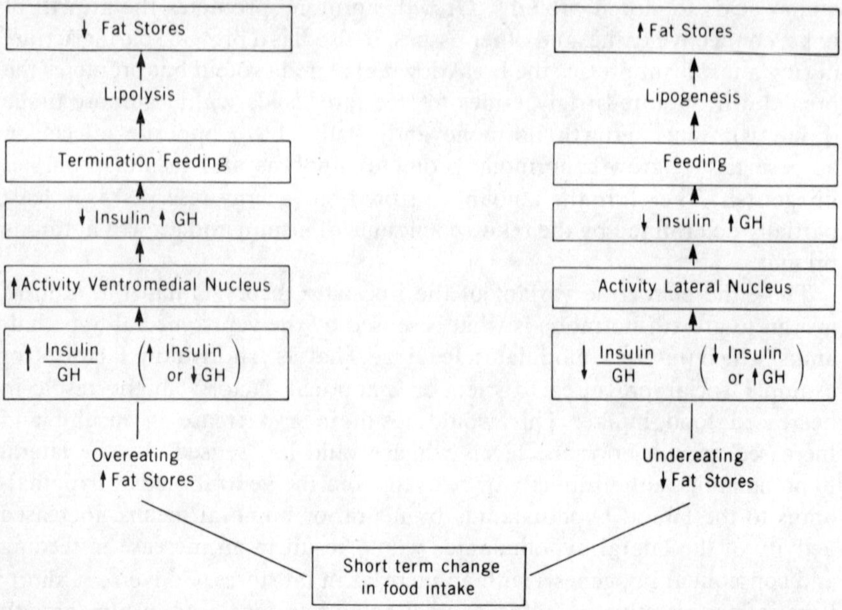

Figure 5.3. Lipostatic theory: Changes in insulin/growth hormone ratio may be the peripheral signal.

must be postulated. Perhaps the VMN is "set" at a higher level and does not sense hyperinsulinemia or decreased growth hormone levels until this ratio is higher than in normal weight persons. Whether this increase in set point might cause or be the consequence of obesity is unknown.

PHYSIOLOGICAL ROLE OF PLEASURE

Cabanac's[74] work on the physiological role of pleasure has provided the theoretical groundwork for some of the more recent theories of the regulation of weight. He contends that what is useful in maintaining the body's homeostasis is perceived as pleasurable. In other words, pleasure occurs whenever a sensation indicates the presence of a stimulus that helps to correct internal trouble, and conversely, displeasure occurs whenever a stimulus is present that does not correct internal trouble. For example, cold is pleasurable during hyperthermia and unpleasant during hypothermia. To describe this phenomenon, Cabanac coined a neologism "allesthesia" which means that a given external stimulus can be perceived as either pleasant or unpleasant depending upon internal body signals.

Cabanac and co-workers demonstrated this principle in relationship to taste and the regulation of weight. Three experimenters acting as subjects evaluated the taste of sweet solutions before and after ingestion of 200 ml of glucose and found, as expected, that the sweet solution was more pleasant before ingestion of the glucose than afterwards. These same experimenters then reduced their weight by 10% and found that the pre-load of glucose did not decrease the judged pleasantness of the sweet solution. This was interpreted as allesthesia: i.e., the sweet solution continued to be perceived as pleasant even after pre-ingestion of glucose because the subjects were below their normal homeostatic body weight and increased intake of sweet solutions was useful to correct the deficit in body weight. Although this experiment is really anecdotal, with all the flaws that can occur when experimenters use themselves as subjects, it does suggest new possibilities regarding weight regulation.

Nisbett[58] has articulated the set point theory of obesity based on the concept of allesthesia. Perhaps more importantly, at least in terms of possible emotional features in the etiology of obesity, is that Cabanac has called attention to the fact that people who overeat may or may not eat to reduce anxiety or tension, but may overeat because it is more pleasurable for them to eat than it is for normal weight persons. This may seem obvious, but in fact, most psychodynamic theories of the pathogenesis of obesity are based on the assumption that overeating decreases displeasure rather than increases pleasure; either reason, or both, may be operative in any given individual obese person.

SET POINT THEORY ("PONDEROSTAT")

The set point theory described by Nisbett[58] is attractive because it accounts, at least in part, for many of the findings in spontaneously obese persons and experimentally obese animals. Essentially the theory states that the central nervous system operates to defend different set points in different individuals. Again, the analogy to a thermostat in a house is appropriate: if the thermostat is set at 70°F and the system is operating correctly, the temperature of the house will be in a healthful and comfortable range. On the other hand, if the thermostat is set at 90°F, the furnace will continue to warm the house past the comfortable temperature range. Likewise, according to the set point theory, the "ponderostat," thought to be in the hypothalamus, in obese persons is set too high and the body operates to maintain body stores above the ideal weight in terms of either health or aesthetics. Overnutrition during the critical periods of increase in fat cell number might result in an increase in adipose cell number which might account for the upward shift in the set point within the hypothalamus. Consequently an elevated level of fat stores becomes the person's natural state. Therefore, reasons Nisbett, when an obese person diets he is below his natural set point for weight and the patient subjectively undergoes the rigors of starvation.

The set point theory really combines elements of the psychosomatic view of obesity and the "externality" theory of Schachter.[75] According to the psychosomatic view, some obese individuals have learned to misuse food and eat in response to "psychogenic hunger" triggered by uncomfortable emotional states rather than in response to physiological needs; i.e., these theorists contend that the obese are neurotic with a variety of underlying emotional conflicts that interfere with correctly distinguishing between emotional states such as anger and physiological states such as hunger. The act of eating is somehow thought to reduce underlying tensions and is thereby reinforced. However, Schachter proposes an "externality" theory of obesity. He hypothesizes that the obese are more sensitive to food-related environmental cues than are normal weight individuals, and therefore they are more likely to eat when presented with tempting, highly palatable food and almost as likely to eat such food immediately after a big meal as before. Furthermore the obese individual would rather miss a meal than eat an unpalatable meal since he responds to external cues rather than the internal state of hunger.

As will be discussed in Chapter 8, there is evidence for and against both theories. As Miller[76] wryly pointed out: "Taken together, the research shows that obese subjects do (Conrad, 1970) and don't (Abramson, 1971) exhibit psychogenic hunger. Eating does (Conrad, 1970) and doesn't (Schachter, 1971) reduce anxiety." And, it might be added, the obese are (Schachter, 1971[75]) and aren't (Singh, 1973[77]) more sensitive to external cues than normal weight individuals. Some of the differences in these findings are explained by subject selection. Most of the research validating the psychosomatic-neurotic view of obesity has been performed in medical clinics with patients who were grossly obese whereas much of the research by Schachter and followers was with mild to moderately obese college students.

Nisbett agrees that the obese do not know when they are hungry, but says this may be because they are always hungry, rather than because they never feel hungry. Furthermore, people who are below their set point (due to dieting for health or aesthetic reasons) and animals who are below their ad libitum weight (e.g. VMH lesioned animals in the "dynamic" phase) are more sensitive to external and environmental food cues. For example, both groups are more finicky about food. Furthermore, Nisbett agrees that the obese are more neurotic than normal weight individuals but believes this is because they are striving to maintain their weight below their physiological set point.

Perhaps the most attractive aspect of the set point theory is that it implies that the obese are not gluttons, but rather are fighting a constant uphill battle against a physiologically high set point. Physicians and nutritionists with such viewpoints might be better able to empathize with obese patients and secure their full cooperation in formulating a treatment plan.

However, there are a number of problems with the set point theory. For example, as Miller[76] has noted, why should someone who is at set point, so far as is known, suddenly become grossly obese following a traumatic experience as in reactive obesity? Or, why do some grossly obese individuals never stabilize at any weight? Are they below some astronomically high set point?

Rodin and colleagues[78] have investigated the set point theory and failed to confirm some of its major predictions. They compared three groups of subjects, divided into normal weight, overweight, and obese groups. Obese and mildly overweight subjects found increasingly sweet solutions more pleasant than did normal weight subjects. After weight loss by dieting, there was no increase in judged sweetness as would be predicted since the subjects were further from their set point. In another group, weight loss due to intestinal bypass surgery did result in altered ratings of pleasantness of glucose solutions so that the subjects' ratings were similar to ratings given by normal weight individuals. Loss of adipose tissue stores following bypass surgery did not result in an increase in perceived pleasantness of sweet taste as would be predicted by the set point theory. Also, these same authors challenge Schachter's assumption that taste is an external environmental cue since internal alterations (loss of fat stores secondary to bypass surgery) alter taste responsiveness.

MULTIPLICITY OF FACTORS

There are many factors involved in the etiology and pathogenesis of obesity and an understanding of the interaction of these factors might provide a basis for a rational treatment program. One way of conceptualizing the interaction between these factors is a feedback diagram[79] which can be used to derive mathematical relationships between various factors. Figure 5.4 shows an example of this method. The small letters are constants. A positive sign means that the two variables being compared are directly related. For example, the positive sign of the constant "a" between hunger and eating, means that as hunger (a variable) goes up, eating (a variable) goes up. The negative sign of the constant "b" means that as eating goes up, hunger goes down. Formulas relating any number of variables can then be mathematically derived. The arrows originating and terminating at the same variable mean that that variable may influence its own occurrence; for example, eating *per se* may tend to increase eating whether or not one is hungry or under any social pressure to eat. The advantage of this system is that it emphasizes the fact that there are a great number of variables which contribute to the regulation of weight, and that a change in one, or more likely changes in some combination of variables, can result in a change of

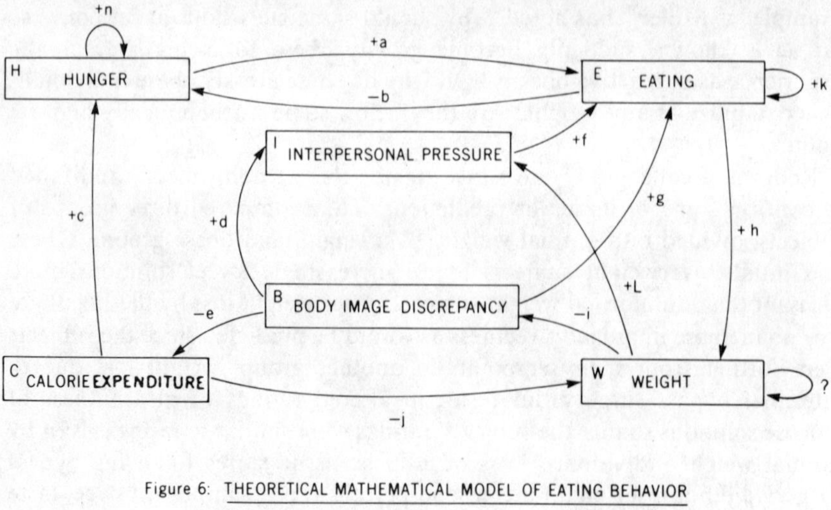

Figure 6: THEORETICAL MATHEMATICAL MODEL OF EATING BEHAVIOR

[box] = a variable

+ sign : variables directly related

− sign : variables indirectly related

+k : increase in variable results in further increase by a constant (k) amount

Figure 5.4. Theoretical mathematical model of eating behavior.

weight. If this diagram is correct, then a mathematical formula which includes the various factors impinging upon eating would be:

$$E = k + aH + fI + gB$$

In words, this means that eating is the sum of the tendency of eating itself to result in an increase in eating plus the increase of eating due to an increase in hunger, plus the increase in eating due to an increase in social pressure to eat, plus the increase in eating due to an increased discrepancy in body image. The discrepancy in body image is in turn affected by a number of variables including weight and interpersonal pressure. The diagram is simplistic and does not include all the relevant variables (for example, palatability) nor are the relationships necessarily correct. However, the advantage of this system is that it emphasizes the fact that there are a great number of variables that contribute to the regulation of weight and that a change in any one, or more likely changes in some combination of variables, can result in a change in eating behavior.

For an individual patient, the important point is that several factors probably contribute to his obesity, and identification of as many factors as possible is most likely to be helpful in devising a treatment strategy. In contrast, concluding that a patient is obese because he overeats is just about as helpful as saying that a hemophiliac will bleed after minor trauma. Neither statement includes the host of factors known to be important in the pathogenesis of the condition.

References

1. Passmore R, unpublished lecture cited in Hervey GR: Regulation of energy balance. Nature 222: 629–631, 1969.
2. Magendie, Tidewald, Milne-Edwards cited in Mayer J, Thomas DW: Regulation of food intake and obesity. Science 156: 328–337, 1967.
3. Mayer A: Essai sur la Soif. Paris, Felix Alcan, 1901.
4. Monello LF, Mayer J: Hunger and satiety sensations in men, women, boys, and girls. Am J Clin Nutr 20: 253–261, 1967.
5. Cannon WB, Washburn AL: An explanation of hunger. Am J Physiol 29: 441–454, 1912.
6. Carlson AJ: The Control of Hunger in Health and Disease. Chicago, Univ of Chicago Press, 1916.
7. Wangensteen OH, Carlson HA: Hunger sensations in a patient after total gastrectomy. Proc Soc Exp Biol Med 28: 545–547, 1931.
8. Stunkard AJ, Koch C: The interpretation of gastric motility: I. Apparent bias in the reports of hunger by obese persons. Arch Gen Psychiatry 11: 74–82, 1964.
9. Stunkard AJ, Fox S: The relationship of gastric motility and hunger. Psychosom Med 33: 123–134, 1971.
10. McCance RA: Food, growth and time. Lancet 2:671–676, 1962.
11. Cohn C, Joseph D: Influence of body weight and body fat on appetite of "normal" lean and obese rats. Yale J Biol Med 34: 598–607, 1962.
12. Liebelt RA, Ichinoe S, Nicholson N: Regulatory influences of adipose tissue on food intake and body weight. Ann NY Acad Sci 131: 559–582, 1965.
13. Chlouverakis C, Hojnicki D Lipectomy in obese hyperglycemic mice (ob/ob). Metabolism 23: 133–137, 1974.

14. Sims EAH, Goldman RF, Gluck CM, et al: Experimental obesity in man. Trans Assoc Am Physicians 81: 153–170, 1968.
15. Sims EAH, Danforth E, Horton ES, et al: Endocrine and metabolic effects of experimental obesity in man. Recent Prog Horm Res 29: 457–487, 1973.
16. Kreisberg RA, Boshell BR, DePlacido J, et al: Insulin secretion in obesity. N Engl J Med 276: 314–319, 1967.
17. Hetherington AW, Ranson SW: The spontaneous activity and food intake of rats with hypothalamic lesions. Am J Physiol 136: 609–617, 1942.
18. Brobeck JR: Mechanism of the development of obesity in animals with hypothalamic lesions. Physiol Rev 26: 541–559, 1946.
19. Mayer J, French RG, Zighera GF, et al: Hypothalamic obesity in the mouse: production, description and metabolic characteristics, Am J Physiol 182: 75–82, 1955.
20. Anand BK, Brobeck JR: Hypothalamic control of food intake in rats and cats. Yale J Biol Med 24: 123–140, 1951.
21. Delgado JMR, Anand BK: Increase of food intake induced by electrical stimulation of the lateral hypothalamus. Am J Physiol 172: 162–168, 1953.
22. Bray G: The Obese Patient. Philadelphia, WB Saunders Co, 1976, p 54.
23. Anand BK, Chhiha GS, Sharma KN, et al: Activity of single neurons in the hypothalamic feeding centers: effect of glucose. Am J Physiol 207: 1146–1154, 1964.
24. Oomura Y, Ooyama H, Yamamato T, et al: Reciprocal relationship of the lateral and ventromedial hypothalamus in the regulation of food intake. Physiol Behav 2: 97–115, 1967.
25. Pfaff D: Histological differences between ventromedial hypothalamic neurones of well fed and underfed rats. Nature 223: 77–78, 1969.
26. Ban T: Fiber connections in the hypothalamus and some autonomic connections in central neural control of eating and obesity. Pharmacol Biochem Behav (Suppl), Volume 3, 1975, pp 3–13.
27. Hustvedt BE, Løvø A: Correlation between hyperinsulinism and hyperphagia in rats with ventromedial hypothalamic lesions. Acta Physiol Scand 84: 29–33, 1972.
28. Bouman PR, Martin JM, Bouhuys AL, Roerdink FH: Studies on the cause and significance of hyperinsulinism in hypothalamic hyperphagia. International Conference on Regulation of Food and Water Intake, Cambridge, England, 1971.
29. Kennedy GC: The regulation of food intake. Adv Psychosom Med 7: 91–99, 1972.
30. Teitelbaum P: Senory control of hypothalamic hyperphagia. J Comp Physiol Psychol 48: 156–163, 1955.
31. Bray GA, York DA: Studies on food intake of genetically obese rats. Am J Physiol 233: 176–179, 1972.
32. Miller NE, Bailey CJ, Stevenson JAF: Decreased "hunger" but increased food intake resulting from hypothalamic lesions. Science 112: 256–259, 1950.
33. Schachter S: Obesity and eating. Science 161: 751–756, 1968.
34. Mayer J: Inactivity as a major factor in adolescent obesity. Ann NY Acad Sci 131: 502–506, 1965.
35. Marks HE, Remley NR: The effects of types of lesion and percentage body weight loss on measures of motivated behavior in rats with hypothalamic lesions. Behav Biol 7: 95–111, 1972.
36. Marshall JF, Turner BH, Teitelbaum P: Sensory neglect produced by lateral hypothalamic damage. Science 174: 523–525, 1971.
37. Panskepp J: Central metabolic and humoral factors involved in the neural regulation of feeding. Pharmacol Biochem Behav (Suppl) 3: 107–119, 1975.
38. Fonberg E, Delgado JM: Avoidance and alimentary reactions during amygdala stimulation. J Neurophysiol 24: 651–664, 1961.
39. Morgane PJ, Kosman AJ: Relationship of the middle hypothalamus to amygdalar hyperphagia. Am J Physiol 198: 1315–1318, 1960.
40. Ungerstedt U: Adipsia and aphagia after 6-hydroxydopamine induced degeneration of the nigrostriatal dopamine system. Acta Physiol Scand (Suppl) 367: 95–122, 1971.
41. Panskepp J, Nance DM: Effects of para-chlorophenylalanine on food intake in rats. Physiol Psychol 2: 360–364, 1964.
42. Ritter S, Stein L: Self-stimulation of noradrenergic cell group (A6) in locus coeruleus of rat. J Comp Physiol Psychol 85: 443–452, 1973.

43. Davies R, Nakajma S, White N: Enhancement of feeding produced by stimulation of the ventromedial hypothalamus. J Comp Physiol Psychol 86: 414–419, 1974.
44. Panskepp J: Hypothalamic regulation of energy balance and feeding behavior. Fed Proc 33: 1150–1156, 1974.
45. Mayer A (1939), cited in Mayer J, Thomas DW: Regulation of food intake and obesity. Science 156: 328–337, 1967.
46. Adam JM, Best TW, Edholm OG: Weight changes in young men. J Physiol (Lond) 156: 38, 1961.
47. Edholm OG, Fletcher JG, Widdowson EM, et al: The energy expenditure and food intake of individual men. Br J Nutr 9: 286–300, 1955.
48. Edholm OG, Adam JM, Healy MJ, et al: Food intake and energy expenditure of army recruits. Br J Nutr 24: 1091–1107, 1970.
49. Garrow JS: Energy Balance and Obesity in Man. New York, American Elsevier Publishing Co, 1974.
50. Janowitz HD: Role of the gastrointestinal tract in regulation of food intake. In: Handbook of Physiology, Section 6, Volume I, Control of Food and Water Intake. Code CF (ed). Washington DC, American Physiological Society 1967, pp 219–224.
51. Janowitz HD, Grossman MI: Some factors affecting food intake of normal dogs and dogs with oesophagostomy and gastric fistulas. Am J Physiol 159: 143–148, 1949.
52. Berkun MM, Kessen ML, Miller NE: Hunger reducing effects of food by stomach fistula versus food by mouth measured by a consummatory response. J Comp Physiol 45: 550–554, 1952.
53. Snowden CT: Gastro-intestinal sensory and motor control of food intake. J Comp Psychol 71: 68–76, 1970.
54. Smith GP, Gibbs J: Cholecystokinin: a putative satiety signal. Pharmacol Biochem Behav (Suppl 1) 3: 135–138, 1975.
55. Hagan RL: Theories of obesity: is there any hope for order? In: Obesity. Williams BJ, Martins, Foreyt JP (eds). New York, Mazel, Inc, 1976, pp 3–19.
56. Cabanac M, Ducleaux R: Obesity: absence of satiety aversion to survive. Science, 168: 496–497, 1970.
57. Wooley OW, Wooley SC: Appetite for palatable food as a function of the caloric density of the previous meal. Paper presented at Eastern Psychological Association, April 19, 1974.
58. Nisbett RE: Hunger, obesity and the ventromedial hypothalamus. Psychol Rev 79: 433–458, 1972.
59. Mellinkoff SM, Frankland M, Boyle D: Relationship between serum amino acid concentration and fluctuations in appetite. J Appl Physiol 8: 535–538, 1956.
60. Rogers QR, Leung PMB: The influence of amino acids on the neuroregulation of food intake. Fed Proc 32: 1709–1719, 1973.
61. Vrba R, Cannon W: Assimilation of glucose in rat brain and metabolic activities of various groups of brain proteins. In: Protein Metabolism of the Nervous System. A Lajtha (ed). New York, Plenum Press, 1977, pp 219–237.
62. Bray GA, Gallagher TF Jr: Manifestations of hypothalamic obesity in man: a comprehensive investigation of eight patients and a review of the literature. Medicine (Baltimore) 54: 301–330, 1975.
63. Bruch H: Eating Disorders: Obesity, Anorexia Nervosa and the Person Within. New York, Basic Books, 1973.
64. Mayer J: Glucostatic mechanism of regulation of food intake. N Engl J Med 249: 13–16, 1953.
65. Wagner JW, DeGroot J: Changes in feeding behavior after intracerebral injections in the rat. Am J Physiol 204: 483–487, 1963.
66. Brobeck JR: Food intake as a mechanism of temperature regulation. Yale J Biol Med 20: 545–552, 1948.
67. Hamilton CL, Brobeck JR: Food intake and activity of rats with rostral hypothalamic lesions. Proc Soc Exp Biol Med 122: 270–272, 1966.
68. Mecklenberg RS, Loriaux DL, Thompson RH, et al: Hypothalamic dysfunction in patients with anorexia nervosa. Medicine (Baltimore) 53: 147–159, 1974.
69. Goodner CJ, Oglivie JT, Koerker OT: The metabolism of glycerol by hypothalamic and pituitary tissues in vitro in the rat. Proc Soc Exp Biol Med 143: 616–622, 1973.

70. Woods SC, Decke E, Vasselli JR: Metabolic hormones and regulation of body weight. Psychol Rev 81: 26–43, 1964.
71. York DA, Bray GA: Dependence of hypothalamic obesity on insulin, the pituitary and the adrenal gland. Endocrinology 90: 885–894, 1972.
72. Hoebel BG, Teitelbaum P: Weight regulation in normal and hypothalamic hyperphagic rats. J Comp Physiol Psychol 66: 189–193, 1966.
73. Powley JL, Keesey RE: Relationship of body weight to the lateral hypothalamic feeding syndrome. J Comp Physiol Psychol 70: 25–36, 1970.
74. Cabanac M: Physiological role of pleasure. Science 173: 1103–1107, 1971.
75. Schachter S: Some extraordinary facts about obese humans and rats. Am Psychol 26: 129–144, 1971.
76. Miller C: New perspectives on obesity. Paper presented at Florida Psychological Association Meeting Miami, Florida, May 1974.
77. Singh D: Role of response habits and cognitive factors in determination of behavior of obese humans. J Pers Soc Psychol 27: 220–238, 1973.
78. Rodin J, Moskowitz HR, Bray GA: Relationship between obesity, weight loss, and taste responsiveness. Physiol Behav 17: 591–597, 1976.
79. Cobb L, Denker M: Linear and non-linear models for counterproductive behavior. In preparation 1979.

CHAPTER

6

Etiology and Pathogenesis of Obesity: Energy Expenditure

Energy is expended in three major ways: basal metabolism, "specific dynamic action" of food, and physical activity. The energy expended by the body can be obtained from food ingested or from stored energy, primarily adipose tissue. The energy content of food, as well as that stored as fat, glycogen, or protein is expressed in terms of available calories. A calorie is defined as the quantity of heat required to raise 1 g of water from 15° to 16°C. The energy obtained from the combustion of food stuffs or from the catabolism of food stores is used by the body to maintain homeothermia and to perform metabolic and physical work.

In his classic experiments, Lavoisier[1] demonstrated that the quantity of heat produced during metabolism of stored energy (i.e., fat) is the same as that produced by oxidizing the same amount of fat or other source of energy outside the body. Carbohydrates produce approximately 4 calories for every gram oxidized. Fats yield approximately 9.1 calories per gram of triglyceride oxidized completely to carbon dioxide and water. Each gram of protein yields approximately 4 calories.

TOTAL ENERGY EXPENDITURE

DIRECT CALORIMETRY

The methods for measuring total energy expenditure are complex. Direct calorimetry[2] requires placing a subject in a chamber which will measure all the heat released in the form of thermal energy, radiant energy, and energy from vaporization of water from the lungs as well as the uptake of oxygen and the production of carbon dioxide.

The experimental procedure for using the Atwater calorimeter is exacting. A team of observers is required to keep records of the temperature of the walls of the calorimeter, of the cooling water, of the air pumped through the calorimeter, and the temperature of the subject (by rectal thermometer). By a series of ingenious devices, each step of which is subject to error, a constant temperature is maintained in the calorimetry chamber with a zero temperature gradient across the walls. Oxygen entering the chamber is determined. Carbon dioxide production is calibrated by the change in weight of soda lime absorbers. The composition of the gas in the calorimeter is analyzed and the subject's clothing and bedding weighed to correct for changes in humidity. These measurements are tedious and the calculations after obtaining the measurements are also laborious. Corrections must be made for the thermal mass of the calorimeter, for the thermal mass and temperature of all food entering and leaving the chamber, and for changes in barometric pressure. Thus the method of direct calorimetry is extremely time-consuming. Also, an airtight system is not well suited to high metabolic rates because air must be circulated through the system rapidly to prevent a rise in carbon dioxide concentration from rebreathing air. The major advantages of direct calorimetry is that in skilled hands it is very precise and can be used to evaluate the precision of indirect methods.

INDIRECT MEASURES

Indirect methods rely on the observation that there is a close relationship between gaseous exchange and heat production. Gaseous exchange is measured using a variety of techniques (ventilated hood systems, Douglas bag, etc.), and energy expenditure is calculated using a method described by Weir. This calculation depends on experimentally determined values of calories released by oxidation of various food stuffs and on a number of theoretical assumptions regarding the oxidation of protein. The regression equation devised by Weir[3] is:

$$K = 3.941\ O_2 + 1.106\ CO_2 + 2.17\ UN$$

K = total heat output in kilocalories (kcal) in a given time
O_2 = the volume of liters of oxygen consumed in that time (O_2 consumption)
CO_2 = carbon dioxide produced
UN = Urinary nitrogen in grams (gm)

Using this equation, estimation of oxygen consumption is the most critical factor. For example, an error of 10% in the estimate of oxygen consumption would result in an error in the answer equivalent to an error of 35% in carbon dioxide estimation. Several experiments have compared direct calorimetry to indirect methods which measure gas exchange and then calculate total heat output by Weir's formula.

In 1957, Swift[4] found an average difference of only 4.4% between direct and indirect calorimetry, suggesting that the formula will provide reasonably accurate estimates of total energy expenditure based on gaseous exchange. However, Swift's study involved only a few young adults, and the calculation may be invalid in other age groups or in differing nutritional states.

Other indirect measurements of total energy expenditure have not been widely used. For example, heart rate has also been used to estimate oxygen consumption but is very inaccurate except under rigidly controlled conditions.[5]

BASAL METABOLIC RATE

DETERMINATION OF BMR

The methods noted above determine total energy expenditure. Determining the portion of energy used in the basal metabolic rate is also fraught with difficulty.

The conditions for measuring basal metabolic rate are as follows. A cooperative patient is evaluated in a neutral thermal environment 12 to 18 hours after a meal, at mental and physical rest. Even minor disruptions can cause a change of 10% in the oxygen uptake of a subject at rest. Strictly speaking, the time of day of the measurement should also be specified since oxygen consumption falls in the morning, whether or not the person is asleep. Furthermore, in women this circadian rhythm is maintained, but a cyclical variation in oxygen uptake is superimposed. Oxygen uptake is lower post-menstrually than pre-menstrually.[6] Therefore, the day of the menstrual cycle as well as the time of day should be specified. Suffice it to say that in most studies comparing basal metabolic rates between obese and normal weight subjects, these conditions have not been met.

BMR INCREASE WITH WEIGHT GAIN

It is known that basal metabolic rate rises with increasing body weight. It has been observed that the basal metabolic rates of rats, of mice and of elephants, and of species of intermediate size, are fairly similar when related to their surface area.[6] Therefore, it has been argued that the increase in surface area results in an increase in heat loss and consequent rise in basal metabolic rate to correct for the heat loss. However, that this is not the whole story is demonstrated by the fact that the basal metabolic rate does not rise if the subject lies spread-eagled presenting the greatest surface area for heat loss compared to lying curled up in a small volume. Therefore, increases in basal metabolic rate associated with increases in weight cannot be accounted for solely on the basis of change in surface area. Ideally, the metabolic rate should be related to lean body mass since the maintenance of these tissues probably requires more energy than maintenance of adipose tissue stores which are thought to be relatively metabolically inert. However, as noted in Chapter 1, measurement of lean body mass is also quite difficult.

HIGHER BMR IN MEN

Other factors well known to alter basal metabolic rate include age, sex, temperature, drugs, hormones, and nutritional status. Men have a higher BMR than women when compared by body weight or surface area.[6] However, when compared on the basis of lean body mass there are no significant differences in basal metabolic rate between men and women.[7] The differences can be accounted for by differences in fat content. Women have more fat which is less metabolically active and thus have a lower basal metabolic rate when corrected for body weight. But, the metabolic requirements for lean body tissue are the same for both men and women.

BMR DECREASES WITH AGE

Age also has an effect on metabolic rate. Rapidly growing children have greater caloric needs. At birth, caloric requirements are approximately 120 kcal/kg and decline to 100 kcal/kg by the end of the 1st year. Over the next 10 years the caloric requirements are approximately 80 kcal/kg until adolescence when they decline to 50 kcal/kg for boys and 35 kcal/kg for girls (Recommended Dietary Allowances, 1974).[8] With advancing age, there is probably also a decrease in basal metabolic rate, but only 1–2% per decade.[9] Since the percentage of fat content increases slightly with age, even if weight remains constant, the decrease in basal metabolic rate may be due to the fact that adipose tissue is less metabolically active than lean body tissue.

EFFECT OF CLIMATE ON BMR UNCERTAIN

Changes in deep body temperature also affect BMR. If body temperature is raised by 1°C, either by fever or by warming the body externally at a rate greater than the possible rate of heat loss, the basal metabolic rate rises by approximately 12%. Conversely, if body temperature is reduced, basal metabolic rate falls. However, it is still questionable whether climate affects basal metabolic rate. Buskirk *et al*[10] studied the resting metabolism of soldiers at Fort Churchill, Canada, where the ambient temperature was −25°C, at Yuma, Arizona, 34°C, at Natick, Massachusetts, 22°C, and on Mt. Washington, New Hampshire, −4°C. They found no significant relationship between resting metabolism and ambient temperature.

THYROID HORMONES, GROWTH HORMONE, AND EPINEPHRINE—CALORIGENIC

Thyroid hormones, growth hormone, glucagon, and epinephrine increase basal metabolic rate and are termed calorigenic. Thyroid hormones increase oxygen consumption and a deficiency of thyroid hormone decreases metabolic rate.[11] There is a characteristic delay of action on basal metabolic rate. After an injection of tri-iodothyronine (T_3) into a hypothyroid patient, the metabolic rate is not immediately affected and peak activity occurs 1 to 5 days later. With thyroxine (T_4) the delay is even longer with peak activity occurring 8 to 18 days later. The delay in effect implies an indirect action, perhaps on protein synthesis. If protein synthesis is inhibited by either actinomycin D, puromycin, or starvation, the calorigenic effect of thyroid hormones is abolished.[12]

Another recent theory is that thyroid hormones may increase the rate of ionic transport across cell membranes.[13] Since perhaps half of the total basal metabolism is involved in maintaining ionic equilibrium between intracellular compartments, an increase in ionic transport across cell membranes would result in an increase in basal metabolic rate. There has been a large number of studies of thyroid hormone activity in the obese, some of which were initially interpreted as abnormal. However, these studies of thyroid activity depended on estimates of basal metabolic rate, which is affected by a variety of other factors, including nutritional status. Thyroid function in the great majority of spontaneously obese patients is usually normal.

Growth hormone is also calorigenic. It produces a small, but significant, increase in basal metabolism in man and animals.[14] In obese humans, the normal rise in growth hormone to insulin-induced hypoglycemia is blunted. Also, response to arginine stimulation is blunted.[15] Furthermore, growth hormone concentrations at rest and after exercise are lower than normal in obese patients.[16,17] Bray[14] demonstrated that growth hormone has a calorigenic effect in obese humans. He gave 5 mg/day of growth hormone for 8 days to obese patients and noted an increase in oxygen consumption of 10%.

Glucagon is also calorigenic, at least in experimental animals. Carcass analysis of rats given injections of glucagon had stored less energy in the form of adipose tissue than normal controls.[18] The difference between the rats treated with glucagon and the control rats was that the treated rats had an increase of oxygen consumption.[19] It is not known whether glucagon secretion in obese patients is abnormal.[20]

Epinephrine injection produces a significant, rapid, but short-lived increase in metabolic rate.[21] In large doses, though, epinephrine depresses oxygen consumption. The exact nature of the relationship between emotional factors and energy expenditure is not known, but epinephrine is one possible endocrine link. However, even documenting the relationship between energy expenditure and emotional factors is difficult, to say nothing of demonstrating that epinephrine might mediate any difference found. The energy cost of lying, sitting, and standing for psychiatric inpatients was compared to the energy cost for normal subjects.[22] The more disturbed patients had a decrement in oxygen used when they stood up, but no significant difference from normal in energy cost of lying or sitting. One study[23] showed that the resting metabolic rate of subjects in a metabolic chamber without a face mask was substantially less than the metabolic rate of the same subjects wearing face masks. This difference may be due to an increased "vigilance," both physical and emotional, when wearing a face mask compared to lying comfortably in a metabolic chamber. Conceivably, this "vigilance" could be due to secretion of epinephrine.

EFFECT OF DRUGS ON BMR

A variety of drugs is known to influence metabolic rate; these include dinitrophenol, salicylate, caffeine, and reserpine. Dinitrophenol causes an increase in basal metabolic rate by uncoupling oxidative phosphorylation (i.e., by uncoupling oxygen utilization from the production of adenosine triphosphate in the mitochondria).[24] This drug was used to treat obesity but because of its serious and potentially lethal side effects, its use has been discontinued. Aspirin (salicylate) also uncouples oxidative phosphorylation, thereby increasing oxygen consumption in both lean and obese patients.[25] However, the dose required to produce these effects is in the toxic range which produces tinnitus and other toxic side effects. Garrow[26] reports that reserpine decreases metabolic rate. Therefore, various drugs are known to influence oxygen consumption.

In summary, basal metabolic rate is difficult to measure and is influenced by a number of factors including nutritional status, sex, age, temperature, time of day, hormones, and probably emotional stress. Studies that have attempted to compare basal metabolic rate in obese subjects to basal metabolic rate in normal weight subjects have often not controlled for these variables. Furthermore, comparing BMR in obese and normal subjects by correcting for surface area is probably invalid. There is evidence, however, that basal energy expenditure rises with increasing body weight, but that the BMR of the lean body mass is the same in normal and obese subjects.

PHYSICAL ACTIVITY

Despite all the difficulties in determining basal metabolic rate, it is relatively easy to determine in comparison with measuring energy expended by physical activity. Estimates of the percentage of energy expended by physical activity are approximately 30% for normal persons, but there are marked differences in activity levels among normal weight individuals.

Various techniques have been used to measure the energy cost of physical activity. Some investigators have used pedometers to obtain semi-quantitative estimates of activity[27] and others have sampled serial motion pictures[28] to estimate activity levels.

Activity diaries have also been used to estimate energy expenditure, and these are widely used in the treatment of obesity. The principle is as follows. The energy cost of various activities is determined (usually by indirect calorimetry). The time spent in that activity is recorded by the subject, and the energy cost per day of that activity is calculated by multiplying the number of minutes in the activity by the experimentally determined energy cost per minute. For example, if the calories expended in riding a bicycle are estimated to be 8 cal/min, and the subject rides for 10 minutes, the energy cost of the activity for that day is 80 cal. The energy cost for the various activities are tallied and this is assumed to account for energy expended in physical activity. This technique has been widely used, but is subject to a number of errors, not the least of which is that the energy cost of an activity under controlled experimental conditions may not be the same outside the laboratory.

It has been suggested that the decrease in physical activity in our sedentary society accounts for the rise in obesity. This seems plausible, but currently available methods for documenting this hypothesis have yielded conflicting results. Most studies have attempted to compare activity levels of obese subjects with those of normal weight subjects. This, of course, does not answer the question of whether decreased activity results in obesity or whether obesity causes a decrease in physical activity. Despite the limitations of this method, however, several studies[28, 29] have shown that obese teenage girls spend less energy in physical activity than normal weight girls. Furthermore, men in more strenuous occupations weigh less than those in more sedentary jobs.[30] Although this is a long way from proving that a decrease in physical activity causes obesity, undoubtedly it is an important factor in the context of the myriad other influences that promote obesity.

"SPECIFIC DYNAMIC ACTION" OF FOOD (THERMIC EFFECT)

The specific dynamic action of food refers to the observation that resting oxygen consumption increases after each meal. Initially, this effect was thought to be specific to protein (hence "specific") but the increase in oxygen consumption after a meal occurs whether it is protein, fat, or carbohydrate. Therefore, the term "thermic effect" is more appropriate. Probably, however, protein produces a greater "thermic effect" than carbohydrates or fats. Students who were fed 122 gm of protein daily had a 6.3% greater heat production than when they were fed an equicalorie diet with 34 gm of protein per day.[31] However, although high protein diets have a somewhat larger thermic effect than equicalorie low protein meals, the increase in oxygen consumption appears earlier after a carbohydrate meal than after a meal of protein or fat. The thermic effect lasts for several hours after the meal and is enough to increase the basal metabolism by 20% for a few hours. Although these observations are on fairly firm experimental ground, it is important to remember that resting metabolic rate shows variations in the same individuals of about 5% from one day to another, thereby producing an uncertainty of about 25% in the magnitude of the thermic effect.

LUXUS KONSUMPTION

Basal metabolism, physical activity, and the "specific dynamic action of food" (thermic effect) are the three major ways that energy is expended. A fourth controversial contribution to energy expenditure is "luxus konsumption." This term refers to a postulated ability to burn off excess calories after overeating. Ostensibly, inability to activate such a mechanism could result in obesity. This theory really has its origin from widespread anecdotal observations that some individuals seem to eat enormous amounts, exercise no more than their peers, yet maintain their weight within a normal range.

In 1902, Neumann[32] measured his food intake and body weight over 3 years, and although his weight remained constant his average daily calorie intake each year varied by several hundred calories. Gulick[33] performed essentially the same experiment during 1 year and also found that his body weight remained constant despite wide fluctuations in calorie intake. In an experimental overfeeding study, Sims and colleagues[34, 35] found that the calories stored as fat over the course of several months of overfeeding were substantially less than calculated from the number of calories ingested. Although luxus konsumption could be the operant mechanism, it may be that growth *per se* requires energy that is difficult to measure.

Miller and Mumford[36] noted that the thermic response (SDA) to a meal increases with the size of the meal. Also exercising after a meal increases this thermic response. They concluded that luxus konsumption is a form of dietary thermogenesis over and above the specific dynamic action of food. (See Figure 6.1)

In a careful study of overfed humans, Passmore and colleagues[37, 38] made calculations that accounted for all of the ingested calories, thus offering strong evidence against the concept of luxus konsumption. However, this study had only three subjects, who were only overfed 2 weeks. Luxus konsumption might be a long-term mechanism. In any case, there are several human and many animal studies in which subjects have eaten excessively for long periods, but gained much less weight than predicted. The reason for

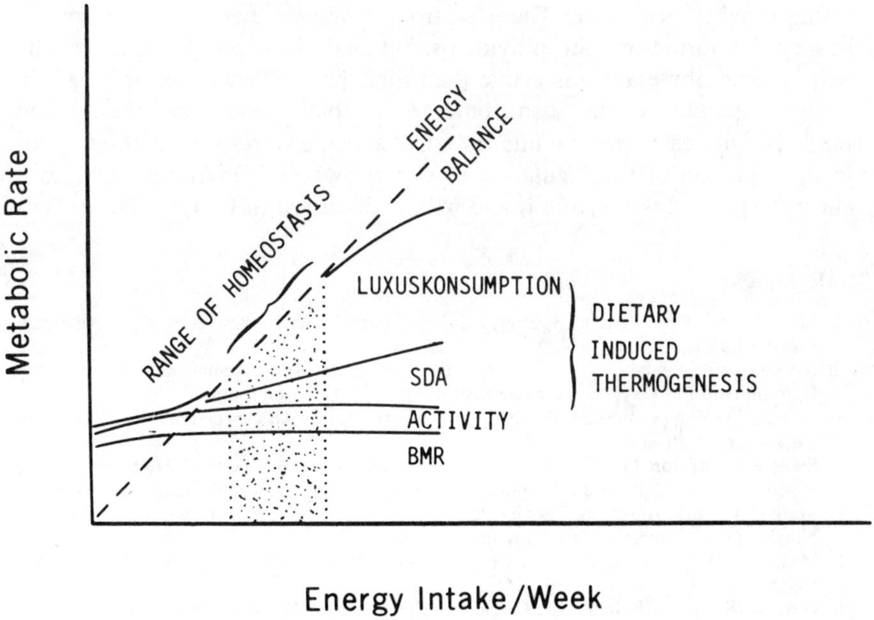

Figure 6.1. Energy expenditure: Distribution of calories between various metabolic compartments. Luxuskonsumption, if it exists, would be a form of dietary-induced thermogenesis. (Reprinted with permission from Miller and Mumford: Luxuskonsumption, in Apfelbaum (Ed) Régulation de l'équilibre énérgetique chez l'homme. Energy Balance in Man. Paris, Masson, 1973.)

this is not clear, and experiments ruling out the possibility of luxus konsumption have not yet been performed.

PERCENTAGES OF ENERGY EXPENDED

In summary, there are at least four possible sources of energy expenditure: basal metabolism, physical activity, the "specific action of food," and possibly luxus konsumption. Probably basal metabolism accounts for approximately 50–60% of calories expended. Physical activity accounts for 25–35%, and the thermic effect of food (either SDA and luxus konsumption) 5–10%. (See Figure 6.1)

Theoretically, the energy cost of any of these factors might be decreased and predispose to obesity. Since basal metabolism of lean body tissue is approximately the same in obese and normal weight subjects, this factor does not appear to be etiologic. However, once obesity is established, the fact that the energy cost of maintaining fat stores is less than the energy cost of maintaining lean body tissue might account for some of the difficulty in losing weight once obese. There is strong evidence that the obese are less active than normal weight individuals, but again little proof that those who will become obese are less active than their peers. Therefore, decreases in energy expenditure may contribute to the pathogenesis of obesity and potentiate increases in food intake. Adipose tissue stores are the third factor in the equation of the regulation of energy balance (energy intake minus energy expended = fat stored) and will be discussed in Chapter 7).

References

1. Lavoisier, cited by Garrow JS: Energy Balance and Obesity in Man. New York, American Elsevier Publishing Inc, 1974.
2. Atwater WP, Benedict FG: A Respiration Chamber with Appliances for the Direct Determination of Oxygen. Carnegie Institution of Washington, publ 42, 1905.
3. Weir JB De V: New methods for calculating metabolic rate with special reference to protein metabolism. J Physiol (Lond) 109: 1–9, 1949.
4. Swift RW, Barron GP, Fisherkit, et al: Relative Dynamic Effects of High versus Low Protein Diets of Equicaloric Content; cited in Garrow JS: Energy Balance and Obesity in Man. New York, American Elsevier Publishing Co. Inc, 1974, p 72. Department of Animal Nutrition, Pennsylvania State Univ, pub no 232, 1957.
5. Mayfield ME: The indirect measurement of energy expenditure in industrial situations. Am J Clin Nutr 24: 1126–1138, 1971.
6. Garrow JS: Energy Balance and Obesity in Man. New York, American Elsevier Publishing Inc, 1974.
7. Behnke AR: The relation of lean body weight to metabolism and some consequent systematizations. Ann NY Acad Sci 56: 1095–1142, 1953.
8. Recommended Dietary Allowances. National Academy of Sciences, Washington DC, 8th revised edition, 1974.
9. Keys A, Taylor HL, Grande F: Basal metabolism and age of adult man. Metabolism 22: 579–587, 1973.
10. Buskirk ER, Iampietro PF, Welch BE: Variations in resting metabolism with changes in food, exercise and climate. Metabolism 6: 144–153, 1957.
11. Pitt Rivers R, Tata JR: The Thyroid Hormone. Callow RK, Campbell PN, Datta SP, Engel LL (eds). London, Pergamon Press, 1959.
12. Tata JR: Advances in metabolic disorders. In: Basal Metabolic Rate and Thyroid Hormones. Levine R, Luft R (eds). New York, Academic Press, 1964, pp 153–189.
13. Edelman IS, Ismail-Beigi F: Thyroid thermogenesis and active sodium transport. Recent Prog Horm Res 30: 235–257, 1974.
14. Bray GA: Calorigenic effect of human growth hormone in obesity. J Clin Endocrin Metab 29: 119–122, 1969.
15. Londono H, Gallagher TF, Bray GA: Effect of weight reduction, triiodothyronine and diethylstilbestrol on growth hormone in obesity. Metabolism 18: 986–992, 1969.
16. Hanson JS: Exercise responses following production of experimental obesity. J Appl Physiol 35: 587–591, 1973.
17. Henneman PH, Forbes AP, Moldawerm M, et al: Effects of growth hormone in man. J Clin Invest 39: 1223–1238, 1960.
18. Salter JM: Metabolic effects of glucagon on the Wistar rat. Am J Clin Nutr 8: 535–539, 1960.
19. Davidson IWF, Salter JM, Best CH: The effect of glucagon on the metabolic rate of rats. Am J Clin Nutr 8: 540–546, 1960.
20. Kalkhoff RK, Gossain VV, Matute ML: Plasma glucagon in obesity: response to arginine, glucose and protein. N Engl J Med 289: 465–467, 1973.
21. Himms-Hagen J: Sympathetic regulation of metabolism. Pharmacol Rev 19: 367–461, 1967.
22. Melville PH, Mezey AG: Emotional state and energy expenditure. Lancet 1: 273–274, 1959.

23. Tremolière J, Carre L, Naon R: Interrelations between body weight, level of vigilance and energy expenditure in subjects on various diets. In: Energy Balance in Man. Apfelbaum M (ed). Paris, Masson, 1973, pp 125–134.
24. Tainter ML, Stockton AB, Cutting W: Dinitrophenol in the treatment of obesity: final report. JAMA 105: 332-336, 1935.
25. Smith MJH, Dawkins PO: Salicylates and enzymes. J Pharm Pharmacol 23: 729–744, 1971.
26. Garrow JS: Energy Balance and Obesity in Man. New York, American Elsevier Publishing Inc, 1974, p 169.
27. Chirico AM, Stunkard AJ: Physical activity and human obesity. New Engl J Med 263: 935–940, 1960.
28. Bullen BA, Reed RB, Mayer J: Physical activity of obese and nonobese adolescent girls, appraised by motion picture sampling. Am J Clin Nutr 14: 211–223, 1964.
29. Johnson ML, Burke BS, Mayer J: The prevalence and incidence of obesity in a cross-section of elementary and secondary school children. Am J Clin Nutr 4: 231–238, 1956.
30. Mayer J, Roy P, Mitra KP: Relation between caloric intake, body weight and physical work: studies in an industrial male population in West Bengal. Am J Clin Nutr 4: 169–175, 1956.
31. Swift RW, Barron GP, Fisher KH, et al.: Relative Dynamic Effects of High versus Low Protein Diets of Equicaloric Content; cited in Garrow JS: Energy Balance and Obesity in Man. New York, American Elsevier Publishing Co. Inc, 1974, p 149. Department of Animal Nutrition, Pennsylvania State Univ, pub no 232, 1957.
32. Neumann RO: Experimentelle Beiträge zur Lehre von dem täglichen Nahrungsbedarf des Menschen unter besorderer Berücksichtigung der notwendigen Eiweifsmenge. Arch für Hygiene 45: 1–87, 1902; cited by Bray GA: The Obese Patient. Philadelphia, WB Saunders, 1976.
33. Gulick A: A study of weight regulation in the adult human body during over-nutrition. Am J Physiol 60: 371–395, 1922.
34. Sims EAH, Goldman RF, Gluck CM, et al: Experimental obesity in man. Trans Assoc Am Physicians 81: 153–170, 1968.
35. Sims EAH, Danforth E, Horton ES, et al: Endocrine and metabolic effects of experimental obesity in man. Recent Prog Horm Res 29: 457–487, 1973.
36. Miller DS, Mumford PM: Luxus konsumption. In: Energy Balance in Man. Apfelbaum M (ed). Paris, Masson, 1973, pp 195–207.
37. Passmore R, Meiklejohn AP, Dewar AD: Energy utilization in overfed thin men. Br J Nutr 9: 20–26, 1955.
38. Passmore R, Meiklejohn AP, Dewar AD: An analysis of the gain in weight of overfed thin young men. Br J Nutr 9: 27–37, 1955.

CHAPTER 7

Anatomy of Obesity

It is only in the last three decades that scientists have undertaken exhaustive studies of adipose tissue. Research into the growth and development of adipose tissue cellularity is one of the most active and interesting areas in the recent study of obesity. It is widely known that treatment of obesity is exceedingly difficult and relapse usually occurs. The current adipose cellularity theories may account for these treatment failures and, more importantly, offer a rational scientific basis for designing sound preventive measures in early childhood. In this chapter, the composition and histology of the fat cell will be described. The current studies investigating the relationship between fat cell size and fat cell number will be summarized in relationship to the validity of the adipose cellularity hypothesis of obesity.

COMPOSITION OF ADIPOSE TISSUE

Fat is relatively anhydrous compared to lean body tissue. Less than 10% of adipose tissue is water. As noted in Chapter 1, this provides a tremendous advantage in terms of efficient energy storage, the major function of adipose tissue. Martinsson[1] has evaluated the composition of subcutaneous adipose tissue in humans and found that lipids represent just over 90% of the total weight of adipose tissue. These lipids include triglycerides, cholesterol, and phospholipids. Triglycerides are by far the predominant lipid component comprising 86% of the wet weight of adipose tissue. Cholesterol is 0.16% and phospholipids 0.15% of the wet weight (See Table 7.1). Martinsson notes that the deoxyribonucleic acid (DNA) content of fat cells is positively correlated with nitrogen content but negatively correlated with total lipids.

Table 7.1

Wet Weight	100%
Dry Weight	91%
Total lipid	90%
• Triglycerides	86%
• Cholesterol	0.16%
• Phospholipid	0.15%
Nitrogen	0.26%
Deoxyribonucleic acid	0.0074%
Water	9%

Composition of subcutaneous human adipose tissue (adapted from Martinsson[1]).

This implies that an increase in the size of a fat cell is associated with an increase of lipid (primarily triglyceride) but not with an increase in DNA, a conclusion compatible with the storage function of adipose tissue.

The fat droplet of adipocytes is almost entirely triglycerides. Triglycerides are three fatty acids attached to a molecule of glycerol in an ester linkage (Fig. 7.1). The fatty acids most commonly found in triglycerides have 16 to 18 carbons and may be unsaturated (i.e., with double bonds between carbons) or saturated. Fatty acids with a chain length between 10 and 16 are usually saturated, but those with a chain length 18 or more are usually unsaturated.

Twenty-two fatty acids have been identified in the adipose tissue triglycerides. Six of these fatty acids—palmitic, myristic, palmitoleic, stearic, oleic, and linoleic acids—account for 95% of the 22 identified.[2] The dietary effects on the fatty acid composition of adipose tissue are slow. Only when human subjects were fed formulas rich in corn oil more than 160 weeks were slow

$$
\begin{array}{c}
H_2\text{-C-O-}FA_1 \\
| \\
H\text{-C-O-}FA_2 \\
| \\
H_2\text{-C-O-}FA_3
\end{array}
$$

FA_1, FA_2, FA_3 represent different fatty acids

Figure 7.1. Structure of triglycerides.

changes in adipose tissue seen.[3] In contrast, several isotope studies have demonstrated a rapid turnover of fatty acids in depot fat.[2] To account for these discordant findings, it has been postulated that there are two metabolic compartments within adipose tissue. The larger compartment may serve as a relatively inert storage site, and the smaller pool, turning over more rapidly, may be in close metabolic relationship to dietary, serum, and liver lipids.

Various investigators have studied fatty acid content in obese subjects compared to normal weight subjects. Hirsch and colleagues[4] found that the ratio of monosaturated to saturated fatty acids was higher in obese subjects. However, Heffernan[5] found that the ratio of saturated to unsaturated fatty acids was similar in obese and normal subjects.

LIPOGENESIS AND LIPOLYSIS

LIPOGENESIS

Lipogenesis is the formation of triglycerides from free fatty acids and glycerol and lipolysis is the breakdown of triglycerides into free fatty acids and glycerol. There are three major sources of free fatty acids used in the synthesis of triglycerides (See Fig. 7.2). First, fatty acids which circulate in the plasma bound to albumin can be incorporated into adipose tissue triglycerides.[6] Second, triglycerides and cholesterol from the diet are absorbed from the small intestine and transported via the lymphatics to the bloodstream in large particles called chylomicrons. Chylomicrons are one of the major classes of lipoproteins. These lipoproteins are the second source of free fatty acids. Lipoprotein lipase is an essential enzyme in the process of breaking down lipoprotein into free fatty acids and glycerol. The resultant free fatty acids, but not the glycerol, are incorporated into the lipid droplet within the adipocyte. The glycerol used in the reesterification of the triglyceride within the adipocyte is derived from other sources. The third possible source of fatty acids is de novo synthesis within the adipocyte. Although there is clear evidence that some animals rapidly synthesize fatty acid within adipose tissue,[7] human data are conflicting. Bray's[8] in vitro studies of adipose tissue from obese subjects fed high-calorie diets demonstrated that carbon atoms from glucose or pyruvate were converted into fatty acids. However, in vivo evidence for fatty acid synthesis within human adipocytes is lacking.

Glycerol used in the synthesis of triglycerides within adipose tissue is derived from glucose which is converted to glycerol 3-phosphate, an essential metabolic precursor of glycerol. In the absence of glucose, pyruvate carbons can be converted to glycerol.

LIPOLYSIS

Lipolysis, the breakdown of triglycerides to glycerol and free fatty acids, can be divided into basal lipolysis and hormone-stimulated lipolysis. Basal

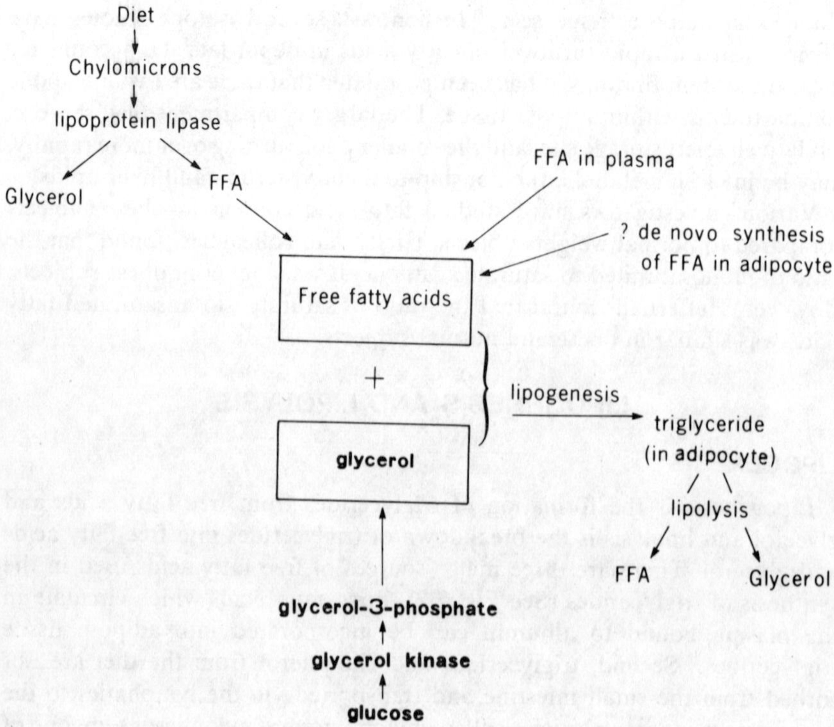

Figure 7.2. Lipogenesis. Three sources of free fatty acids: diet, free fatty acids in plasma, and possibly de novo synthesis in adipocyte.

lipolysis occurs in the absence of added hormones and under experimental in vitro conditions results in one molecule of glycerol and three molecules of free fatty acids. If glucose is present in the medium, the free fatty acids can be recoupled to glycerol 3-phosphate to form new triglyceride molecules, so the measured level of free fatty acids is less than anticipated. However, since glycerol kinase, an enzyme which is essential for the phosphorylation of glycerol is absent from adipose tissue, measurement of glycerol is the best indicator of lipolysis.

METABOLIC CONSEQUENCES OF LARGE FAT CELL

The size of the fat cell, which is determined primarily by its lipid content, has important consequences on both lipogenesis and lipolysis. However, as Salans and co-workers[9] have noted, the fat cell size is only one of many factors that influence lipogenesis.

Smith and Levine[10] found that as fat cell size increased, insulin levels rose. In adults, the larger the fat cell size, the less sensitive it is to insulin.[11] Large fat cells in adults are thus less sensitive to the lipogenic effect of insulin. Glucose intolerance and elevated insulin levels are common findings in obese adults; those who lose weight show diminished insulin levels and an improvement in glucose tolerance. Distention of the adipocyte membrane by increased lipid content may alter its transport mechanism for glucose and thereby decrease its sensitivity to insulin. In obese children, however, in vitro studies of adipose cells have not demonstrated insulin insensitivity.[12] There is a correlation between fat cell size and glycerol release: larger adipocytes release more glycerol than smaller adipocytes.[13] Therefore, large fat cell size is associated with increased lipolysis and decreased lipogenesis.

EMBRYOLOGY OF ADIPOCYTE

The origin of the adipose cell is an important unresolved issue. The methods for identifying adipose cells in human subjects all rely on identifying cells with some lipid content. Presumably, at some point in the development of the adipose cell there is no lipid present, and current methods fail to detect these "pre-adipocytes." Furthermore, some mature adipocytes may be devoid of lipid and available for later energy storage; these cells are also not identified by available techniques. In fact, at present, the sole identifying characteristic of the adipocyte is the presence of lipid.

One theory of the origin of the adipocyte is that it arises from unspecialized cells of connective tissue. Flemming[14] initially posited this hypothesis and Clark and Clark[15] provided some experimental evidence in favor of the theory. Clark and Clark observed the formation of fat cells in transparent chambers built into rabbit ears. Adipose cells regularly formed at chamber sites entirely separated from the adipose cells present in the original ear tissue. Individual cells were observed to change from an elongated to a rounded shape and fat droplets increased in number and size and eventually coalesced to form a single lipid droplet. Prior to this transformation, the cells were indistinguishable from fibroblasts. It is possible that these cells resemble fibroblasts, but were actually specific cells of a primitive type that were destined to become mature adipocytes.

More recently, it has been postulated that adipose tissue develops from a specialized anlage, the cells of which spread throughout the body and accumulate fat. Wassermann[16] contends that in the embryo no conversion of connective tissue into adipose tissue occurs. Rather, he suggests that lentiform areas of characteristic structure are separated from surrounding connective tissue by a thin capsule, and in these areas adipose tissue is deposited. These lentiform areas consist of a network of capillaries and mesenchymal cells and it is in these cells that fat appears. His argument is based primarily on animal studies. However, Napolitano[17] has presented electron microscopic evidence that even at a very immature stage of development, adipose cells have special structural features and can be distinguished from fibroblasts. Furthermore, adipose cells from animals in extreme nutritional depletion do not revert to their original spindle-shaped form, which resembled a fibroblast, but remain irregularly rounded with abundant cytoplasm.[18]

BROWN ADIPOSE TISSUE

There are two types of adipose tissue—white and brown. They are structurally different, have very different functions, and probably arise from different embryological origins.[2] In man, most adipose tissue is white. Brown adipose tissue is clearly present in the human fetus, and the normal adult has small amounts in the regions of the neck and chest. Brown adipose tissue occurs only at certain body sites and new areas do not develop after birth. Brown adipose tissue is not primarily an energy reservoir; rather, it is a heat producing tissue.[2] Structurally it varies from a reddish-brown in color, when depleted in fat, to a light tan, when fat concentration is high. The color is due to the high concentration of cytochrome in the mitochondria of these cells. Some of the color may be hemoglobin since the tissue is highly vascular. A normal mature brown adipocyte contains a number of small fat droplets in contrast to a white adipose cell which contains only one large lipid droplet (See Fig. 7.3). Furthermore, unlike white adipose cells, brown fat is highly innervated and brown adipocytes are frequently in close approximation to non-myelinated axons. It has been argued that the brown fat cell is actually an immature white cell, because with advancing age the lipid in brown fat cells becomes localized into one lipid droplet. However, this is probably not the case, because when overfed animals are placed on a restricted diet brown adipose cells revert to and keep their multivacuolar form, whereas white adipose cells rapidly lose their entire fat content. Since structure, function, and embryological origin appear to be entirely different, the remainder of this chapter on the adipose cell will focus on white fat cells.

HISTOLOGY OF WHITE ADIPOSE TISSUE

Adipocytes range from 100 to 120 μm in diameter. Every mature fat cell contains one large drop of fat which can be stained with osmium tetroxide or Sudan Black. In hematoxylin and eosin staining the fat is lost during preparations and the single fat cells are seen as little holes and adipose tissue appears as a net. Under the light microscope with an osmic acid stain, the adipocyte contains a large central lipid droplet surrounded by a ring of

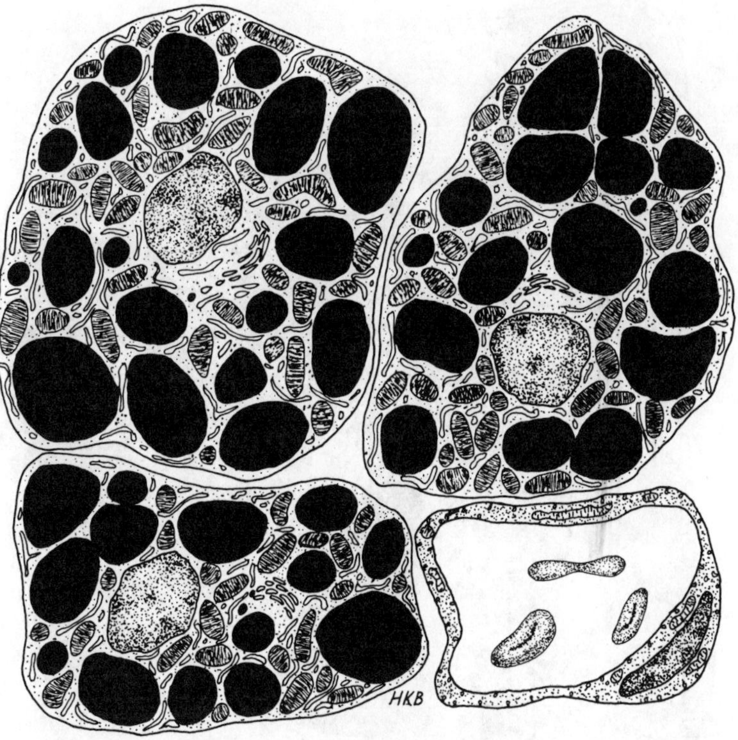

Figure 7.3. Brown adipose tissue. Illustration of electron micrograph with multi-vacuolar lipid content (Drawn by H. Keith Brown, PhD, Department of Anatomy, Medical School, University of South Florida, Tampa, Florida).

cytoplasm with the nucleus flattened and displaced to the periphery of the cell. The appearance of the cell in cross-section (if the section passes through the section of the nucleus) is of the signet ring worn on a finger of fat; the ring is the rim of cytoplasm and the nucleus is the signet.[19]

During lipogenesis, the fat droplets increase in number and eventually fuse into one droplet, displacing the nucleus and resulting in the classic signet ring appearance.[20] Because of the unusually large size of these cells, the plane of the histological section may include the nucleus of only a few cells. With the Sudan Black stain, the peripheral cytoplasm is not stained and only the large round lipid vacuole is visible. When adipose cells are crowded, they are compressed into various polygonal forms.

The nature of the fat cell itself has hindered studies of its fine structure. The disproportionate content of lipid relative to the amount of cytoplasm has hampered preparation of adipose tissue for study with the electron microscope. However, the ultrastructural characteristics of the fat cell are similar to that of other living cells. Figure 7.4 shows an illustration of an

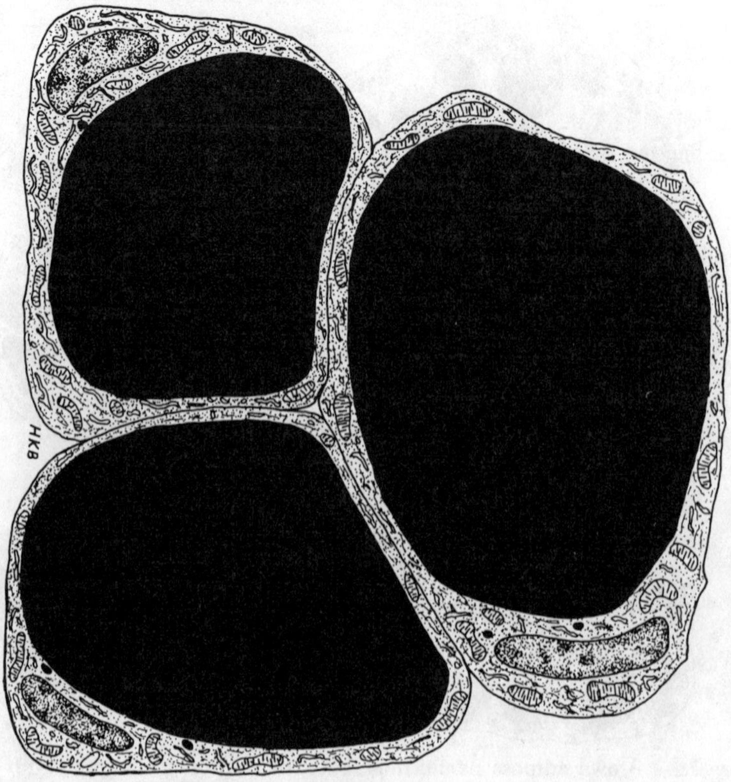

Figure 7.4. White adipose tissue. Illustration of electron micrograph with univacuolar lipid content (Drawn by H. Keith Brown, PhD, Department of Anatomy, Medical School, University of South Florida, Tampa, Florida).

electron micrograph of a white fat cell. White fat cells contain numerous mitochondria and have an extensive network of smooth endoplasmic reticulum. Rough endoplasmic reticulum and free ribosomes are only occasionally present. In adipose tissue that is rapidly synthesizing lipid from glucose, there are numerous discontinuous profiles of smooth endoplasmic reticulum in close proximity to small, presumably newly-synthesized, lipid droplets which fuse with the central lipid droplet.

White adipose tissue is divided into ill-defined lobules by thin connective tissue septa. In addition to these septa, there are delicate reticular fibers that form networks that surround the capillaries. Approximately 50% of the cells of adipose tissue are cells of the stroma. Although white adipose tissue has been described as poorly vascularized, each fat cell, despite its large size, is in contact with at least one capillary. The metabolic activity of the fat cell is confined to the narrow rim of cytoplasm surrounding the large lipid droplet.

If the ratio of capillary surface to volume of active non-lipid protoplasm is calculated, the capillary bed in proportion to active cytoplasm is as extensive as in skeletal muscle. Thus, despite an apparently poor vascular supply, white adipose tissue actually has an adequate blood supply to support a very active metabolism.

CELL NUMBER AND SIZE AS DETERMINANTS OF SUBSEQUENT OBESITY

Obese humans may have a normal or increased number of fat cells. This distinction was initially noted by Bjurulf in 1959[21] and later elaborated by Hirsch, Knittle, Salans, and Bjorntörp. The adipose cell theory of obesity is that obesity may be accompanied by an excessive number of adipocytes, possibly caused by overnutrition in infancy and childhood, and that this excessive number of fat cells remains constant despite weight loss and somehow causes a drive to maintain the obese state. Although there are numerous valid criticisms of the theory (to be discussed below), it has stimulated fruitful research into the growth and development of adipose tissue. Furthermore, it has focused scientific attention on the distressing fact that obese individuals usually regain any weight that they lose. Perhaps more importantly, a corollary of the theory is that prevention of overnutrition in infancy may prevent later severe obesity. Although the fat baby does not necessarily become the fat adult, probably a large majority (80%) of obese youngsters do remain fat throughout life. Measures which might significantly alter this outcome are well worth pursuing.

The following generalizations about fat cells in obesity seem justified on the basis of the experimental work to be reviewed. In all human obesity there is hypertrophy (enlargement) of fat cells. Hyperplasia (an increase in fat cell number) may or may not be present. The maximum fat cell size is approximately twice the normal size and this is achieved only when weight is in excess of 170% of the ideal height-weight standards. Hyperplasia is more evident with severe obesity. The increase in number of fat cells is proportional to an increase in weight when weight exceeds 170% of normal. Severe obesity and hyperplasia characterize early onset obesity. Usually there are two periods of rapid increase in the number of adipocytes—the perinatal period and adolescence. During childhood, fat cells do replicate, but at lower rates than at these critical periods. Presumably, in adult life adipocytes increase in size but not in number. However, occasionally individuals with adult onset obesity also have an increase in fat cell number.

The experimental data supporting these generalizations about the growth and development of adipose tissue are from several sources. There are extensive animal studies, particularly in rodents, which have documented that some strains of genetically obese mice do have critical growth periods during which nutritional changes result in altered fat cell numbers. Several cross-sectional and retrospective studies of obese humans have been interpreted to validate the theory. However, longitudinal studies of children are only now beginning to appear in the literature. Studies of infants are particularly difficult for technical and ethical reasons. Therefore, the validity of the cell number-cell size hypothesis as a causal explanation of the fetus-infant-child-adult progression of obesity is not yet firmly established.

Initially, it might seem impossible that fat cell hypertrophy without an increase in fat cell number could account for the degree of obesity seen in some patients with adult onset obesity. However, a small increase in fat cell diameter results in a dramatic increase in fat cell volume. Bjorntörp[22] studied a cohort of randomly selected middle-aged men in Sweden with an average fat cell diameter of about 100 μm and an average body fat content of 16 kg. Bjorntörp notes that an increase of the average fat cell diameter to 140 μm, a value often seen in obese subjects, would increase body fat by a factor of about three, or to about 50 kg. Therefore, hypertrophy of fat cells could be responsible for very marked obesity without an increase in fat cell number.

METHODOLOGY OF DETERMINING FAT CELL NUMBER

There are two major methods for measuring fat cell number and size, and they share the common failure of only counting adipocytes that contain lipid. Thus, "empty" fat cells are not counted. The osmium tetroxide method[23] (See Fig. 7.5) which has been used extensively by Hirsch and collaborators is as follows. After a preliminary wash, tissue fragments are dried and fixed. A cell suspension is prepared and freed of tissue debris by filtration through nylon sieves. The cell suspension is mixed with a previously known volume of saline, and aliquots are removed by a Coulter electronic counter to give determination of the number of cells per unit volume of cell suspension. The fat spherule is what is counted rather than actual cells. In a separate aliquot the lipid content is determined by chemical methods. Then the average lipid content per cell is calculated as an estimate of fat cell size. Calculation of adipose cell number is estimated by dividing the average cell lipid content into the total amount of lipid present in all adipose tissue. Total body fat is calculated from the body density determined by underwater weighing, or from skinfold measurements, or indirectly from total body water or potassium (See Chapter 1).

In the second method, frozen sections are cut and the mean volume and weight of cells in the adipose tissue are determined from their diameter measured under the microscope. This method also requires that the average lipid content be determined by chemical means in a separate aliquot.

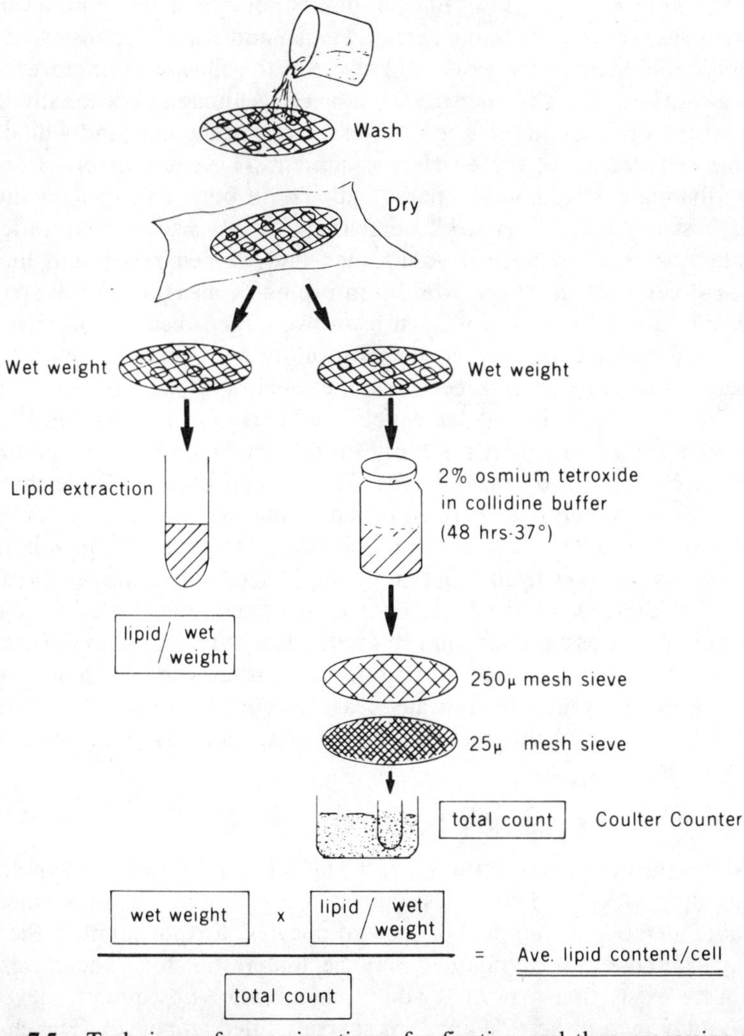

Figure 7.5. Technique of preparing tissue for fixation and then processing for a determination of average cell size in terms of average lipid content. Note that fat spherules rather than cells are what are counted by the Coulter counter (adapted from Hirsch and Knittle[23]).

SOURCES OF ERROR IN METHODOLOGY

SAMPLING ERRORS

There are a number of possible technical errors in both methods. For example, only approximately 20 mg of adipose tissue are obtained from the biopsy site and the results are extrapolated to the entire body, which may contain 100 kg or more of fat. Fat cell number and fat cell size may vary in different sites even in the same person. Hirsch and Knittle[23] considered this possibility in their early work and compared cell size from three sites (buttocks, arms, and abdomen) in 23 subjects. Although occasionally there was marked variation in cell size at different sites in the same individual, the average cell size in the three sites was similar. This study involved only a few individuals, and data compared cell size in only a few subcutaneous sites. Sjöström and colleagues[24] compared fat cell size in four different subcutaneous sites in normal young men and women and found limited statistical variation in fat cell size. Bjorntörp and colleagues[25] compared fat cell size in normal men and women from two large subcutaneous sites and found no difference. In another study Bjorntörp and Sjöström[26] found little variation in cell size from three subcutaneous sites in obese subjects. However, there are also visceral fat depots. Goldrick and McLoughlin[27] have shown that statistically there is a fairly strong correlation between the size of subcutaneous cells and omental cells. Thus, these results indicate that the differences in fat cell size between different sites in the groups of subjects compared are small. However, in an individual there were frequently large variations in cell sizes from different depots. Therefore, if individual values are needed, these should be based on averages from several sites.[28]

Therefore, the assumption that the individual sample obtained is representative of average adipose cell size thus far rests on scanty evidence. Other technical problems include accurate measurement of body fat. As discussed in Chapter 1, any of the available methods are tedious and subject to a variety of errors.

"EMPTY" FAT CELLS NOT COUNTED

Perhaps the most telling criticism of the fat cell number-cell size hypothesis is that adipocytes that contain less than 0.01 mg of lipid are not counted by available methods. If "empty" or "pre-adipocytes" are not counted, the thin person's adipose cell population may be underestimated. Therefore, the possibility exists that a normal adult subject who subsequently develops obesity may recruit these "empty" or sparsely-filled adipocytes. Hirsch and Batchelor[29] have found in a detailed cross-sectional study of obese adults that some subjects with severe obesity beginning in adulthood have an increased fat cell number. Usually, however, adult onset obesity was associated with an increase in fat cell size rather than an increase in fat cell number. Bray and Gallagher[30] reported one patient with onset of obesity in adult years related to hypothalamic dysfunction caused by a lipoma in the interpeduncular fossa: this patient had hypercellularity.

OTHER CRITICISMS

Widdowson and Shaw[31] report that piglets underfed from 10 days of age and weighing 5–6 kg at 1 year of age rather than the normal 200 kg, have no detectable fat cells by the methodology currently in vogue. Yet these animals become extremely fat as abundant food is available. The longer the period of food deprivation, the fatter they become. This finding is opposed to the hypothesis that an excessive number of fat cells can occur only during a critical growth period in early life. These authors also contend that recovered marasmic children have an excessive body fat content, a finding incompatible with the adipocyte proliferation hypothesis. However, studies of actual fat cell number in these children are not available. It is possible that the increase in fat content is due to an increase in fat cell size.

Measurement of fat cell diameter to estimate fat cell size may result in paradoxical findings. Ashwell and Garrow[32] studied an obese 24-year-old man before and after a 12-kg weight loss. They measured fatfolds and took adipose tissue biopsies from the triceps, abdominal wall, and gluteus. After weight loss, there was a decrease in fat thickness at all sites and at all sites modal cell size decreased. But because there was also a decrease in the number of small cells, the mean cell diameter showed a paradoxical increase at all sites. Conversely, a normal 44-year-old man was studied before and after a weight gain of 8 kg during a period of experimental overfeeding. The increase in fatfold thickness was greater in the abdomen than in the other sites, but the mean cell size at all sites decreased with weight gain. Apparently this was because very small cells were recruited, particularly in the abdominal area. Although these anedoctal examples may not be generally applicable, they serve to emphasize the need for caution in interpreting studies of fat cell size and number.

ANIMAL DATA AND THE ADIPOCYTE PROLIFERATION THEORY

Animal studies, particularly of rats, initially provided the impetus for extensive studies of the growth and development of human adipose tissue. Although the early extrapolation of this research data to humans was probably overly enthusiastic, an animal model can be valuable. In the normal rat, fat depots continue to grow in adult life, but this is due to an increase in cell size rather than an increase in cell number. Fat cell multiplication seems to be limited to the first few weeks of life.[33] This normal growth and development can be modified by nutritional manipulation.[34] Caloric deficiency causes a decrease in fat cell size in the adult rat and a decreased rate of multiplication in the young rats. However, during refeeding of the calorie-deprived young rat, there is a rapid fat cell multiplication that compensates for the prior deprivation. Overfeeding has different consequences at different times during the rat's life span. Prior to weaning, overfeeding causes fat cell hyperplasia, apparently by increasing the rate of fat cell multiplication. However, later in life even extreme overfeeding following hypothalamic lesions causes only an increase in fat cell size. Thus, the total number of fat cells seems to be constant in the adult animal, indicating that fat cells once formed remain or destroyed fat cells are replaced by newly formed fat cells at the same rate.

In addition to early overnutrition, genetic factors are important in the development of later obesity. Zucker and Zucker[35] described a strain of rat with a recessive gene for obesity (fa). The obese rats (fa/fa) do not breed. Therefore, it is necessary to breed heterozygous lean rats (Fa/fa) to produce the homozygous recessive genotype. In litters from such matings (Fa/fa × Fa/fa) obese young rats (fa/fa) occur 25% of the time while the remaining offspring are lean, either heterozygous or homozygous (Fa/fa and Fa/Fa). There have been extensive studies of the growth and development of adipose tissue in these obese Zucker rats (fa/fa). Greenwood and Johnson[36] report that by 9 weeks of age the obese Zucker rats are heavier than their lean counterparts. The difference in weight is due to an increase in fat tissue. The growth and development of adipose tissue was studied by sampling fat pads at different ages. In the lean young rats, there is an increase in fat cell number until 20 weeks of age when fat cell number remains constant. Fat cell size in lean rats of this strain continue to increase in size until 14 weeks of age. In the obese Zucker rats, fat cells continue to increase in number and size beyond 20 weeks of age. Therefore, the obesity found in these rodents begins early and is both hyperplastic and hypertrophic. Bell and Stern[37] found that body fat was elevated in the obese Zucker rat by 13 days of age.

By contrast, in the Danforth or yellow mouse, genetic influences result in obesity later in life, and this obesity is exclusively hypertrophic, with no increase in fat cell number.[38] Thus, it appears that either overnutrition early in life in normal rats or genetic influences operating in early life can result in hyperplastic obesity.

Rodents have also been studied in an attempt to clarify the embryology of the adipocyte. Greenwood and Hirsch[39] conclude that in the Sprague-Dawley rat adipocyte development begins with a stage of rapid cellular replication in the early weeks of postnatal life. Although these rapidly proliferating cells are indistinguishable from the stromal cells of adipose tissue, radioactively labeled ^{3}H-thymidine incorporated into the "adipoblasts" can be measured. Later analysis of label incorporated into the adipocytes yields an estimate of the subsequent development of adipose tissue in these animals. In 3 to 5 weeks most of the proliferation has ceased, but a bed of "pre-adipocytes" containing no lipid exists. These pre-adipocytes slowly fill during the ensuing weeks, and the full complement of adipocytes is achieved by 12 to 14 weeks of age. Apparently, no new adipocytes are added since there is no turnover of adipocyte DNA. These ^{3}H-thymidine studies have provided useful data but are tedious, and, of course, can never be applied to humans. Further, most stromal cells take up the thymidine label as well as adipocytes and their precursors. Separating the two classes of cells requires that the fat cell, liberated by collaginase, contain enough fat to float.

Because of the limitations of the thymidine-labeling technique, other methods are under investigation. For example, Cleary and colleagues[40] have reported that thymidine kinase, one of the enzymes that provides precursors for DNA synthesis, is an accurate monitor of pre-adipocyte division. The activity of thymidine kinase is elevated in young obese Zucker rats compared to lean rats. However, after 26 weeks of age, there is no detectable difference in thymidine kinase activity level between obese and normal Zucker female rats. This finding supports the hypothesis that adipocyte multiplication responsible for the Zucker rat obesity occurs only during early life.

CRITICAL PERIODS IN ADIPOSE CELL DEVELOPMENT IN HUMANS

There is now a voluminous literature exploring the growth and development of adipose tissue in obese and lean rodents. The obvious question is whether this information is applicable to humans. Several lines of investigation suggest that in childhood there are critical periods of fat cell multiplication and that the full complement of fat cells is normally obtained by the end of adolescence.

The pioneering work by Hirsch and Knittle[23] was a cross-sectional study of adult obese subjects. They then studied 19 previously obese subjects who had each lost approximately 50 kg and who had a persistently elevated adipose cell number but marked reduction in cell size. They divided the 20 obese subjects into groups by age of onset of obesity determined by the patient's history and family photographs. The obese group with the highest adipose cell numbers contained predominantly individuals with the earliest onset of obesity. Combining the results of these experiments with their work on animals, Hirsch and Knittle proposed their hyperplastic-hypertrophic theory of obesity.

Experimental overfeeding of non-obese human volunteers[41] has provided corroboration for the idea that adult onset obesity results in an increase in fat cell size but no increase in fat cell number. In these normal subjects, alterations in the fat depot was mediated solely by changes in cell lipid content. There was a dramatic increase in fat cell size with increasing weight, but no increase in fat cell number.

PERINATAL SENSITIVE PERIOD

Human studies elucidating the early development of adipose tissue are inconclusive. In addition to the work by Hirsch, Knittle, and collaborators, Brook[42] compared adipose cell development in normal and obese children.

Adipose cell number increased until puberty in normal subjects. The obese children were divided into two groups—those obese from infancy and those who became obese after age 1. Only the children with the onset of obesity in infancy had an increase in number of fat cells. Children whose obesity began after age 1 had adipose cell numbers similar to those of the control group. Brook postulated that there is a sensitive period for multiplication of adipose cells beginning about the 5th month of gestation and continuing to the end of the 1st year of life. Therefore, there should be predictable changes in adipose cell number depending on the ages at which adverse influences occur. The earlier the events occur during the sensitive period, the more severe the effects. When the sensitive period ends, adipose cell growth in number would theoretically be resistant to adverse circumstances.

To evaluate these hypotheses, children with an isolated deficiency of growth hormone from birth were compared to those who developed a deficiency of growth hormone later in life due to a craniopharyngioma. These groups were compared to light-for-dates children (LFD). The LFD children had birth weights below the 5th centile when allowance was made for length of gestation and parity. Theoretically, the LFD children should have the fewest adipose cells since the adverse effects occurred early in the sensitive period, in utero. The children with an isolated growth hormone deficiency at birth would be expected to have fewer than normal adipose cells, but more than the LFD children because growth in utero would presumably be normal and the adverse effects did not start until birth. Children who develop a growth hormone deficiency later in life, after the sensitive period, following removal of a craniopharyngioma, would be expected to have a normal complement of adipose cells. Brook's findings confirmed these predictions. However, the numbers of children studied were small, with less than 20 in the LFD and growth hormone-deficient groups. Also, the osmium tetroxide method for determining adipose cell number was used, and this method does not count cells without lipid. Therefore, this interesting and well-designed study suggests, but does not prove, the existence of a perinatal sensitive period for adipose cell number growth.

ADOLESCENCE

The evidence for a second critical period of increase in adipose cell number is even less conclusive. It is well known that there is a growth spurt in adolescence beginning earlier in girls than boys, and it is theorized that adipose cells participate in the general increase in growth in number and size. Animal data (usually of the Zucker rat) have been extrapolated to humans. Also, clinical reports of an increased incidence of obesity in adolescence, particularly in girls, have been used to support the concept of a critical period during adolescence. Knittle and colleagues[43] have started longitudinal studies on normal and obese children ranging in age from 2 to 26 years. Their initial report indicates that none of the non-obese children attained their full complement of fat cells until at least age 12, nor was the adult size attained until then. However, in the obese children studied, they noted a rapid increase in fat cell number between ages 5 and 7, whereas normal children had an increase in fat cell number between ages 8 and 12, with little or no change between ages 2 and 8. Their conclusion is that there is normally a second period of rapid proliferation of adipose cells, but that it begins before puberty (usually between ages 10 and 12) and ends sometime after age 12.

In the obese children studied there was a very different pattern. At all age levels studied, obese children had larger than average cells, although there was some overlap. However, all non-obese children had cell sizes below adult values, but most of the obese children had adult fat cell sizes. At all ages the obese children had a greater number of adipocytes. In some obese children a rapid increase in cellularity began between ages 2 and 8, a period when there is normally only a moderate increase in fat cell number. Furthermore, at all ages studied decreases in body fat were the result of decreases in fat cell size rather than a reduction of fat cell number. Thus when a particular cell number is achieved, whatever the age, apparently it cannot be decreased by dietary restriction alone.

NORMAL PATTERN

Probably the most reasonable interpretation of the currently available human data is as follows. The normal growth and development of adipose tissue begins about the 5th month of gestation. There is a rapid proliferation in number until the end of the 1st year when adipose cell number increase continues but at a very slow rate. Just before or during puberty there is a second period of rapid increase in the adipose cell number, and an associated increase in fat cell size. Usually by the late teens or early 20's there is no change in adipose cell number.

POSSIBLE ABNORMAL PATTERNS

By contrast, obese children may have a different pattern of growth and development. One possibility is that overnutrition during the sensitive perinatal period may cause an increase in fat cell number that persists even if subsequent adipose cell proliferation is normal (Fig. 7.6). Another possibility is that proliferation may be normal during infancy, but adverse effects during childhood (e.g. emotional trauma) may result in overnutrition and consequent increase in the rate of proliferation of fat cells during the normally relatively quiescent period from ages 2 to 10. This possibility fits

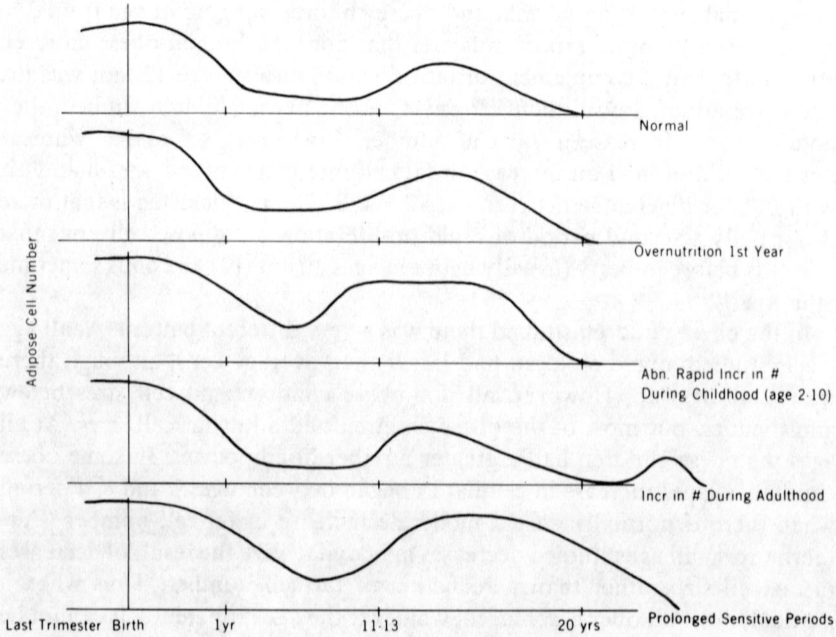

Figure 7.6. Possible patterns of abnormal growth in adipose cell number.

with the clinical observation that obesity following a significant emotional loss in childhood often begins between ages 4 and 7. The third possibility is that some individuals may have other periods in adult life when adipose cell proliferation can occur; physical or emotional stresses at these times in vulnerable individuals might result in adipose cell proliferation in adult life. Theoretically, this could account for those individuals who develop hyperplastic obesity in adult life. A fourth possibility is that some individuals might have an abnormally prolonged period when adipose cell proliferation could occur. In summary, there are several possible patterns of abnormal growth and development of adipose cells which theoretically could account for the hyperplastic obesity seen in some individuals.

CRITICISMS OF THEORY

One observation that has cast doubt on the adipocyte proliferation theory is that approximately 20% of obese infants outgrow their "baby fat." If the number of fat cells is largely determined before the first birthday, how do these youngsters and adults manage to remain slim? A possible answer to this question is provided by Knittle.[43] He studied obese 6-year-olds and found that they could be divided into two groups: (1) youngsters with marked hypercellularity exceeding normal adult values; and (2) youngsters with modest increases in cell number relative to non-obese subjects of the same age. Perhaps the obese children who have exceeded normal adult values for cellularity will retain their obesity whereas those with normal cellularity, but large size, may outgrow the obesity. However, longitudinal studies elucidating this point are still pending.

A less cogent criticism of the theory is that it is fatalistic. It is argued[44] that if the die is cast early in life then fatness is inevitable and treatment is either futile or ineffective. Furthermore, non-obese adults may believe themselves immune from later obesity. This criticism is invalid on two counts. First, the validity of a theory does not depend on whether we like the consequences of a theory. For example, even though we might wish to increase the number of brain cells later in life, our wish does not alter the fact that the entire complement of brain cells is attained early in life. It is foolhardy to reject a theory because its implications are not to our liking. Second, it may have been incorrectly assumed that prevention of childhood obesity prevents adult obesity, but as noted earlier in this chapter, an increase in the average size of fat cells can also produce obesity.

References

1. Martinsson A: On the composition of human adipose tissue. Acta Med Scand 182: 795–803, 1967.
2. DasGupta TK: Tumors and tumor-like conditions of the adipose tissue (monograph). Curr Probl Surg 7: 2–60, 1970.
3. Hashim SA: Metabolism of body fat. NY State J Med 61: 1339–1344, 1961.
4. Hirsch J, Farquhar JW, Ahrens EH, et al: Studies of adipose tissue in man: a microtechnic for sampling and analysis. Am J Clin Nutr 8: 499–511, 1960.
5. Heffernan AGA: Fatty acid composition of adipose tissue in normal and abnormal subjects. Am J Clin Nutr 15: 5–10, 1964.
6. Galton DJ, Wilson JPD: The effect of starvation and diabetes on glycolytic enzymes in human adipose tissue. Clin Sci 41: 545–553, 1971.
7. Jeanrenaud B, Hepp D (eds): Adipose Tissue: Regulation and Metabolic Functions. New York, Academic Press, 1970.
8. Bray GA: Effect of diet and triiodothyronine on the activity of sn-glycerol-3-phosphate dehydrogenase and on the metabolism of glucose and pyruvate by adipose tissue of obese patients. J Clin Invest 48: 1413–1422, 1969.
9. Salans LB, Knittle JL, Hirsch J: The role of adipose cell size and adipose tissue insulin sensitivity in the carbohydrate intolerance of human obesity. J Clin Invest 47: 153–165, 1968.
10. Smith M, Levine R: Obesity and diabetes. Med Clin North Am 48: 1387–1397, 1964.
11. Salans LB, Bray GA, Cushman SW, et al: Glucose metabolism and the response to insulin by human adipose tissue in spontaneous and experimental obesity: effects of dietary composition and adipose cell size. J Clin Invest 53: 848–856, 1974.
12. Ginsberg-Fellner F, Knittle JL: Adipose tissue cellularity and metabolism in newly diagnosed juvenile diabetics. Diabetes 22: 528–536, 1973.
13. Bjorntörp P, Karlsson M, Hovden A: Quantitative aspects of lipolysis and re-esterification in human adipose tissue in vitro. Acta Med Scand 185: 89–97, 1969.
14. Flemming W: Weitere mittheilungen zur physiologie der fettzelle. Cited in Das Gupta TK: Tumors and tumor-like conditions of the adipose tissue (monograph). Curr Probl Surg 7: 2–60, 1970.

15. Clark ER, Clark EL: Microscopic studies of the new formation of fat in living adult rabbits. Am J Anat 67: 255–286, 1940.
16. Wassermann F: The concept of the "fat organ." In: Fat As a Tissue. Symposium Monograph. Rodhal K, Issekut ZB (eds). New York, McGraw-Hill Book Co, 1962, pp 22–40.
17. Napolitano L: The differentiation of white adipose cells: an electron microscope study. J Cell Biol 18: 663–679, 1963.
18. Hull D, Segall MM: Distinction of brown from white adipose tissue. Nature 212: 469–472, 1966.
19. Greep RO, Weiss L: Histology. Ed 3. New York, McGraw-Hill Book Co, 1973, pp 162–170.
20. Ham AW: Histology. Ed 7. Philadelphia, JB Lippincott Co, 1974, pp 226–231.
21. Bjurulf P. Atherosclerosis and body-build. Acta Med Scand [Suppl] 349: 21–54, 1959.
22. Bjorntörp P: Disturbances in the regulation of food intake. Advan Psychosom Med 7: 116–147, 1972.
23. Hirsch J, Knittle JL: Cellularity of obese and non-obese human adipose tissue. Fed Proc 29: 1516–1521, 1970.
24. Sjöström L, Smith U, Krotkiewski M, Bjorntörp P: Cellularity in different regions of adipose tissue in young men and women. Metabolism 21: 1143–1153, 1972.
25. Bjorntörp P, Bengtssen C, Blohmé G, et al: Adipose tissue fat cell size and number in relation to metabolism in randomly selected middle-aged men and women. Metabolism 20: 927–935, 1971.
26. Bjorntörp P, Sjöström L: Number and size of adipose tissue fat cells in relation to metabolism in human obesity. Metabolism 20: 703–713, 1971.
27. Goldrick RB, McLoughlin GM: Lipolysis and lipogenesis from glucose in human fat cells of different sizes. J Clin Invest 49: 1213–1223, 1970.
28. Salans LB, Cushman SW, Weismann RE: Studies of human adipose tissue. Adipose cell size and number in non-obese and obese patients. J Clin Invest 52: 929–941, 1973.
29. Hirsch J, Batchelor B: Adipose tissue cellularity in human obesity. Clin Endocrinol Metab 5: 299–311, 1976.
30. Bray GA, Gallagher TF: Manifestations of hypothalamic obesity in man: a comprehensive investigation of eight patients and a review of the literature. Medicine (Baltimore) 54: 301–330, 1975.
31. Widdowson EM, Shaw WT: Full and empty fat cells (letter to the editor). Lancet 2: 905, 1973.
32. Ashwell M, Garrow JS: Full and empty fat cells (letter to the editor). Lancet 2: 1036–1037, 1973.
33. Hirsch J, Han PW: Cellularity of rat adipose tissue: effects of growth, starvation and obesity. J Lipid Res 10: 77–82, 1969.
34. Knittle JL, Hirsch J: Effect of early nutrition on the development of rat epididymal fat pads: cellularity and metabolism. J Clin Invest 47: 2091–2098, 1968.
35. Zucker LM, Zucker TF: Fatty, a new mutation in the rat. J Hered 52: 275–278, 1961.
36. Greenwood MRC, Johnson PR: Adipose tissue cellularity and its relationship to the development of obesity in females. Curr Concepts Nutr 5: 119–135, 1977.
37. Bell GE, Stern JS: Development of obesity and hyperinsulinemia in the Zucker obese rat (fa/fa). Fed Proc 35: 657, 1976.
38. Bray GA: The Obese Patient. Philadelphia, WB Saunders, 1976, p 165.
39. Greenwood MRC, Hirsch J: Postnatal development of adipocyte cellularity in the normal rat. J Lipid Res 15: 474–483, 1974.
40. Cleary MP, Greenwood MRC, Brasel JA: Thymidine kinase as a measure of adipocyte proliferation in normal and obese rats. Fed Proc 34: 908, 1975.
41. Salans LB, Horton ES, Sims EAH: Experimental obesity in man: cellular character of the adipose tissue. J Clin Invest 50: 1005–1011, 1971.
42. Brook CGD: Evidence for a sensitive period in adipose cell replication in man. Lancet 2: 624–627, 1972.
43. Knittle JL: Basic concepts in the control of childhood obesity. Curr Concepts Nutr 3: 135–140, 1975.
44. Mann GV: The influence of obesity on health. N Engl J Med 291: 226–232, 1974.

CHAPTER

8

Psychiatric Considerations in Obesity

For centuries, physicians have suspected a relationship between obesity and emotions, but it was not until Freud[1] that a coherent, theoretical framework for this relationship was possible. Freud's orality theory, as applied to obesity, is not currently in vogue in many scientific circles, in part because later theorists developed the idea to the point of absurdity and rigidly applied it to all obese patients. However, the theory probably has validity for some obese patients and has stimulated the development of interpersonal theories of the eating disorders.

In the last two decades, there has been a burgeoning interest in the role of psychological factors in the development of obesity, but the results of the studies have been confusing. Emotional and cultural factors do play a crucial role in the development and maintenance of obesity in many patients, particularly those who have been obese since childhood, but the nature of these emotional and cultural factors varies widely among patients. A sizable proportion of patients has symptoms of anxiety, depression, or other emotional disturbances. Apparently some patients have no identifiable emotional problems except the behavioral disturbance of overeating or underactivity. The failure to identify neurotic traits in some obese patients may be because their obesity protects them from emotional conflict. This idea is supported by reports of depression, anxiety, and occasionally psychosis following weight loss.

There is a marked negative social attitude toward obese people, particularly female adolescents. Monello and Mayer[2] have even compared the obese to a disadvantaged minority group. Thus, some experts have concluded that the psychiatric symptoms are the consequence of hostile condemnation of obese patients by their family and society. While it is true that negative attitudes toward obesity facilitate psychological symptoms, particularly body image disturbances in female adolescents, this finding does not exclude the possibility of other contributing emotional factors.

The research studying the psychological aspects of obesity is confounded by the erroneous assumption that obesity is a uniform condition. Often the significance of some well-described observation is rejected as invalid because it cannot be demonstrated in all cases of obesity. Also, if one etiological factor is identified, it is often assumed to be the only factor operant, even though it is well known that many factors may contribute to the development of obesity in one individual.

As Stunkard[3] has repeatedly emphasized, there are two major findings in obesity. The first is hyperphagia (overeating). This symptom is observed in most, but not all patients. Some obese people apparently eat the same number of calories as their slim peers, but expend fewer calories in physical activity.[4] However, if hyperphagia is defined as excessive intake of calories relative to energy expenditure, all obese subjects overeat or have overeaten in the past. A host of psychological explanations have been proposed to account for this hyperphagia and include psychoanalytic, interpersonal, and learning theories. These will be discussed in detail later in this chapter. The second major finding in some obese subjects is a disturbance in body image, commonly found in patients who have been obese since adolescence.

BODY IMAGE

Body image is the inner mental picture of one's body and the sum of emotional attitudes toward one's body. The mental picture is a kind of blueprint representing one's body as a whole, as well as its parts, including their size, shape, and spatial relationships. This neurological or *perceptual aspect* of body image, including all the physical properties of one's body, has been extensively studied, particularly in relationship to the phantom limb phenomenon.

The *emotional feelings and attitudes* toward one's body are the second major component of body image. These attitudes and feelings may actually influence the accuracy of the inner mental blueprint representing the physical parameters of one's body. Cultural and familial attitudes toward an individual's body influence body image. The interaction between the perceptual aspects of body image, and the emotional, familial, and sociological aspects of personality development were recognized early in this century, both by Freud and neurologists Head[5] and Schilder.[6] Interpersonal influences that impinge on the development of body image were initially studied in seriously disturbed schizophrenic patients. It has only been in the last 10 to 20 years that the marked body image disturbances in anorexia nervosa and some patients with obesity have been recognized.

PERCEPTUAL ASPECTS OF BODY IMAGE

Initial Studies of Phantom Limb

Ambroise Paré, a 16th century surgeon, wrote the first description of the phantom limb phenomenon.[7] Following a traumatic or surgical loss of a limb, the patient may continue to experience the perceptual sensations of the lost limb; that is, the inner mental blueprint of the body does not immediately change even though the part has been lost. Paré advised surgeons not to allow this phantom limb phenomenon to prevent proceeding with additional necessary surgery.

Anosognosia

Neurologists have since identified other dramatic examples of disturbances in the perceptual aspects of body image. For example, some patients are unaware of hemiplegia of sudden onset and they pay no attention to the paralyzed side. If the patient's attention is directed to the affected limb, he may remain indifferent or claim that someone else is in his bed. This particular perceptual defect is most likely to occur following disease in the parietal or parietal-occipital region in the non-dominant hemisphere. A patient with left hemiplegia denied that the limbs were hers and when the connection to her body was shown, she stated:

> "But my eyes and my feelings don't agree, and I must believe my feelings. I know they look like mine, but I can feel they are not, and I can't believe my eyes" (p 506).[8]

Both the phantom limb phenomenon and the unawareness of hemiplegia are examples of what Babinski[9] termed "anosognosia" and are dramatic examples of disturbance in the perceptual aspects of body image.

Importance of Kinesthetic and Tactile Senses

Although all the senses contribute to the perceptual aspects of body image, the kinesthetic and tactile senses are the most important. In the example just cited, accurate optic stimuli were not sufficient to correct the disturbance in body image. The primary importance of touch and kinesthesia are consonant with observations of the embryology of the nervous system.

Sensory pathways subserving the tactile kinesthetic senses are the first to complete myelinization.[10] The hand-to-mouth movements appearing early in utero are precursors of the complex face-hand relationship subserved primarily by touch. Furthermore, the earliest stages of ego development in the infant are intimately associated with tactile sensations. In the feeding process, touch is the first sense to provide information to the infant and activity is initially organized around these tactile impressions as the baby locates the nipple and begins sucking. From about the 12th week after birth, the developing hand-to-mouth relationship accelerates and the baby begins to use both hands and arms to grasp and knead the mother's breast. Then the infant begins to use his hands to explore his own body and to contact others. These initial tactile impressions form the most important part of the body image.

Other sensory modalities including those subserving optic, olfactory, auditory, thermal, and pain stimuli contribute to the development of the perceptual aspects of body image, but are less important than the tactile and kinesthetic senses. This is a very important point because many studies that purport to measure body image in patients with eating disorders rely on the use of visual sensory data by the subject. These techniques have provided some very interesting and illuminating findings, but do not elucidate the role of touch in body image disturbances.

Schizophrenia

In schizophrenic patients, the major disturbances in body image have generally been categorized as defects in ego boundaries; for example, the patient may be unaware of the limits of his own body, particularly in relationship to important people in his life. Chapman[11] has described a number of characteristic perceptual disturbances that may occur early in the course of schizophrenia and may involve body image. For example, some patients may perceive parts of their body as larger or smaller than they really are (macropsia or micropsia). This misperception may involve other people or objects as well. In addition to these disturbances in the perceptual aspects of body image, many schizophrenic patients also have negative attitudes toward their own bodies which they may describe as loathesome or grotesque.

EMOTIONAL ASPECTS OF BODY IMAGE

Some of the early neurologists were fascinated with the emotional influences on body image. Schilder[6] broadened the concept of body image to include interpersonal and sociological aspects as well as the perceptual aspects of body image.

The emotional quality of the interpersonal relationship between mother and child is the cornerstone for the development of later attitudes toward one's body. A positive, mutually satisfying emotional transaction between mother and child is crucial. A defect in these transactions is thought by some, notably Bruch,[12] to provide the basis for the body image disturbances seen in anorexia nervosa, developmental obesity, and some patients with schizophrenia.

Bruch's theory posits that there are two types of behaviors in a child—those that originate from the child and those in response to external stimuli.

In a family producing a disturbed patient, with either anorexia nervosa or developmental obesity, the behavior originating from the child is ignored or discouraged and the child acts only in response to others. Therefore, the person grows up unaware of his own perceptions, feelings, and thoughts as reflected by a disturbance in body image.

Typically, both anorexia nervosa and developmentally obese patients overestimate their size. The attitudinal aspect of body image is also disturbed. The obese patients may believe they are repulsive and fatter than they actually are. The anorexia nervosa patients usually highly prize an emaciated starved appearance (See Fig. 8.1). Bruch's theory, while interesting, has yet to be fully documented. For example, although she maintains that the core problem of schizophrenia, anorexia nervosa, and developmental obesity is the same, and that some patients with these eating disorders go on to develop schizophrenia, other authors have not found this to be the case.[13]

CULTURAL INFLUENCES ON BODY IMAGE

Cultural and social factors also impinge upon the development of body image. The socialization process begins in the family and the attitudes of the parents leave an indelible impression on the child's concept of himself and his body and its functions. Certain aspects of body development are valued while others are denigrated. For example, muscle strength and prowess are generally emphasized and prized in the body development of boys but criticized in girls. This is but one example of a current prevailing cultural body standard.

Certain cultures value obesity as a symbol of success and economic

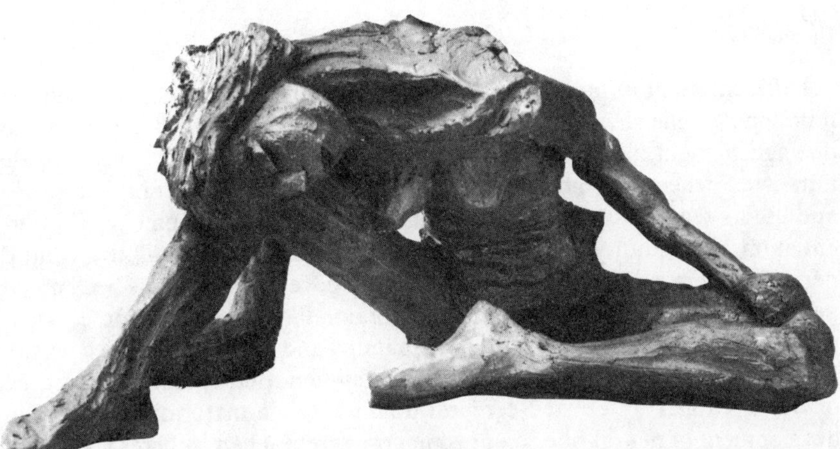

Figure 8.1. This anorexia nervosa patient posed as a model for art classes. She highly prized her emaciated appearance (sculpture by Ursula Mahlendorf).

security. Aga Khan was weighed yearly and increments in weight were hailed as a tribute to the success of Islamic religion. If obesity is prized, a disturbance in body image in obese individuals is probably much less common.

Henry VIII of England was massively obese by current American standards, but was so emulated by peers of the realm that the chairs in Parliament had to be enlarged to accommodate their enlarged girth. Probably these individuals did not have a disturbance in bódy image. Perhaps those whom we might consider normal size had negative attitudes toward their body size. In any case, societal attitudes toward body size and shape have important consequences for the development of body image.

In the United States and many industrialized countries obese persons are denigrated and ridiculed. A svelte figure is particularly valued among members of the upper and middle socioeconomic classes, those groups to whom food is most easily and abundantly available. Although an obese individual is subject to criticism at any age, an adolescent is exquisitely sensitive to any remark about his or her body.

EARLY DEVELOPMENT OF BODY IMAGE

The development of an accurate body image begins during fetal life with the embryogenesis of the nervous system. The newborn begins to explore the surface of his body and quickly gains the concept of body orifices including mouth, nose, ears, and anus. This exploration initially tactile, and soon involving the other sensory modalities, is the basis of awareness of the body, its parts, and its spatial interrelationships.

Laterality

Differentiation of laterality (right-left orientation) is one easily identified milestone in the development of body image. Children usually begin to distinguish right and left after age 3 but the skill is usually not complete until age 5 when the youngster can differentiate right and left in themselves and others regardless of spatial orientation. The full development of differentiation of laterality requires the continuing maturation of the central nervous system. Confusion may occur during development as has been noted particularly in children with minimal brain damage (MBD) or crossed-cerebral dominance (the patient is left-handed and right-eyed or vice versa). In MBD, as the name implies, the nervous system itself is thought damaged or dysfunctional. In crossed-cerebral dominance[14] a maturational delay in development of neural fibers connecting the cerebral hemispheres is thought to account for the lag in achieving right-left orientation accurately.

Influence of Culture on Laterality

Cultural influences are important in the development of laterality. There is a long cultural heritage identifying the left side as evil or bad, and the right side as good. Even the derivation of the word left is from the Latin word "sinister." This value differentiation of the left and right side may emerge during a psychotic regression. Hirsch,[15] for example, has reported on a series of psychotic patients who equated those parts of their personality they considered "bad" with the left side of their body and considered the "good" parts of their personality as part of the right side of their body. Recently, a psychotic patient presented to our clinic with the delusion that the right side of his brain controlled all his laudatory behavior, and that the left side caused all of his unacceptable behavior, thoughts, and fantasies. Right and left differentiation is, thus, an integral part of body image that requires adequate neurological maturation and is influenced by emotional and cultural experiences.

Language and Body Image

The interrelationship between neural substrate and cultural influence on body image has been studied by Wright.[16] He analyzed the names of parts of the body that occur most in literature and found a correspondence between the extent of sensory-motor cortical representation of that part and the frequency that the name of the part occurred in literature; e.g., the hand is mentioned frequently in literature and has extensive cortical representation.

Valued and Devalued Physical Characteristics

As the child matures he comes to value or devalue parts of his body during the socialization process initiated by his parents. When the child fails to meet the expectations of those around him, realistic or not, he will develop derogatory attitudes toward his body and a variety of defense mechanisms may be used to obscure the defect from himself or others. Thus a boy who is shorter than his family expects boys to be may try to compensate by participating in particularly aggressive sports. Or a girl who is more muscular than the current fashion dictates may refuse to participate in athletics. Similarly, a stout child may refuse to go to parties with youngsters his age to avoid being teased about his size or shape.

In other families, certain body characteristics may be overvalued and relied on for security. For example, a very beautiful girl may be admired only for her appearance or a very agile boy for his athletic prowess. A person who relies predominantly on body attractiveness or activity for his or her security is particularly vulnerable to any condition (including obesity) that disrupts their body image.

BODY IMAGE DISTURBANCES IN EATING DISORDERS

Major Findings

For years, disturbances in body image have been noted in the eating disorders, particularly anorexia nervosa. Unlike the neurological conditions that result in anosognosia, the body image disturbances that occur in the eating disorders are less dramatic. There is usually an overestimation of actual size and shape coupled with derogatory attitudes toward the misperception. In anorexia nervosa the grossly emaciated patient often considers herself fat, to the astonishment of observers. Contrary to expectation, not all obese patients have a distorted body image. In fact, probably fewer than half the obese population have disturbances of either the perceptual or attitudinal aspects of body image. Patients with early onset of obesity that persists through adolescence and who are condemned by family and peers because of their obesity are most vulnerable. Associated psychological disturbances in an obese person increase the likelihood of an inaccurate body image. Furthermore, weight reduction *per se* does not alleviate the body image disturbance.

The studies supporting these findings are reviewed below. There are numerous limitations with all the studies discussed, but a major one is that no two studies defined obesity in the same way. Also very few studies had control subjects and fewer yet had controls matched for age, sex, absence of psychological disturbances, etc.

Normal Girls Inaccurate

The age at which a child can give accurate estimates of size and shape is not known. One study[17] reported that normal weight adolescent girls tend to overestimate body width and underestimate body length. The younger the girl the greater the overestimate of body width. Although this relatively large scale study of 86 subjects attempts to evaluate normal development, it relies on visual sense to estimate the various widths of the body (face, chest, waist, hips). Visual estimates may provide some information, but tests utilizing tactile and kinesthetic sensory modalities are more likely to be valid since vision can be intact and body image still be grossly disturbed. However, it is important that even apparently normal young adolescent girls overestimate their widths.

Body Image Disturbance and Obesity

Stunkard and co-workers[3, 18] initiated detailed studies of body image disturbances among the general obese population. In their first report,[3] 70 obese subjects were randomly selected from general medical and psychiatric clinics. One-hour interviews with each subject elicited information about their self-esteem as well as their attitudes toward the view of themselves in a mirror. These workers found that not all obese subjects had derogatory attitudes toward their bodies. Furthermore, not all patients with obesity and emotional disturbances had disturbances in body image, although emotional disturbance was present in all patients who had a distorted body image. In other words, emotional disturbance was a necessary but insufficient condition for a distorted body image.

Even some massively obese persons have no body image disturbance. E.g., "Baby" Francis Hope Grove, who weighed 826 pounds, not only reportedly thanked God for every pound she weighed, but had a successful career spanning several decades as Queen of the circus fat ladies and had been married with several children. Perhaps she had an emotional disturbance and harbored an intensely negative body image, but if so, it was not apparent.[19]

ADOLESCENCE CRITICAL FOR BODY IMAGE

Stunkard and co-workers[3] found that obese subjects most likely to have a body image distortion are those with juvenile onset of obesity. Stunkard posits that disturbances in body image originate during adolescence when obese teenagers incorporate derogatory views of peers and parents into enduring attitudes of the self. In an additional attempt to verify this hypothesis,[18] 189 obese adults were evaluated in an attempt to locate subjects who had been obese in childhood and adulthood, but of normal weight in adolescence. If such subjects were free of body image disturbance, the hypothesis that obesity during adolescence is a necessary condition for a disturbed body image would be supported. However, only two obese adults who were obese as children had a normal weight during adolescence. Although both were free of body image disturbances, the frequency of such subjects was too scant to be conclusive.

Other lines of evidence have provided support for the theory that adolescence is critical in the development of body image. Although parts of the body retain their general spatial relationships and articulations throughout life, it is not until late adolescence that the final size and shape of most body parts are attained. With the exception of trauma and senile changes, the parts of the body remain constant after adolescence. Furthermore, it is during adolescence that sexual drives are intense. Body attractiveness and functioning are extremely important for teenagers as they begin heterosexual involvement. Adolescents are very sensitive to remarks about their appearance. Thus, it is reasonable to assume that adolescence is a critical period in the development of body image, particularly in the attitudes toward the self.

However, there are probably other critical periods during which a faulty body image may develop. Perhaps the perceptual aspects of body image are more vulnerable during childhood.

One of the difficulties with much of the work on body image is that there is frequently a confounding of the perception of the physical appearance of the body with the thoughts, attitudes, and feelings about the body. Perhaps this is inevitable, since both aspects of body image develop in concert with each other and influence each other. It is important to remember that Stunkard's conclusions were based on the evaluation of the attitudinal aspect of body image rather than on direct perceptual measures.

Analogy to "Imprinting"

Concepts borrowed from animal studies have been applied to the development of body image. "Imprinting" is a term initially used by Lorenz[20] to describe the attachment behavior that goslings develop toward their mother or a mother substitute during critical times in their life cycle; this attachment behavior continues through life. Body image has been said to be "imprinted" during adolescence. Appealing as this idea is, the extrapolation from animal studies to humans may not be valid.

Teenagers with Body Defects

Other evidence favoring the hypothesis that adolescence is crucial derives from studies of children and teenagers with body defects. For example, MacGregor and associates[21] conclude that facial deformities should be corrected before puberty, if possible, to prevent deleterious psychological consequences. Schonfeld[22] found that the psychological repercussions of gynecomastia during adolescence were greater than during childhood or adult life.

PLASTICITY OF BODY IMAGE

There is an impressive array of evidence that body image is variable, plastic, and subject to constant revision. A series of anorexia nervosa subjects and normal control subjects were evaluated before and after carbohydrate and non-carbohydrate meals.[23] The anorexia nervosa patients, as a group, reported an increase in their body widths following a carbohydrate meal, but not after a non-carbohydrate meal. The normal subjects, and one recovered anorexia nervosa patient, showed no major change after a carbohydrate meal.

Stunkard and Mendelson[3] noted in their evaluations of a group of obese patients with disturbances in body image that the intensity of the disturbance varied widely, even over short periods of time. When the patient had no particular difficulty in his life, he might not be troubled by his body image disturbance. However, if depressed or functioning poorly in any area of his life, the patient became highly critical of his body. Sometimes obesity even becomes the explanation and symbol of his unhappiness, thereby setting up a vicious circle which fosters a lowering of self-esteem. Thus, ingestion of ambivalently valued food (carbohydrate) by anorexics and negative life experiences in obese subjects can produce rapid changes in body image.

The effects of wearing inverted prisms are well known.[24] Although the visual fields are inverted, the person rapidly revises his concept of the relationship between what he sees and what he feels and does. Apparently the brain reinterprets what is seen so that the visual field is no longer perceived as inverted. This relatively rapid adjustment suggests that body image can be revised constantly.

Metamorphosia

Various drugs are known to produce temporary, usually reversible, disturbances in body image. LSD, marijuana, psilocybin, and peyote cause dramatic and unusual distortions. The size of limbs may be misperceived as larger or smaller than in reality, distances may be misjudged or objects may appear slightly distorted. This metamorphosia depends upon a disturbance in the judgement of spatial relationships.

One problem highlighted by metamorphosis is the conceptual confusion in most studies between perception of one's own body and the perception of external objects. Many studies of body image have not defined this issue clearly, although several studies of anorexia nervosa indicate the need for such clarification. At younger ages, the normal subjects in one study overestimated the size of a block of wood but their estimates improved by age 17 or 18.[17] Conversely, however, one study[23] of anorexia nervosa patients demonstrated that although the patients overestimated their own widths, they correctly estimated the size of a block of wood.

Schizophrenic patients may have distortions in perceptions of their own bodies as well as of external objects or other people. Temporal lobe pathology may result in similar perceptual abnormalities. Micropsia or macropsia may occur in temporal lobe epilepsy. Certain toxic conditions such as encephalitis may also result in illusions (misperceptions based on an actual sensory stimulus). Illusions or hallucinations experienced in these conditions are all examples of perceptual abnormalities and may involve perception of the body or its parts or external objects. That these disturbances are often temporary lends credence to the idea that body image is highly variable.

Sudden Changes Not Immediately Incorporated into Body Image

On the other hand, sudden major changes in the body are not immediately incorporated into the body image. The rapidity with which changes in the body occur is very influential in the development of perceptual distortions in body image. Surgical or traumatic loss of a limb is more likely to result in the phantom limb phenomenon than loss of the limb from a gradual process such as leprosy.[25] Furthermore, as the phantom limb disappears, it usually does so in a predictable way. With the extremities, the parts which recede first are the upper arms and thighs. Next the lower arm or calf disappears, followed by the joints and parts of the hands and feet. The large toe, thumb, and index finger and little finger disappear last. This sequence follows the well-known neurological homunculus.[26] Those parts with the richest sensorimotor innervations (for example, the thumb) are retained the longest in the phantom limb phenomenon. Apparently when a limb is lost, relearning is required for an accurate perception of body image. In the case of leprosy, reabsorption of the digits or limbs is very gradual, thus permitting an ongoing perceptual reorganization of body image.

There are several other conditions in which a phantom limb is not reported. Those conditions in which a phantom limb is not reported include aplasias of the body part (a congenital defect) or amputations during infancy or early childhood. As body image develops in these youngsters, the schema that develops probably incorporates their actual appearance, including absence of the body part. Another cause of failure to report a phantom limb after amputation is psychological denial. This unconscious defense mechanism may be used to cope with overwhelming feelings of anger, guilt, or sadness about the loss of the body part, and the patient may deny the presence of a phantom limb. An adolescent or adult patient who denies the phantom limb after the sudden loss of a limb may be using denial.

Body Image Change in Pregnancy

During pregnancy a dramatic change in body size is normal. Slade[27] studied 40 pregnant women at approximately 4 months duration and retested 16 of the subjects at 8 months. At 4 months, these women overestimated their body widths, although less than a group of previously tested anorexia nervosa patients.[28] At 8 months, the 16 women who were retested tended to improve in their estimate of body dimensions. Although their actual size and weight were greater at 8 months, their estimates of body widths improved.

The initial 40 women were subdivided on the basis of history of weight changes during the preceeding 12 months. The subgroup with stable weights during the prior year were found to overestimate their width significantly more than the subgroup whose weight had varied, although both groups overestimated more than the control group. The subjects estimated several different body dimensions. The two that were associated with the greatest degree of overestimation were waist width and stomach depth. Since these are the areas most affected by pregnancy, this is not a surprising finding.

This study of pregnant women was undertaken to elucidate the cause of body image disturbances in the eating disturbances, particularly anorexia nervosa. Two explanations have been proposed. The first posits that the patient with the body image disturbance is abnormally sensitive to her physical size. The alternative explanation proposed by Crisp and Kalucy[23] is that it reflects a "failure to adapt" to a change in physical size. Although Slade's study can be used to support either explanation, the most important aspect of this work is that normal pregnant women also have body image disturbances. Probably body image disturbances are more common than previously suspected, and they occur in a variety of conditions.

Summary

Although body image is highly variable and plastic, changes that occur quickly are more likely to result in distortion. Furthermore, the fact that perceptual accuracy improves in pregnant women near term as their actual size increases supports the notion that adaptation of the body image to a new reality requires time. Glucksman and Hirsch[29] studied a group of massively obese subjects who continued to overestimate their body width long after they had lost significant amounts of weight and had corresponding changes in size and shape. This continued perceptual distortion was more common among those patients who had been obese since childhood. Also, patients who suffer a sudden or traumatic loss of a limb are more likely to develop a phantom limb. As the phantom limb gradually disappears, perceptual accuracy is restored. Thus, after young childhood, any sudden change in body shape is likely to result in a distorted body image percept which may resolve with time. If the abnormality (obesity, loss of a limb, disfigurement, etc.) occurs during adolescence in association with condemnation by peers or family, spontaneous resolution of the distorted body image is unlikely.

PSYCHOTHERAPY TREATMENT FOR BODY IMAGE

Stunkard[18] believes the presence of a body image disturbance in an obese patient is a clear indication for psychotherapy. Traditional insight psychotherapy has been the most widely used treatment, but newer techniques may prove useful as part of a holistic treatment plan. For example, dance therapy, although extremely difficult to evaluate objectively, holds promise as an adjunctive treatment method. Desensitization procedures to a new thinner size may help prevent relapse in previously obese patients. These issues will be discussed more thoroughly in Chapter 12. Suffice it to say that a body image disturbance in obesity probably requires specific treatment in conjunction with a change in eating or exercise patterns.

MEASUREMENT OF BODY IMAGE

Simple Office Procedures

Several methods have been devised to evaluate body image. The simplest is to ask the patient to describe his body and his feelings about his body. A recent patient with bulimia responded as follows:

> "Although I know intellectually that I now weigh 125 pounds compared to 145 pounds 3 months ago, it's as though I've really only reduced from about 375 pounds to 225 pounds. I'm so fat I can barely get through the door. I'm so heavy I can't walk well. I'm so fat, ugly, grotesque, and bad. Just thinking about eating a piece of cake gives me nightmares."

This patient describes both a perceptual and attitudinal disturbance in body image.

In screening obese subjects for a study[30] we asked each potential subject to describe his body. The following are responses from obese subjects who probably didn't have a body image disturbance:

> "I don't feel really obese or unpresentable but I do feel large and awkward at times and worry about the threat of overweight to my future health, especially since it runs in both sides of the family"
>
> "I love it, but it needs an overhaul."

The following responses from several different subjects are typical of patients with body image disturbances:

> "I think I look horrible and I dislike being fat. My body is ugly."
>
> "Too fat. Avoid mirrors. Hate my body."
>
> "Am very unhappy with the way I now look. Feel very unattractive bodywise. Feel ungainly. Hard to see myself as I really am."
>
> "It is very repulsive to me—I pant and puff when I have to tie laces and when I try on clothes I'm depressed for weeks."

Levy[31] suggested a method of evaluating body image in children. While the child is still undressed at the end of an ordinary physical examination, he is asked to play the role of the doctor and examine his own body. The physician asks him to comment on the parts of his own body and asks if he has noticed any differences between himself and others. The child is also asked what he would like his body to look like when he grows up. He may be asked about the importance of height, weight, strength, and appearance. Levy noted a number of discrepancies between the children's attitudes toward their body parts and their actual physical appearance. This simple office procedure can be useful for the child before adolescence. During adolescence, youngsters are so intensely sensitive about their bodies, that a clear demarcation between the physical examination and psychiatric interview is wise.

Simonson[32] has described another office procedure for estimating disturbances in perception of body image. The patient is asked to open a door just wide enough to allow him to pass through it unobstructed. Patients with gross disturbances in body image will often open the door much wider or narrower than actually necessary.

Draw-A-Person Test

The Draw-A-Person test described by Machover[33] has been used to evaluate body image disturbances in a wide variety of conditions. It is a projective technique designed to elicit unconscious attitudes and percepts of body image. It is easily administered and often provides valuable information about an individual patient. The subject is asked to draw a person and to comment on the person drawn. Then the subject is asked to draw a person of the opposite sex. Various scoring techniques have been used but the method described by Harris[34] is best known. In this method, the more accurate, detailed, and sexually differentiated the drawing, the higher the score. Although there is a debate about what psychodynamic conclusions can be inferred from figure drawings,[35] there is general agreement that they reflect developmental change as they become more detailed and accurate with age.[35, 36]

Nathan[37] studied the male and female figure drawings of 36 obese and 36 normal weight children, with 12 children at each age level of 7, 10, and 13. The control children scored significantly higher than their age-matched obese peers. The obese children tended to omit some essential body parts (for example, shoulders, necks, fingers, feet). The drawings by the obese youngsters were generally less differentiated. Some obese children at all ages drew 1-dimensional stick figures, whereas none of the normal weight children, even in the 7-year-old group, drew stick figures. Also, the obese children tended to draw very similar male and female figures, whereas the drawings of normal weight children showed sexual differentiation. Several obese children submitted bizarre, distorted drawings. Interestingly, none of the obese children drew obese figures. These findings are shown in Figure 8.2. Although this study is of relatively few obese children, it does suggest that the development of body image may be defective prior to adolescence. Again, these obese subjects were brought for evaluation of a weight problem at a medical clinic and, therefore, may not be representative of obese children in general.

Hilde Bruch's classic study[12] of the Draw-A-Person test revealed marked body image disturbances in both anorexia nervosa and developmental

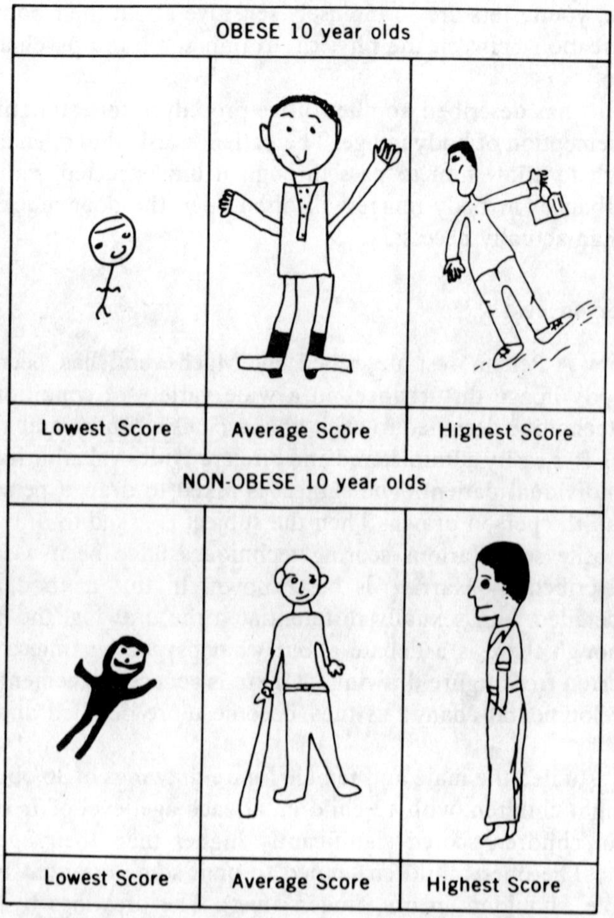

Figure 8.2. Draw-A-Person Test with obese and non-obese children. Upper panel, drawing from obese 10 year olds with lowest, average and highest scores; lower panel, drawings from non-obese 10 year olds with lowest, average and highest scores. (Reprinted with permission from S Nathan: J Pers Assess 37: 456–463, 1973.)

obesity. She noted that the patients often drew pictures of themselves that were grossly misshapen or larger than their actual size. Also, they made more derogatory, derisive remarks about their bodies. Her work has stimulated research for two decades, and therefore, has been invaluable. However, the patient sample is skewed since obese patients who present to a psychiatrist are more likely to have emotional problems, and, therefore, more likely to have body image disturbances.

The use of the Draw-A-Person test depends on the assumption that the individual's spontaneous drawing of a human figure represents an accurate projection of his own body image. To date, there have been no external criteria validating this point; in fact, the Draw-A-Person test has been used as a standard against which to compare other tests that measure aspects of body image.

Bailey and co-workers[38] compared figure drawings of 105 college students, 38 of whom were considered obese (10% or more overweight). The obese subjects drew significantly larger figures. Since the authors do not provide a correlation between the figure size and actual body size, this finding may or may not represent a distortion in the perception of body size.

Examples of Draw-A-Person Test

Although the validity of the Draw-A-Person test has not been established with certainty, it can be useful in providing rapid preliminary information about body image. For example, the figure drawings of two obese adults are shown in Figure 8.3. The first subject (Fig. 3, drawing on left) had mild emotional disturbances as reflected in a marital maladjustment. She was

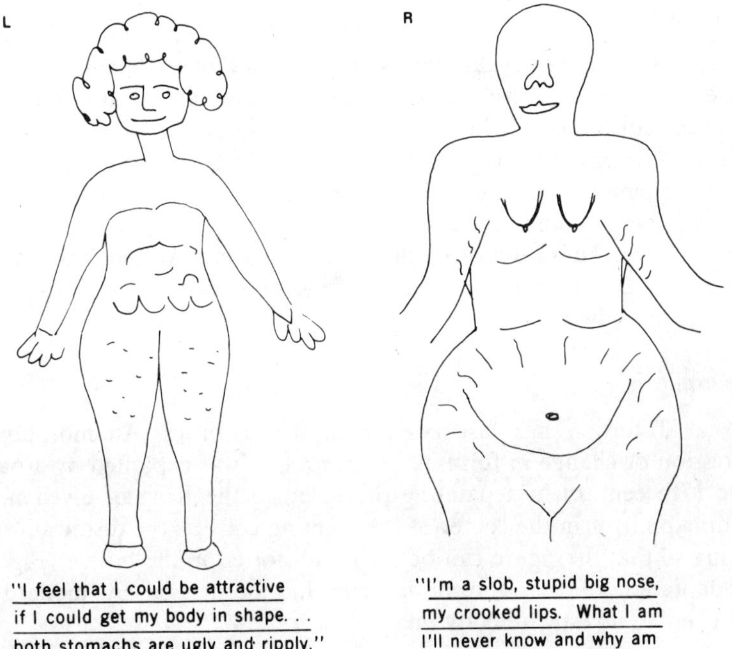

Figure 8.3. Draw-A-Person Test from obese adults. Left, mild disturbance in attitudinal aspect of body image; right, severe disturbance in attitudinal and perceptual aspects of body image.

mildly obese during adolescence and currently weighs 175 pounds and is 5 feet 6 inches tall. Her figure drawing was accurate and well differentiated, suggesting an accurage perception of her body. Her remarks about her body suggest only a mild disturbance in the attitudinal aspects of body image:

> "I feel I could be attractive if I could get my body in shape" and "my stomachs are ugly . . . legs are ugly and ripply."

By contrast, the second obese subject has been obese since childhood, currently weighs 220 pounds and is 5 feet 4 inches. She has serious psychiatric problems especially with dependency. Her drawing (Fig. 3, right) is incomplete with no eyes and only rudimentary arms and legs suggesting a disturbance in body percept. This patient described her body as follows:

> "I am a slob, stupid, big-nosed, my crooked lips. What I am, I'll never know and why I am here."

In reality she is an attractive woman. Thus, her drawing suggested disturbances in both perceptual and attitudinal aspects of body image.

Clay Modeling

A related method of evaluating body image is clay modeling. The patient is asked to form a figure out of clay and to comment on the figure. One theoretical advantage of this technique is that it may allow the subject to render a 3-dimensional projection of his body image, which might provide more information than the 2-dimensional Draw-A-Person test. Also, clay modeling depends not only on visual cues (as many of the techniques to be discussed later), but also on accurate tactile sensation. Although this method has not been as well documented as the Draw-A-Person test, it holds promise in studies of body image.

Anamorphosis

Visual distortion has fascinated man for centuries. Anamorphosis, a progression or change in form, is a concept that was exploited by a painter in the 17th century in a painting presented to the King of Sweden. The cylindrical mirror in the center of the painting corrects the distortion in the painting so that the figure can be seen undistorted in the mirror (Fig. 8.4). An adaptation of this ancient concept has been used by modern day researchers to investigate body image.

Adjustable Body-Distorting Mirror

The adjustable body distorting mirror[39] has been used to evaluate visual perception of the body. A special full length mirror is used which can be

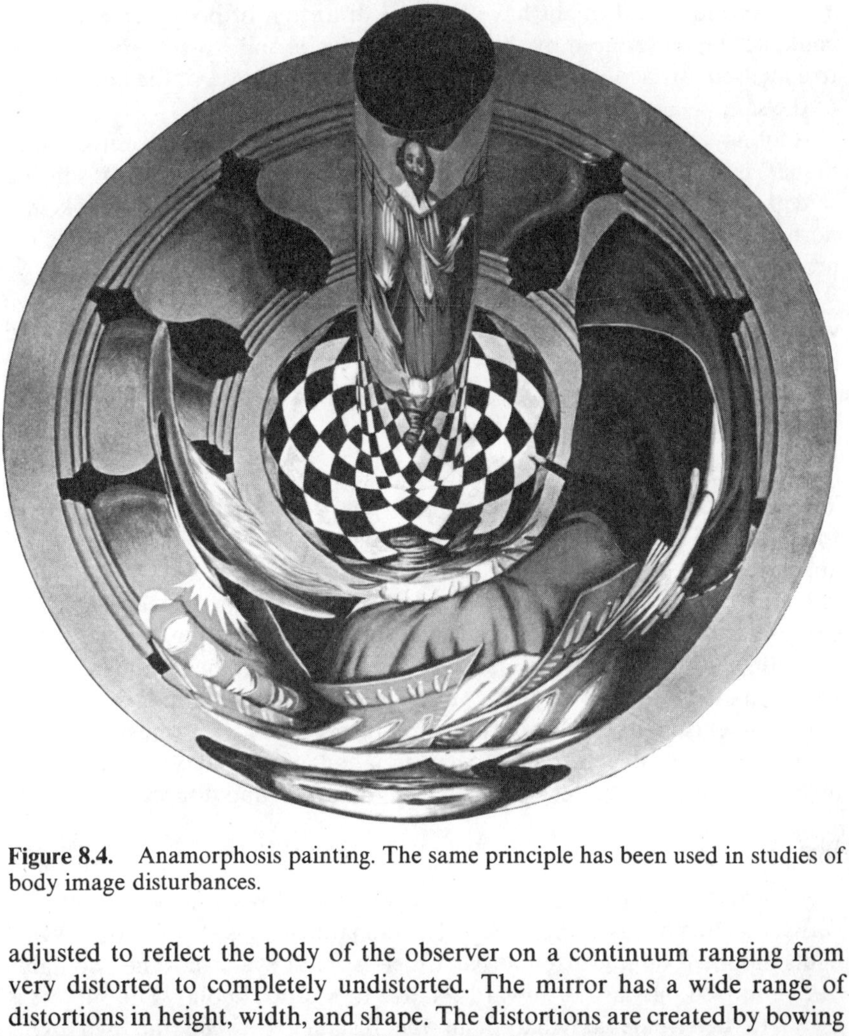

Figure 8.4. Anamorphosis painting. The same principle has been used in studies of body image disturbances.

adjusted to reflect the body of the observer on a continuum ranging from very distorted to completely undistorted. The mirror has a wide range of distortions in height, width, and shape. The distortions are created by bowing a mirror in a concave or convex direction with a motor under the control of the observer. The observer is allowed a series of trials to learn how to use the equipment and is then asked to adjust the mirror until it matches his appearance. This fascinating approach to the study of body image is still in the experimental stages.

There are several problems with the method. First, it only measures the visual perceptual aspects of body image. Second, height as well as width and shape are distorted and there is preliminary evidence that estimates of height are usually correct,[17] even if there is a distortion in width and shape. Also, only a limited assortment of distortions is provided by the instrument.

Thus, an individual might have a visual distortion of body percept which could not be reproduced by the instrument. Slade and Russell[28] believe that this method erroneously assumes a generalized distortion of the body image of the same magnitude for all parts of the body.

Another interesting complication noted with the distorted mirror technique[39] is that after several minutes of adjusting the mirror, many subjects said they had forgotten what they looked like. Some asked to look in a normal mirror before continuing and others examined themselves before proceeding (re-emphasizing the importance of touch and kinesthesia).

Finally, as with all the instruments thus far devised, it is not known whether what the subject finally produces is an accurate representation of his mental image.

Distorting Photograph Technique

A distorting photograph technique has been used to evaluate body image. The method utilizes a variable anamorphic lens capable of distorting a standardized slide photograph of the subject by 20% in the direction of appearing thin or fat.

Garner and colleagues[40] evaluated 18 subjects with primary anorexia nervosa and 16 subjects with juvenile onset obesity using this distorting technique. They found that, statistically, both groups overestimated their size compared to control groups. Although a given obese or anorexic subject might underestimate size, overestimation of size was a very unusual finding among control subjects. Thus, overestimation of size may occur and be objectively measured in certain people who have eating disorders.

Body Width Estimate

Slade and Russell[28] devised an instrument that allows a subject to estimate various widths of his or her body. This apparatus consists of two movable lights mounted on a horizontal bar which is set at eye level. The two lights can be moved outward or inward relative to a central point. The subject is asked to determine at what point the distance between the two lights corresponds to the distance across a particular part of the body. The result is a measure of "perceived size" of that part. "Real size" is determined by measurement and a body perception index calculated using the following formula:

$$\text{body perception index} = \frac{\text{perceived size} \times 100}{\text{real size}}$$

Various body widths have been measured, but they usually include face (between zygomas), chest (across axilla), waist (at narrowest point), and hips (at widest point). The subject is also asked to estimate the width of an inanimate object, usually a vase. Using this technique, the authors have shown that anorexia nervosa patients and normal pregnant women overestimate various widths compared to control groups. Garner and colleagues[40] have been unable to replicate these findings with anorexia nervosa patients using the instrument designed by Slade and Russell.

Glucksman and Hirsch[29] also used a visual size estimation apparatus to measure perceived width of specific body regions. In contrast to Slade and Russell, they found no significant differences between groups using this technique, and they concluded that the distorting photograph technique may be a more sensitive measure of one's perceptions and feelings about overall appearance. Although conflicting results are being reported with this technique, it is being studied in several eating disorder clinics across the country.

Psychological Tests

Various psychological tests have been used to assess body image. Although the findings may relate to body image disturbances in the eating disorders, most were designed to elucidate schizophrenia or brain disease.

For example, Bender's[41] study of double simultaneous stimulation of nonsymmetrical areas of the body, has shown differences between normal and schizophrenic subjects. Although this test measures tactile and kinesthetic perception, its relevance to the eating disorders is not known.

Asch and Wilkin[42] have studied perception as related to the postural image of the body. In this work, subjects were placed in a small tilted room and asked to adjust a rod to the true upright. Striking individual differences have been found, but whether the technique will clarify the disturbance of body image seen in obesity is not known. This technique has promise since there is a heavy reliance on touch rather than vision.

Fisher and Cleveland[43] have correlated the concept of boundary definiteness with responses from subjects to the Rorschach ink blot stimuli. Other projective techniques including various word association tests have also been used to assess body image. Other investigators have attempted to relate various personality variables to body image disturbances.

SUMMARY

In summary, body image is a term that encompasses many meanings. In the eating disorders, body image disturbance refers to two closely intertwined problems. The first is an inaccurate perception of actual size or shape, and the second is an unrealistic, usually negative, self-appraisal of one's appearance. There is preliminary evidence that fewer than half the obese population suffer from body image disturbances. Apparently, emotional disturbance is a necessary, but insufficient, condition for body image disturbance. It is most likely to occur in individuals who have been obese during adolescence, probably because teenagers are so self-conscious about their bodies and any deviation from their peers. Reduction in weight is probably insufficient to correct a co-existing body image disturbance. Transient emotional upsets may intensify negative attitudes towards one's body. Various instruments used to evaluate body image in obesity have focused primarily on body percept. Still urgently needed are studies which evaluate the major aspects of body image disturbance in the context of the obese person's entire life.

ABSENCE OF ONE PERSONALITY TYPE ASSOCIATED WITH OBESITY

The psychiatric literature is replete with studies investigating the relationship between obesity and personality characteristics. Although correlations between obesity and various measures of neuroticism have been demonstrated, it is by no means clear that the neurosis is the cause of the obesity. No one personality trait has been found to be characteristic of all, or even most, obese persons. Early theorists attempted to link certain personality profiles to specific body illnesses. Obesity was considered a psychosomatic illness and an immature "oral" personality was thought to be characteristic. Although this may be true for some obese patients, it is probably not correct for a large majority of patients.

Several problems have interfered with studies of neuroticism among obese patients. The major one has been repeatedly emphasized. Obesity is probably a final common pathway for a variety of physiological or pyschological problems. Very few studies have selected obese subjects by the same criteria, and different parameters have been used to assess psychological well-being. Furthermore, the subjects available for study have come from different sources. Most studies by psychiatrists have evaluated patients with severe obesity referred from medical clinics, and most behavioral psychologists have studied mildly obese college students.

OBESITY, MENTAL HEALTH, AND SOCIOECONOMIC CLASS

Stunkard's studies have been an exception to this trend in utilizing broadly based epidemiological techniques beginning with the mid-town Manhattan study in the 1960's. In an early report[44] a striking correlation between obesity and lower socioeconomic status was noted. Obesity was 7 times more common in the lowest socioeconomic class than in the highest in this sample of 1660 persons. The psychological status was evaluated by nine mental health indices. The information was obtained by interviews lasting approximately 2 hours. The obese subjects made more pathological responses on eight of the nine measures. Three of these were statistically significant: "immaturity," "rigidity," and "suspiciousness." This study was controlled for socioeconomic status and higher levels of psychopathology were found among obese persons than among non-obese persons. These correlations do not, however, prove an etiologic relationship between psychopathology and obesity. One problem with this study is that it relies on interpretation of interviews (which may, in fact, be more valid) that are difficult to compare with other measures of psychological functioning, such as the Minnesota Multiphasic Personality Inventory (MMPI) or California Psychological Inventory (CPI).

CONFLICTING RESULTS FROM PSYCHOLOGICAL TESTS

In an in-depth study of 18 obese and 18 non-obese men, a battery of psychological tests was administered including the WAIS (Wexler Adult Intelligence Scale), the CPI, and Draw-A-Man test.[45] No distinctive personality features were found. There were no differences between the groups in level of anxiety. Although dependence problems have been considered a cardinal feature of obesity, this was not confirmed. None of the obese men were found to be more feminine in their interests than non-obese men. Although the authors have been careful in applying their results only to the group of obese men studied, this relatively small scale investigation has been repeatedly hailed as a landmark study documenting the absence of neuroticism among obese subjects. One theoretical problem of this study is that the CPI was designed to measure normal variances of certain personality characteristics, whereas the MMPI (not used in this study) was designed to detect psychopathology. Therefore, studies utilizing the CPI are difficult to compare with the more numerous, but less famous, studies using the MMPI.

Atkinson and Ringuette[46] studied very obese adults using the MMPI and detailed interviews. Again, no one personality factor was identified. However, there was a correlation between high psychopathology scores and early onset of obesity, massive weights by mid-adolescence, and the ability to lose large amounts of weight temporarily. This last observation is consonant with Bruch's belief that the severity of an obese child's weight problem is better measured by fluctuation in weight than by percentage overweight.

In another study,[47] a group of 116 obese subjects at an obesity clinic were given the MMPI. The results were compared to the MMPI profiles of 50,000 patients in a general medical clinic. Although some statistical differences were detected, the authors note the presence of diverse personality patterns among the obese subjects rather than a single personality pattern characteristic of the group. In addition, the presence of a normal or abnormal MMPI profile did not predict success or failure in the weight reduction program.

Pomerantz and colleagues[48] administered the MMPI to 40 patients (20 male, 20 female) drawn at random from an entire patient population of 250 in a weight reduction program. The mean score of the depression scale for men was 69. The mean score on this clinical scale for normal subjects is 60, with a range from 50–70. Therefore, this result suggests that these obese men, as a group, may be more depressed than a normal group. On the masculinity-femininity scale (Mf scale), female patients scored significantly lower than a normal population (i.e., the obese subjects had a very high femininity interest pattern). The male patients had a marginally significant higher mean score. The authors conclude that these scores indicate passivity and non-assertiveness in both groups. The problem with this conclusion is that the Mf scale is perhaps the most controversial of the clinical scales of the MMPI. Recent cultural changes have dramatically influenced interest patterns that once were traditionally male or female.

Are Fat People Jolly?

The notion that fat people are also jolly has an old and respectable history. Recently Crisp and McGuiness[49] documented a correlation between substantial obesity and low levels of anxiety (in men and women) and depression (in men). Their sample of 17 obese men and 18 obese women was drawn from a group practice of approximately 1000 patients in London. The obese men were at least 20% above standard weight and the obese female subjects 40% above standard. The Middlesex Hospital Questionnaire (MHQ) was administered to the subjects. This instrument is a brief, self-rating inventory designed to elicit evidence of neurosis. As a group, the obese patients were much less anxious and the men much less depressed than the rest of the population. The authors note that these findings may support the idea that overeating helps to console some people, especially those who are lonely or insecure. Or obesity itself may protect the individual from awareness of interpersonal problems. This study is valuable because it studies a general population group. However, the use of the MHQ makes comparison with other studies utilizing the CPI or MMPI difficult.

PSYCHOLOGICAL ABNORMALITIES IN OBESE CHILDREN

Studies attempting to document psychological abnormalities in obese children or adolescents are even more difficult to evaluate than studies of adults. Different age groups have been studied defining obesity in very different ways and rarely have the same psychological tests been used. For example, Hammer and colleagues[50] evaluated 10 obese and 10 non-obese adolescents and concluded that the obese were usually a focus of family conflict and were characterized by defective body image development, low self-esteem, physical inactivity, and depression. In contrast, Sallade[51] studied 120 obese and 120 non-obese subjects from grades 3, 5, 8, and 11 and found that overall personality adjustment was unimpaired! These two studies arrive at diametrically opposed conclusions, but probably for very good reasons. The study by Hammer and colleagues was an intensive one and included a complete medical examination, nutrition history, and a battery of psychological tests. Most of the subjects were from middle or upper socioeconomic groups and had been brought to an adolescent clinic for evaluation. By contrast, Sallade's subjects were selected from school, not a medical clinic, and were primarily from lower socioeconomic groups. Her conclusions are based on the results of three psychological tests (none of which were used in the study by Hammer and colleagues). Thus, it is not surprising that the results are so divergent.

CONCLUSION

The most valid conclusion to be drawn from this morass of conflicting data is that obese subjects are a disparate group with a wide variety of personality characteristics. However, this does not mean that there is no relationship between psychological factors and obesity. There may well be certain subgroups of obese patients who have common neurotic features which predispose to obesity. The night-eating syndrome or binge-eating syndrome may be examples. The studies just cited do, however, dispel the notion that all obese subjects are neurotic or "orally fixated." A careful individual appraisal of each obese patient will usually allow the physician to decide whether emotional disturbance is present and the relationship, if any, to his or her obesity.

PSYCHIATRIC SYMPTOMS ASSOCIATED WITH WEIGHT LOSS

Another method of investigating the contribution of psychological factors to obesity has been to study patients who have lost weight by following a diet. Traditionally, overeating has been thought to comfort the eater, and obesity itself to insulate the patient from overwhelming interpersonal difficulties. If reduced obese patients suffer an increase in psychiatric symptoms, the traditional view would be supported, although not proven. The literature on this subject is contradictory for the familiar reason: different studies evaluated many different kinds of patients who had a variety of different treatments. However, certain findings are consistent in different studies.

In a series of studies, Glucksman and Hirsch[52, 53] found that depression occurred frequently following weight loss, particularly in those patients with childhood onset of obesity. Fifteen subjects were closely followed. The 10 subjects with childhood onset of obesity became increasingly sad, pessimistic, and disappointed as the weight loss increased. An associated rise in hostility, irritability, and aggressiveness was noted. Furthermore, these subjects overestimated their size, as though they had not lost weight, a phenomenon the authors label "a phantom-body size." By contrast the five patients with adult onset of obesity did not have signs of depression or a rise in hostility, and perception of their body size was accurate.

In a related report, Hirsch[54] notes that the sense of time passage, which may be a correlate of depression, is impaired in reduced juvenile onset obese subjects. Before and after weight loss, subjects were asked to estimate the duration of a tone that lasted either 1 second or 3 seconds. During and after weight loss the juvenile obese subjects judged the tones as shorter in duration than prior to weight loss.

Several other studies have emphasized the possible dangers of calorie restriction. Bruch has repeatedly warned against the indiscriminate prescription of diets. Robinson and Winnik[55] in Israel described 10 patients who were hospitalized following weight loss. Seven of these patients were psychotic and three had severe neurotic reactions. Nine of the 10 patients responded rapidly to weight gain and antipsychotic medication. Only one patient ascribed his illness to the diet. Four of the 10 subjects had a history of previous psychiatric disorders. Although this study does not demonstrate that the diet or weight loss caused the psychiatric symptoms, it does highlight the need for careful psychiatric evaluation of any patient contemplating a weight reduction program.

A common pattern has been noted in patients who develop emotional problems following dieting. Stunkard and Rush[56] reviewed a study of 25 obese subjects who were referred because of the severity of their obesity or difficulties in management. In half the patients, at the beginning of the diet, there was an early period of euphoria and extravagant fantasies about the benefits that would accrue from weight loss. Then there was an abrupt onset of anxiety which lasted 1 to 3 weeks. This was followed by a depression which lasted for weeks or months. Sleep disturbance, crying spells, and suicidal ideation were frequent symptoms.

One of the difficulties with this approach is that there is a very high dropout rate in most reduction programs. It may be that the patients who drop out do so to avoid disabling depression or anxiety. For example, although Shipman and Plesset[57] concluded that successful dieting lowered anxiety and depression in 38 subjects, 74% of the initial 151 subjects dropped out. Stunkard and Rush[56] advanced the view that the very high dropout rate in weight reduction clinics may really be a highly adaptive coping mechanism for some obese subjects and the physician should commend their good sense rather than criticize the patient.

PSYCHOANALYTIC THEORY OF OBESITY

BASIS OF THEORY

The psychoanalytic theory of obesity holds that overeating by obese persons is a fixation or regression to the oral stage of psychosexual development. Although Freud's theory of personality development has been severely criticized, often with justification, it remains the most comprehensive theory currently available. Many new theories modify or elaborate the traditional Freudian viewpoint. Even theories that initially appear radically different (e.g. learning models) have been compared with, and even incorporated into, the psychoanalytic model of personality development.

The classical stages of psychosexual development are the oral, anal, and genital phases. The pivotal point of the theory is that libidinal (sexual or erotic) drives predominate at all stages, although the focus normally progresses from the oral area to the anal area and culminates in a mature genital sexuality. Various coping mechanisms originate during various stages. These defense mechanisms serve to protect the person from awareness of frustration of sexual or pleasurable drives or instincts. As maturity is achieved the person can relinquish the more primitive defense mechanisms that were suitable for earlier stages of development.

The normal individual retains the capacity to utilize a wide variety of defense mechanisms in stressful situations. By contrast, in neurosis, the defense mechanisms that are appropriate in early stages (for example, denial or projection) may be retained or the person may substitute less mature erotic satisfaction for an unattainable mature sexual gratification. In 1932, Freud wrote " ... instinctual impulses from one source can join onto instinctual impulses from another and share their further vicissitudes and ... the satisfaction of one instinct can be substituted for the satisfaction of another."[58] The aim of satisfaction, i.e., libidinal pleasure, remains unchanged, but the means by which the goal is achieved is substituted. That is, eating is substituted for genital sexual satisfaction. Overeating and obesity may follow if the substitution occurs regularly and inappropriately.

The orality theory of obesity was further clarified by Hamburger.[59, 60] Mouth activities play an important role in early infant development. The infant nurses at his mother's breast and comes to equate receiving of food with love. The feeding process and the intimacy of the mother-child relationship become fused. Certain children may fail to develop psychosexually beyond this point; i.e., they become fixated at the oral stage either from a deficit or excess of maternal love. Later in life these individuals may have excessive oral receptive needs and are dependent, child-like and demanding. If this need for love and security is not satisfied, eating may be used as a substitute because of the unconscious association of food with love. Thus, overeating may fulfill unmet dependency needs. Furthermore, in infancy, all oral activity (eating, thumbsucking, etc.) is an erotic activity that merges with the nutritional and nurturing aspects of eating. As the child develops, the nutritional aspect of eating becomes separated from the erotic components which gradually shift to the genital. Hamburger notes that traces of this erotic component persist into adult life and are evidenced by the oral gratification of kissing, smoking, or chewing. In adulthood, stress may precipitate a return to the oral phase (regression) in a predisposed individual in some way fixated at the oral phase. Thus, this psychoanalyst concluded that overeating may reflect either the need for love and support, or disguised erotic wishes.

DREAM ANALYSIS

Analysis of dreams of food and eating is another method of studying the relationship between personality and obesity. Hamburger[60] analyzed the dreams of four patients in long-term psychoanalysis in terms of the manifest and latent content.

The *manifest content* of a dream is the overt theme of the dream, and the *latent content* is the underlying psychodynamic meaning of the dream as inferred from the associations of the patient to elements of the dream.

In the four patients studied, the manifest (apparent) content of the dreams involved food and eating in 10–20% of reported dreams. There was a tendency for this percentage to decrease as analysis proceeded. The technique of free association was used to elicit the unconscious meaning of the dream. Using this method, Hamburger concluded that although food and eating had highly specific symbolic meanings for each patient, two major latent meanings of these dreams were paramount. The dreams either symbolized the need for anaclitic love and affection, or, by unconscious displacement and symbolization, the eating drive was substituted for the sexual drive. The following is an example of a dream about food interpreted by Hamburger to illustrate the use of food as a symbol of love and support:

> Dream—"In a cafeteria line—I was the first person in line—but when I got there the two main dishes were gone."
>
> Associations: She stated that this dream of wanting food and then not getting it is a repetitive theme . . . this dream condenses her attitudes early in analysis. Food and eating symbolize substitute gratifications for love and succor; she feels that all she can do is *passively* wait to receive this . . . " (p 2).[60]

Although this study was carefully documented, the sample size was small and only one of the patients was obese. It is reasonable to conclude that these psychodynamic formulations may apply to some obese patients.

BROAD SCALE PSYCHOANALYTIC STUDY

In the decades since Hamburger's work relating Freud's concept of orality to obesity, psychoanalysis has been subject to vociferous criticism. Arguments favoring psychoanalytic interpretations of obesity have often been based on anecdotal case reports and larger studies have often failed to confirm psychoanalytic hypotheses.

However, recently Rand and Stunkard[61, 62] have completed the first phase of a comprehensive study of obese patients undergoing psychoanalysis.

Eighty-four obese patients were selected and evaluated by questionnaires completed by their analysts. Fifty-three non-obese patients were selected for comparison and were similar on all demographic variables except marital status. More obese patients were single (48%) than were the non-obese (29%). Few of these subjects (6%) sought psychoanalysis because of their obesity. The majority of both obese and non-obese subjects reported anxiety, or depression, or both, as their presenting complaint.

Although most obese subjects had specific psychodynamic constellations associated with weight gain or weight loss, these were markedly different from patient to patient. Few of the comparison non-obese subjects had specific psychodynamics associated with weight loss or weight gain (p 473).[61] The authors cite examples of positive response associated with weight gain:

> "Patient feels huge and imposing compared to more puny-looking mortals; thus, builds up weak ego; being small is being a child and powerless."

A negative response to weight gain was increased feelings of distance and isolation from others. Positive and negative responses to weight loss were also more frequent in the obese group. For example, with weight loss, one patient:

> "feels wonderful about self."

The negative response of one patient was reported as:

> "fear total personality change."

The analysts reported that 47% of their obese subjects ate to avoid sex compared to 7% of their non-obese patients. For example, the following were reported:

> "Single obese woman: when the patient is faced with the possibility of getting close to a man she overeats to get fat and ugly" (p 483).[61]
>
> "Married obese man: after eating the patient feels 'too full' to have sex" (p 484).[61]

This finding provides support for the theory that eating can substitute for more mature sexual gratification. Also the analysts reported that 79% of the obese persons overate under stress compared to 9% of the non-obese group.

The *dreams* of the two groups were also assessed. Obese patients reported dreams less often than the normal weight patients. There was no difference in the frequency of dreams about food and eating. The presence of the patient's own body in dreams was reported by about half of each group. None of the non-obese patients who saw their own body in their dreams saw themselves as fat, whereas 44% of the obese who dreamt of their own body saw themselves as fat. Most of these patients had been obese since adolescence.

Body image disparagement was much more common among the obese group (88%) than the non-obese group (43%). The effect of treatment on the attitudinal aspect of body image was surprisingly beneficial. Psychoanalysis resulted in a decrease in body image disparagement in 21 of the 35 obese patients who had severe feelings of unattractiveness. Furthermore, 47% of the obese patients lost more than 20 pounds during treatment.

This ambitious study of the effect of psychoanalysis on obesity suggests that this form of treatment may be quite effective for obesity in some patients and invaluable in alleviating body image disturbances. However, there are several potential sources for error in the project. First, the evaluation of the patient was second-hand via questionnaires completed by the analysts themselves, and it may be that the analysts tended to overestimate improvement in the patients. Second, although significant weight losses were reported, the patients were not actually weighed and the analysts thought that to do so might interfere with the therapeutic process.

FAMILY INTERACTION

The emotional transactions between family members can dramatically influence eating patterns. The use or misuse of food to control, reward, or punish behavior in childhood can have a lasting detrimental effect. Food can symbolize love and caring and replace other expressions of affection. Transactions between family members during mealtime may be symptomatic of underlying family psychopathology. Although there is little doubt that such problems can cause or contribute to the development and maintenance of obesity, documentation is difficult for several reasons. Family interaction involves a multitude of variables and early workers tried to isolate certain variables and identify them in obese groups selected by widely varying criteria. Later investigators, notably Minuchin and Bruch, tried to identify certain characteristic patterns of family interaction.

PSYCHOSOMATOGENIC FAMILIES

Minuchin[63] has utilized systems theory in his studies of families. Systems theory posits that the characteristics of a group can be studied. Although it is the unique blend of individual characteristics that produce certain patterns of group interaction, the group itself is the focus of study rather than specific members of the group. Minuchin has utilized this model to study families who have one or more members with a psychosomatic illness. Minuchin and colleagues consider obesity and anorexia nervosa examples of psychosomatic illnesses. According to this theory the psychosomatogenic family has three major characteristics: a special family configuration and functioning, involvement of the children in parental conflict, and physiological vulnerability of the child (Table 8.1).

Table 8.1. Psychosomatogenic families (Minuchin).

1. Special Configuration and Functioning
   - enmeshment
   - overprotectiveness
   - rigidity
   - conflict avoidance
2. Child Involved in Parent Conflict
3. Physiologic Vulnerability of Child

The pattern of family functioning is characterized by enmeshment, overprotectiveness, rigidity, and a lack of conflict resolution. *Enmeshment* is a term used to describe the absence of personal boundaries and the overinvolvement family members have in each other's thoughts, feelings, and behavior. The boundaries between the children and the subset of the parents within this system is unclear, resulting in confusion of roles and responsibilities. Autonomy of an individual is severely restricted.

Overprotectiveness describes the over-concern for each other's welfare. If one member of the family is sick, all members of the family become involved in the care of that member and other family conflicts are submerged. Each member of the family feels responsible for every other member's health and welfare.

Rigidity describes the inflexible pattern of interaction that is maintained over years. The family may insist that no change is wanted or needed.

Lack of conflict resolution describes the failure of the family to openly confront disagreements and arrive at solutions. The family may deny any disagreements at all (a family fighting style termed "pseudo-mutuality") or may quarrel continuously without really grappling with the problem ("pseudo-hostility").[64] In any case, conflicts are not negotiated and resolved. The psychosomatically ill child plays a vital role in providing a focus for the family concern and facilitating the avoidance of conflict.

The second major characteristic of families producing a psychosomatically ill child is involvement of the child in parental conflict. Appropriate intergenerational boundaries are not maintained. When unnegotiated parental conflict threatens the integrity of the family, the identified patient is drawn into the spouse dyad to form a rigid triad. The unresolved conflict continues, but family disruption is obviated by focusing on the child's symptoms.

The physiological vulnerability of the child with certain psychosomatic illness is a necessary, but usually insufficient condition, for the development of a psychosomatic illness.

SYSTEMS MODEL APPLIED TO EATING DISORDERS

Minuchin and colleagues[65] have applied this family systems model to the eating disorders, particularly anorexia nervosa. In careful case studies of the families of anorexia nervosa patients, they elucidate the thesis that these "psychosomatic families" are especially likely to avoid open conflict; superficially the family is well-mannered and civil, but resentment and anger lie just below the surface. The anorexic patient becomes the center of family attention in a desperate attempt to keep parental conflict submerged. The third major tenet of the theory, that these youngsters have a physiological vulnerability to anorexia nervosa, is less well-established.

This family systems model has not been as rigorously studied in families with obese youngsters, but is probably applicable to some obese patients. "Developmental obesity" may include patients whose families have the characteristic structure and functioning described by Minuchin. Certainly many obese youngsters come from overprotective families that appear to avoid conflict at almost any cost. The obese youngster is often the target for family concern and is frequently the scapegoat for family hostility. Furthermore, physiological vulnerability to obesity may be more likely than physiological vulnerability to anorexia nervosa. Genetic factors and increased fat cell number may be part of such a physiological vulnerability. Thus, it seems likely that some obese youngsters do come from "psychosomatic families."

IMPORTANCE OF FAMILY

The major contribution of family systems theory is that it directs attention to the family rather than the individual. In any area of medicine, it is well known that treatment of the patient is more likely to be effective if the cooperation of the family is elicited. Understanding the family as a group (i.e., as a social system) will facilitate the treatment of obese subjects who reflect, maintain, or contribute to family psychopathology.

OVEREATING AS AN ADDICTION

Compulsive eating has been considered a type of addiction. Fenichel[66] thought that a compulsive craving for food represented a striving for simultaneous gratification of sexuality and self-esteem. He considered a fixation at an early oral mode of psychosexual development the underlying cause of all addictions including alcoholism and food addiction.

SIMILARITIES TO ALCOHOLISM

In the case of food addiction, Fenichel thought that later stages of development may have added other unconscious meanings to the pathologically craved food. Hamburger[59] elaborated on this idea in his lucid description of eight patients who had compulsive cravings for food often starting in earliest childhood and independent of external precipitating events. One patient compared her compulsive eating to the behavior of an alcoholic. She said she could no more take one bite of food than an alcoholic could take one drink. A patient in our clinic said she would continue eating as long as there was any food available. Rand and Stunkard[61] found that food cravings were more common among the obese than among the non-obese and that most foods craved were of a very high calorie content.

Some of the terms in common usage suggest similar behavior patterns in some overeaters and alcoholics. For example, "carboholic" is a neologism coined to describe a person who overeats carbohydrates. "Overeaters Anonymous" is the name of a group that meets to control overeating; it operates on principles analogous to those of Alcoholics Anonymous.

Swanson and Dinello[67] described a number of similarities between a group of very obese subjects and alcoholics. They studied 25 obese subjects who exceeded ideal weight by at least 50% with a range of weights from 197 pounds to 473 pounds. Fourteen of the subjects were grossly overweight before age 16, and 15 subjects reported significant obesity in at least one member of their immediate family. In these subjects, food was the focus of daily life. They often minimized their food intake like the alcoholic rationalizes his drinking. Food was the source of greatest pleasure, including preparation as well as eating. Sedation and drowsiness were the usual sequelae to overeating. Most of the subjects reported intense cravings for certain foods and were unable to stop eating once they started. Most believed they received some relief from anxiety or frustration by eating. Many spent hours preparing and eating a very high calorie meal. This precluded evening social activities. All had attempted to diet and most had been at least partially successful, but had regained to previous weight. The ability to lose weight on a diet had convinced most subjects that they could control their obesity if absolutely necessary. Very similar behavior has been noted in alcoholics.

The authors concluded that overeating in these obese subjects constituted habituation or addiction. Food was used to such excess that it produced sedation. There was a compulsive use to excess, a tendency to continually increase the amount, a psychological dependence, and detrimental effects on the person and his family. These patients were placed on a starvation diet, but with an adequate intake of fluids and vitamins, and most developed significant psychopathology. This finding is also consonant with the concept of addiction.

CRITERIA FOR ADDICTION

The World Health Organization defines addiction as follows:

> Drug addiction is a state of periodic or chronic intoxication, detrimental to the individual and society produced by the repeated consumption of a drug ... its characteristics include: (1) an overpowering desire or need (compulsion) to continue taking a drug and obtain it by any means, (2) a tendency to increase the dose, (3) a psychic (psychological) and sometimes a physical dependence on the effects of the drug.[68]

Although food is not a drug, the similarities to addiction are clear in some patients. Habituation may be typical of some patients who are obese. This theory, like many others, is probably applicable to some patients and can provide a useful guide to understanding psychodynamics in the context of a comprehensive treatment plan.

LEARNING THEORIES

Learning theories have become prominent in treating a wide variety of disorders, including obesity. Because conventional medical management of obesity had produced discouragingly ineffective results, researchers began to focus on the act of overeating, one common behavioral abnormality in obese subjects.

Ivan Pavlov,[69] the Russian physiologist, and B. F. Skinner, a psychologist, have been the most influential contributors to current learning theories. In classical (Pavlovian) conditioning, a stimulus incapable of eliciting a response prior to training is able to elicit that response after training. For example, Pavlov found that in a hungry animal the presence of food normally elicits the response of salivation; or restated in behavioral terms, an unconditioned stimulus (food) elicits the unconditioned response (salivation). During training, a bell is sounded at the same time as food is presented. The bell is called the conditioned stimulus. After training, the bell alone will elicit salivation, now called the conditioned response (Fig. 8.5). In the case of classical

<u>Before Training:</u> UCS (unconditioned stimulus) → UCR (unconditioned response)
(e.g. food) (salivation)

<u>During Training:</u> CS (conditioned stimulus) + UCS → UCR
(e.g. bell) (e.g. food) (salivation)

<u>After Training:</u> CS → CR (conditioned response)
(bell) (salivation)

Figure 8.5. Classical conditioning.

conditioning, the unconditioned stimulus precedes and elicits the unconditioned response, which is usually considered a reflex.

In operant conditioning, as elaborated by Skinner, the response is emitted, i.e., occurs first, and consequences follow which may increase or decrease the likelihood of the response occurring. Skinner emphasized that inner psychodynamic causes were less important than questions that asked "why the response was emitted in the first place, why it was punished, and what current variables are active."[70]

COMPARISON OF OPERANT CONDITIONING AND PSYCHODYNAMIC MODEL

Stuart,[71] a pioneer in behavioral approaches to obesity, has diagrammed the usual psychodynamic approach to obesity as follows:

PSYCHODYNAMIC MODEL
(Psychoanalytic)

Personality →	Behavior →	Consequences
(e.g. anxiety)	(overeating or underexercising)	(e.g. social ostracism)

That is, various personality factors including feelings or thoughts are presumed to precede the maladaptive behavior—overeating or underexercising—resulting in obesity and various positive or negative consequences.

The behavioral model incorporates the same elements as the psychodynamic model, but the point of entry is different:

BEHAVIORAL MODEL

Behavior →	Consequences →	Thoughts, Feelings
(overeating or underexercising)	(e.g., weight gain)	(e.g., low self-esteem)

TERMINOLOGY

Certain terms are used in operant conditioning programs that have very specific meanings. "*Positive reinforcement*" is any consequence that results in an increase of the preceding response. "*Punishment*" is any consequence that decreases the probability of a preceding response. The term "punishment" in operant conditioning has a very special meaning, and is probably an unfortunate choice since the word conjures up negative feelings in many people.

The following are examples of positive reinforcement and punishment. For example, overeating (the response) might result in larger size (the consequence) believed symbolic of strength and competence (thoughts and feelings) which results in an increase of the frequency of overeating (the response). The larger size believed symbolic of prowess is an example of a *positive reinforcer* because it increases the response of overeating.

In another person, overeating, (the response) might result in a larger size (consequence) perceived as grotesque (thoughts and feelings) which results in a decrease in food intake (the response). This is an example of *punishment* because it decreases the probability of the response (overeating).

Note that large size is the consequence in both examples, but in the first example is a positive reinforcer and in the second it is punishment. The two behaviors identified in obesity (i.e., the responses emitted) are overeating and underactivity. Both contribute to obesity at various times for various individuals. The important point is that although the thoughts and feelings in the two examples are different, it is not necessary to know this to decide whether large size is a positive reinforcer or punishment. Observation of the frequency of the preceding behavior (i.e., overeating or underactivity in the case of obesity) will determine whether the consequence is a positive reinforcer or punishment.

A *negatively reinforcing stimulus* is one that strengthens the response that takes it away. An example of negative reinforcement is as follows. Physical activity (the response) may remove tension (the consequence) and result in an increased frequency of physical activity. Tension is the aversive stimulus that is removed. Punishment differs from negative reinforcement in that it may be presented specifically to suppress a response (for example, spanking a dog who has jumped on the couch is designed to decrease the frequency of the jumping). In punishment, it is possible that no consequence may be apparent to the organism responding. In Figure 8.6, the four possibilities that may occur are diagrammed. A behavior may produce a positive consequence increasing the behavior, i.e., positive reinforcement. The behavior

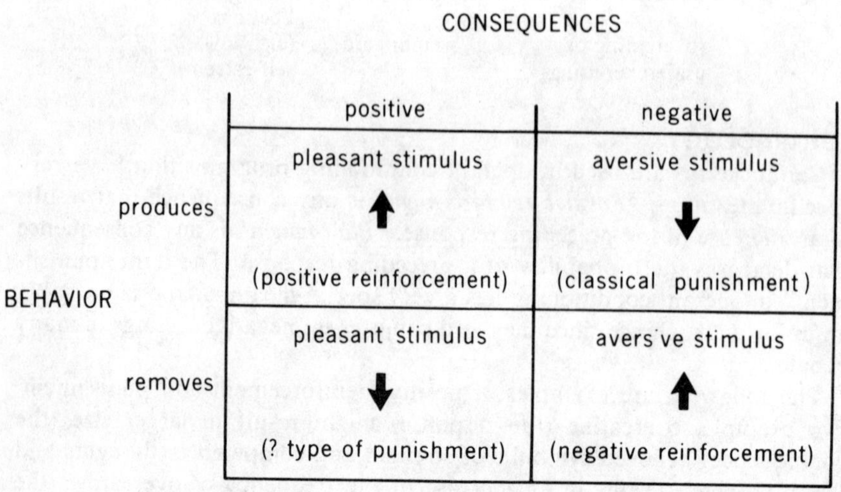

Figure 8.6. Operant conditioning model.

may produce a negative consequence resulting in a decrease in behavior, i.e., punishment. Or a behavior may remove a positive consequence (a type of punishment, but not the classical punishment as described by most behaviorists) and result in a decrease in the behavior. Or, finally, a behavior may remove a negative consequence, resulting in an increase in the behavior, i.e., negative reinforcement.

APPLICATION TO EATING BEHAVIOR

Hagan[72] has applied operant conditioning principles to eating and activity. Figure 8.7 details the possibilities for eating and activity. Eating may produce a positive consequence (for example, good taste) which serves as a positive reinforcement and increases the response, i.e., eating, which may result in obesity. Likewise, eating may produce a negative consequence (for example, abdominal discomfort) and result in a decrease in eating. Eating may remove a positive consequence (for example, feeling alert) and lead to a decrease in eating. Or, eating may remove an unpleasant state (for example, anxiety) and lead to an increase in eating. This last example has dominated the psychoanalytic theories of obesity which postulate that overeating removes tension. Or, in operant conditioning terms, overeating is perpetuated or increased because removal of the unpleasant affective state is a negative reinforcer. As Hagan and others have pointed out, however, there is no reason to presume that this is necessarily the case. It may be that the pleasure of eating is a greater positive reinforcement for obese people than for the non-obese. There is some evidence that obese subjects continue to find sweet foods more palatable after greater consumption than do the non-obese.

In many obese subjects, probably both factors are important to an increase in eating: eating probably produces pleasant feelings that lead to positive reinforcement and removes negative consequences, resulting in an increase in eating.

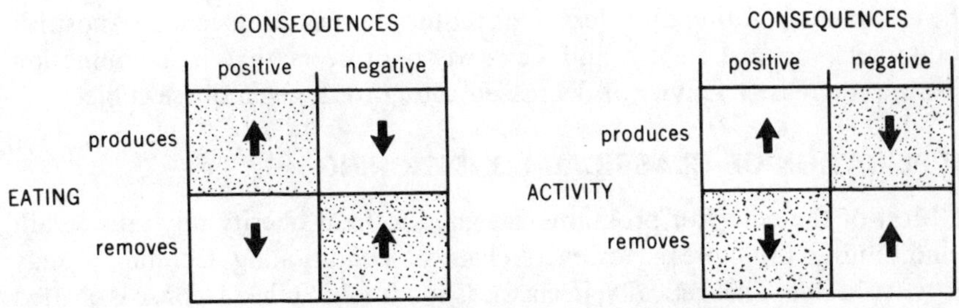

Figure 8.7. Operant conditioning model applied to obesity. Overeating and lack of activity are the two target behaviors in obesity. The diagram illustrates the possible results of positive or negative consequences on eating and activity. The shaded boxes indicate changes in behavior predicted to result in obesity.

APPLICATION TO EXERCISE PATTERNS

Similarly, activity may produce unpleasant consequences for the obese subject (for example, shortness of breath) leading to a decrease in activity and subsequent weight gain. Or, activity may remove some of the positive aspects of an obese person's life (for example, attention, sympathy) leading to a decrease in activity. Conversely, activity may produce positive feelings (for example, sense of accomplishment) resulting in an increase in activity. Or activity may remove an unpleasant, negative consequence (for example, anxiety) and result in an increase in activity.

USEFULNESS OF OPERANT CONDITIONING

In any given obese subject, many of the reinforcers are present, influencing the probability of the major behavioral responses (overeating or lack of activity). The greatest contribution that behaviorists have made is to emphasize actual observation of the patient's target behavior and the consequences that follow. Understanding this aspect of a person's functioning may allow the therapist and patient to be aware of unconscious thoughts or feelings. For example, if a patient states that activity results in positive feelings, yet decreases activity with subsequent weight gain, other reinforcers or punishment are probably operant and must be identified.

Behavior modification has been used extensively in the treatment of the eating disorders as discussed in Chapter 12. Operant conditioning using positive reinforcement to increase adaptive behavior (for example, eating slower) has been the major method investigated. "Punishment" has been largely avoided for several reasons. First, Skinner and others have feared dehumanization if aversive stimuli are used to suppress behavior. Behavior therapy has been thought by some to be a form of "thought control" or "brainwashing" and may indeed have been used as such in certain situations. However, correctly understood in the context of a therapeutic cooperative doctor-patient relationship, behavior modification can be a powerful tool in the treatment of eating disorders. This requires judicious selection of positive reinforcers, "punishment," and negative reinforcers that in combination result in increased activity or decreased eating for a given obese subject.

APPLICATION OF CLASSICAL CONDITIONING

Most of the behavior programs designed to treat obesity rely on operant conditioning principles. However, classical conditioning techniques may prove valuable. Theoretically, in classical conditioning the response is elicited by the stimulus. For example, food in the mouth (stimulus) results in salivation (response). In operant conditioning there are at the beginning no special stimuli which evoke the response; rather, the response is emitted voluntarily and then reinforced or punished. Eating behaviors undoubtedly include both reflex and voluntary responses and both the classical and operant conditioning paradigms may be useful in different situations.

CASE REPORTS

In summary, a variety of factors may contribute to any given patient's obesity, and a careful understanding of possible predisposing psychodynamic factors, maladaptive behavior patterns, and family interactions will enable the physician to design a treatment program tailored to the patient's needs.

CASE 1: OBESITY AND PERSONALITY DISORDER

In some patients, obesity may be but one of many factors contributing to the development of severe psychiatric problems. The following case exemplifies this situation.

Sarah is a 17-year-old obese white girl from a lower middle class family who was admitted to the hospital after complaining that she was frightened of devils and of a "gray man" who wanted her to go with him. She weighs 185 pounds and is 5 feet 2 inches tall. During childhood she was an unpopular girl and suffered "horrible nightmares". In early adolescence (age 11) she had an excessive weight gain, began using drugs, was truant from school, and had a boyfriend who also skipped school and used drugs. At age 12 this boyfriend was killed in a car accident and she withdrew even from dyssocial activities and began blaming others for his accident. She took an overdose of drugs and during a subsequent psychiatric evaluation tried to jump out of her psychiatrist's seventh floor office window. She was hospitalized for 7 months but remembered little of this hospitalization. A few days after discharge she again took an overdose and was readmitted. The pattern of long hospitalizations and quick readmissions continued until age 16 when she states "she received Jesus Christ," found the Pentacostal Church, and started Bible College. During the stormy year at the College she had bizarre activity (e.g. walking down the middle of the highway in a nightgown saying she was waiting to strangle someone) and began to complain of seeing devils. She was eventually hospitalized and during hospitalization she was assaultive to patients and staff and unpredictably one night set fire to her mattress. She was transferred to a state hospital and finally discharged and is currently in long-term intensive psychotherapy and group therapy. The diagnosis was severe hysterical personality with periodic psychotic episodes.[73]

CASE 2: OBESITY SECONDARY TO DEPRESSION

In some patients obesity is clearly secondary to a well-defined psychiatric disorder. Appetite disturbance and weight changes are very characteristic of depression and although it is more likely to result in weight loss, weight gain can occur. The following depressed patient gained 50 pounds following the death of her husband.

Mrs. Smith is a 68-year-old widow whose chief complaint was crying spells. Her husband had died suddenly 2 years earlier a few days after a quarrel during which he threatened to divorce her. At the time he developed chest pain his physician could not be immediately located and there was some delay in getting to the Emergency Room. He died a few hours later. On the day of the funeral Mrs. Smith and her son argued over the disposition of insurance funds. In the ensuing weeks she spent most of her time attending to financial matters and didn't grieve. Two months after her husband's death she started to have difficulty concentrating, woke early in the morning, cried easily and felt sad. She had difficulty getting started in the morning. She noticed that in the evenings when she was alone she would eat more to console herself. Backaches from a previous car injury worsened. She tired easily and stopped going to her usual activities. She began to ruminate about her relationship with her husband and felt guilty about the last quarrel with him. She was angry with their doctor and felt her husband's life might have been saved if the doctor had been available. She wanted her sons to spend more time with her and was resentful and hurt when they stayed with their families. At the time she sought psychiatric help she had gained 50 pounds and weighed 224 pounds. She said she was too religious to kill herself but sometimes wished she would have an accident.

She was briefly hospitalized and started on tricyclics. She began to talk about her feelings about her husband and gradually her mood improved. After several weeks of psychotherapy she was able to participate in her usual activities and had more realistic expectations of her sons. She then began a behavior modification program to lose weight. She arranged to eat her breakfast and dinner with friends and scheduled activities for the evening to prevent overeating. She set weekly weight goals and chose rewards for achieving these goals. After 3 months she has lost 15 pounds. She has fewer backaches and is confident of her ability to continue to lose weight.

In this patient overeating was related to her feelings of loneliness and isolation following the death of her husband. The treatment of her severe depression was of primary importance and only after resolution of the major depressive symptoms was consideration of her obesity appropriate. An increase in appetite may have contributed to her weight gain, but probably the major contributing factor was her need to console herself with food.

REFERENCES

1. Freud S: Three essays on the theory of sexuality (1905). In: The Complete Works of Sigmund Freud, vol 7. London, Hogarth Press, 1953, pp 125–245.
2. Monello LF, Mayer J: Obese adolescent girls. An unrecognized "minority" group? Am J Clin Nutr 13: 35–39, 1963.
3. Stunkard A, Mendelson M: Obesity and the body image. I. Characteristics of disturbances in the body image of some obese persons. Am J Psychiatry 123: 1296–1300, 1967.
4. Mayer J: Inactivity as a major factor in adolescent obesity. Ann NY Acad Sci 131: 502–506, 1965.
5. Head H: Studies in Neurology. London, Oxford Press, 1920.
6. Schilder P: The Image and Appearance of the Human Body. Studies in the Constructive Energies of the Psyche. London, Kegan Paul, 1935.
7. Paré A: The Workes of That Famous Chirurgion, Ambrose Parey, translated out of the Latin and compared with the French by T Johnson. London, Cotes, 1649.
8. Gerstmann J: Psychological and phenomenological aspects of disorders of the body image. J Nerv Ment Dis 126: 499–512, 1958.
9. Babinski, cited in Gerstmann J: Psychological and phenomenological aspects of disorders of the body image. J Nerv Ment Dis 126: 505, 1958.

10. Langworthy OR: Development of behavior patterns and myelinization of the nervous system in the human fetus and infant. Contrib Embryol 443: 1–57, 1933.
11. Chapman J: The early symptoms of schizophrenia. Br J Psychiatry 112: 225–251, 1966.
12. Bruch H: Eating Disorders: Obesity, Anorexia Nervosa and the Person Within. New York, Basic Books Inc, 1973.
13. Mendelson M: Psychological aspects of obesity. Med Clin North Am 48: 1373–1385, 1964.
14. Russell EW, Neuringer C, Goldstein G: Assessment of Brain Damage: A Neuropsychological Key Approach. New York, Wiley-Interscience, 1970.
15. Hirsch SJ: Left, right and identity. Arch Gen Psychiatry 14: 84–88, 1966.
16. Wright GH: The names of the parts of the body: a linguistic approach to the study of the body image. Brain 79: 188–210, 1956.
17. Halmi KA, Goldberg SC, Cunningham S: Perceptual distortion of body image in adolescent girls: distortion of body image in adolescence. Psychol Med 7: 253–257, 1977.
18. Stunkard A, Burt V: Obesity and the body image. II. Age at onset of disturbances in the body image. Am J Psychiatry 123: 1443–1447, 1967.
19. Guinness Book of World Records. Ed 16. McWhirter N. (ed). Des Plaines, Ill. Bantam, 1978.
20. Lorenz K: "Imprinting" the object of instinctive social reactions. In: Instinctive Behavior. Schiller CH (ed). New York, International Universities Press, 1957, pp 102–110.
21. MacGregor FC, Abel TM, Bryt A, et al: Facial Deformities and Plastic Surgery: A Psychological Study. Springfield, Ill, Charles C Thomas, 1953.
22. Schonfeld WA: Gynecomastia in adolescence: effect on body image and personality adaptation. Psychosom Med 24: 379–389, 1962.
23. Crisp AH, Kalucy RS: Aspects of the perceptual disorder in anorexia nervosa. Br J Med Psychol 47: 349–361, 1974.
24. Stratton CM: Vision without inversion of retinal image. Psychol Rev 4: 341–360, 463–481, 1897.
25. Simmel ML: Conditions of occurrence of phantom limbs. Proc Am Phil Soc 102: 492–500, 1958.
26. Kolb LC: Disturbances in the body image. In American Handbook of Psychiatry, Ed 2, vol. 4. S Arieti (ed). New York, Basic Books, 1975, pp 810–837.
27. Slade PD: Awareness of body dimensions during pregnancy: an analogue study. Psychol Med 7: 245–252, 1977.
28. Slade PD, Russell GFM: Awareness of body dimensions in anorexia nervosa: cross-sectional and longitudinal studies. Psychol Med 3: 188–199, 1973.
29. Glucksman ML, Hirsch J: The response of obese patients to weight reduction: the perception of body size. Psychosom Med 31: 1–7, 1969.
30. Powers PS, Holland P, Miller C, Powers HP: Transswitching of conditioned responses to food cues in obese human subjects. In preparation.
31. Levy DM: Method of integrating physical and psychiatric examination with special studies of body interest, overt protection response to growth and sex difference. Am J Psychiatry 9: 121–194, 1929.
32. Simonson M: Lecture at Conference: The Management of Obesity. Johns Hopkins Medical Institutions, Feb 13–16, 1978.
33. Machover K: Personality Projection in the Drawing of the Human Figure. Springfield, Ill, Charles C Thomas, 1957.
34. Harris DB: Children's Drawings as Measures of Intellectual Maturity. New York, Harcourt, Brace & World, 1963.
35. Swensen CH: Empirical evaluations of human figure drawings. Psychol Bull 70: 20–44, 1968.
36. Koppitz EM: Psychological Evaluation of Children's Human Figure Drawings. New York, Grune & Stratton, 1968.
37. Nathan S: Body image in chronically obese children as reflected in figure drawings. J Pers Assess 37: 456–463, 1973.
38. Bailey WL, Shinedling MM, Payne IR: Obese individuals' perception of body image. Percept Mot Skills 31: 617–618, 1970.
39. Traub AC, Orbach J: Psychophysical studies of body image. Arch Gen Psychiatry 11: 53–66, 1974.

40. Garner DM, Garfinkel PE, Stancer HC, Moldofsky H: Body image disturbances in anorexia nervosa and obesity. Psychosom Med 38: 327–336, 1976.
41. Bender MB: Disorders in Perception. Springfield, Ill; Charles C Thomas, 1952.
42. Asch SE, Witkin HA: Studies in space orientation. II. Perception of the upright and displaced visual fields and with body tilted. J Exp Psychol 38: 455–477, 1948.
43. Fisher S, Cleveland SE: Body Image and Personality. Princeton, NJ, D Van Nostrand, 1958.
44. Moore ME, Stunkard A, Srole L: Obesity, social class, and mental illness. JAMA 181: 138–142, 1962.
45. Weinberg N, Mendelson M, Stunkard A: A failure to find distinctive personality features in a group of obese men. Am J Psychiatry 117: 1035–1037, 1961.
46. Atkinson RM, Ringuette EL: A survey of biographical and psychological features in extraordinary fatness. Psychol Med 29: 121–133, 1967.
47. Johnson SF, Swenson WM, Gastineau CF: Personality characteristics in obesity; relation of MMPI profile and age of onset of obesity to success in weight reduction. Am J Clin Nutr 29: 626–632, 1976.
48. Pomerantz AS, Greenberg I, Blackburn GL: MMPI profiles of obese men and women. Psychol Rep 41: 731–734, 1977.
49. Crisp AH, McGuiness B: Jolly fat; relation between obesity and psychoneurosis in general population. Br Med J 1: 7–9, 1975.
50. Hammer SL, Campbell MM, Campbell VA, et al.: An interdisciplinary study of adolescent obesity. J Pediatr 80: 373–383, 1972.
51. Sallade J: A comparison of the psychological adjustment of obese vs. non-obese children. J Psychosom Res 17: 89–96, 1973.
52. Glucksman ML, Hirsch J: The response of obese subjects to weight reduction: a clinical evaluation of behavior. Psychosom Med 30: 1–11, 1968.
53. Glucksman ML, Hirsch J, McCully RS, et al.: The response of obese patients to weight reduction. II. A quantitative evaluation of behavior. Psychosom Med 30: 359–373, 1968.
54. Hirsch J: The psychological consequences of obesity. In: Obesity in Perspective. Bray GA (ed). Fogarty International Center Series on Preventive Medicine. Vol II, Pt 2, Washington, DC, US Government Printing Office, 1976.
55. Robinson S, Winnik H: Severe psychotic disturbances following crash diet weight loss. Arch Gen Psychiatry 29: 559–562, 1973.
56. Stunkard AJ, Rush J: Dieting and depression re-examined: a critical review of reports of untoward responses during weight reduction for obesity. Ann Intern Med 81: 526–533, 1974.
57. Shipman WG, Plesset MR: Anxiety and depression in obese dieters. Arch Gen Psychiatry 8: 530–535, 1963.
58. Freud S: Anxiety and instinctual life. In: New Introductory Lectures on Psychoanalysis, Lecture XXXII. New York, Norton, 1933.
59. Hamburger WW: Emotional aspects of obesity. Med Clin North Am. Philadelphia, WB Saunders, 1951, pp 483–499.
60. Hamburger WW: The occurrence and meaning of dreams of food and eating. Psychosom Med 20: 1–16, 1958.
61. Rand CS, Stunkard AJ: Psychoanalysis and obesity. J Am Acad Psychoanal 5: 459–497, 1977.
62. Rand CS, Stunkard AJ: Obesity and psychoanalysis. Am J Psychiatry 135: 547–551, 1978.
63. Minuchin S: Families and Family Therapy. Cambridge, Harvard Univ Press, 1974, pp 240–243.
64. Wynne LC, Singer MT: Thought disorder and family relations of schizophrenics. Arch Gen Psychiatry 9: 191–198, 1963.
65. Minuchin S, Rosman BL, Baker L, Liebman R: Psychosomatic Families. Cambridge, Harvard Univ Press, 1978.
66. Fenichel O: The Psychoanalytic Theory of Neurosis. New York, WW Norton & Co Inc, pp 381–382, 1945.
67. Swanson DW, Dinello FA: Severe obesity as a habituation syndrome. Arch Gen Psychiatry 22: 120–127, 1970.

68. Expert Commission on Drugs Liable to Produce Addiction. WHO Technical Report Series No. 59, p 9 (cited in Swanson DW, Dinello FA: Severe obesity as a habituation syndrome. Arch Gen Psychiatry 22: 120–127, 1970.)
69. Pavlov IP: Conditioned Reflexes and Psychiatry. New York, International Publishers, 1941.
70. Skinner BF: The Behavior of Organisms. New York, Appleton-Century-Crofts, 1938.
71. Stuart RB, Davis B: Slim Chance in a Fat World: Behavioral Control of Obesity. Champaign, Ill, Research Press Co, 1972.
72. Hagan RL: Theories of obesity: is there any hope for order? In: Obesity: Behavioral Approaches to Dietary Management. Williams BJ, Martin S, Foreyt JP (eds). New York, Brunner-Mazel, Inc, 1976.
73. Powers PS: Weight problems in adolescence. Primary Care 3: 337–352, 1976.

CHAPTER

9

Social and Cultural Factors in Obesity

Cultural, historical, economic and political factors are enormously important in understanding obesity and the regulation of weight. Food and eating are imbued with symbolic meanings that permeate nearly every aspect of our culture: " . . . food is more than just sustenance; it is the crossroads of emotion, religion, tradition, and habit" (p 579).[1] It has been said that the history of man is only intelligible in the context of the history of food. The current abundance of food in developed countries is the consequence of a multitude of social, political, and economic forces that have developed over the centuries. In a society that encourages ever-increasing consumption of all products, including food, it may seem paradoxical that the obese are castigated and encouraged to lose weight. The roots of this paradox are found in our religious and philosophical heritage.

Anthropological studies have highlighted the different cultural attitudes toward food, eating, and obesity, and have illuminated the tenacity of these attitudes. There is abundant evidence that our society has cherished often erroneous beliefs about food, its use, and its symbolic meaning. Food faddism is rampant and myths about food ubiquitous. Projects undertaken by the World Health Organization and the United Nations to decrease malnutrition have demonstrated that changing a traditional food practice is extremely difficult and fraught with unexpected hazards. Understanding the cultural reasons underlying food habits increases the chance of successful intervention. Any major change influences society in numerous, often unpredictable ways. For example, television has dramatically influenced mass communication and drastically altered food preferences, particularly of the young. These cultural influences must be given careful consideration in any plan designed to change the currently escalating prevalence of obesity in our society.

HISTORICAL PERSPECTIVE

Probably the first major change in eating habits occurred in prehistoric times at the close of the Ice Age when man began to produce his food rather than to rely on gathering it. Nomadic tribes apparently began returning year after year to places where wild food plants grew abundantly, and then established permanent settlements. It is not known how early man learned that he could grow crops. One folk tale for children tells of women throwing seeds on the ground to thank the gods for food and then observing the growth of a patch of cereal grasses the next year when they returned to the same spot.[2] Archeologists estimate that the change to food production occurred between 40,000 and 10,000 B.C. Even during this age, when food was probably scarce, there were apparently people who would be considered obese by today's standards. The Venus of Willendorf, estimated to be 20,000 years old, has huge breasts, abdomen, and thighs (See Fig. 9.1). It has even been theorized[3] that Adam was a food gatherer prior to his fall from the Garden of Eden and that he became a food producer after tasting the forbidden fruit of the Tree of Knowledge. The strife between Cain and Abel has been interpreted[3] to symbolize the conflict between food gatherers and food producers.

GREEK INFLUENCE

Classic Greek tradition continues to influence current medical practice. Hygeia was a lovely goddess believed to watch over the health of Athens. She symbolized the belief that man could remain well if he lived according to reason, epitomized in the idea of a healthy mind in a healthy body (mens sana in corpore sana). Although concerned with health, Hygeia was not involved in the treatment of the sick. She was probably more of an abstract concept than a historical person remembered from myths, and did not really capture the imagination of the people. Aesculapius was the first physician, according to Greek legend, and gained fame by surgery and use of herbs, rather than by teaching wisdom in living. He apparently lived about the 12th century B.C. and his popularity grew until he was made a god in the 5th or 6th century B.C. Hygeia was never as popular and was relegated to a lesser role, usually as his daughter or wife. By the 3rd century B.C., Aesculapius was characterized as a young, confident god accompanied by two maidens, Panakeia and Hygeia. Panakeia became omnipotent as a healing goddess through her use of drugs; her cult is alive today in the search

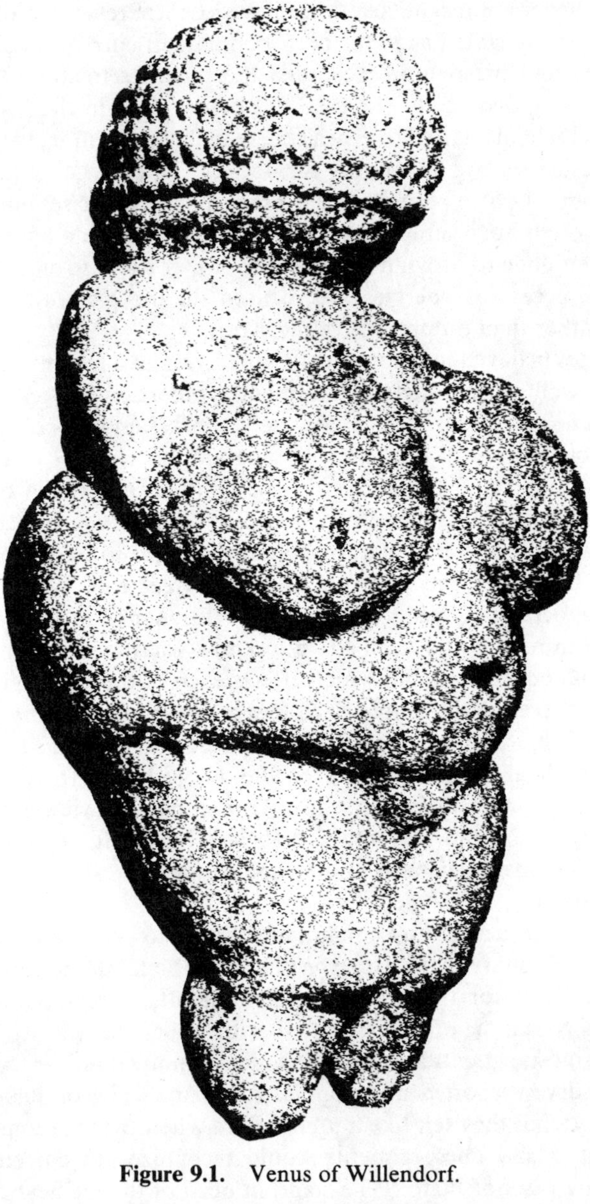

Figure 9.1. Venus of Willendorf.

for a "panacea." Liquid protein diets and "rainbow pills" are but two recent examples of attempts to locate a panacea for obesity.

Hygeia and Aesculapius symbolize two conflicting viewpoints in medicine: prevention versus treatment. Through the centuries, active treatment has always been more popular, perhaps because it is more dramatic, or perhaps because we never appreciate health until we lose it. Prevention of disease by moderation in life style has never been popular. In current medical schools more money and prestige are accorded the faculties treating disease than those preventing disease. In the case of obesity, only in the last few years have medical schools started to give a course in basic nutrition, yet prestigious surgeons lecture on bypass surgery for obesity. The physician in training is taught to counsel obese patients to eat properly and exercise, but little more is said. Although huge sums are spent yearly to investigate anorectic drugs, little has been done to provide facilities for proper exercise or eating. Just as in classic Greece, our energies are focused on the glamorous aspects of treatment rather than on preventive measures.

Hippocrates believed in the virtues of sane living in a healthy environment (Hygeia) as well as the practical treatment symbolized by Aesculapius.[4] In one aphorism, he advises, "eat moderately, work rapidly and drink wine." His was a holistic view of medicine. Throughout his writings he emphasized the need to understand the person in the context of his environment. He believed that disease was caused by a multitude of circumstances and that the sick body calls into play natural forces that tend to restore equilibrium and health. The word "physician" is from the Greek root "nature" and was used by Hippocrates to mean that every practitioner of medicine " . . . was to be skilled in nature and must strive to know what man is in relationship to food, drink, occupation and which effects each of these has on the other" (p 138).[4] Furthermore, he emphasized that a disturbance in any part of the body resulted in a disturbance of the whole person: " . . . to heal even an eye, one must heal the head and even the whole body" (p 138).[4] Perhaps nowhere in current medicine is such a comprehensive view more needed than in the treatment and prevention of obesity. Successful treatment is more likely when the obese person is understood in the context of his family, life style, and culture.

The theory that health can be maintained by following the laws of reason has led to the corollary that disease results from the failure to follow natural laws and accounts for the sense of guilt that often accompanies disease. Obesity is a condition often associated with guilt and a sense of shame. Many, if not most, patients assert that they lack "motivation" or "willpower." In a recent survey reported in a popular magazine,[5] 81% of 30,000 respondents reported that they felt like a total failure when they ate something not on their diet. Many obese patients would recognize our current society's attitude in the work of Plato:[6] "To stand in need of the medical art through sloth and intemperate diet . . . obliging the skillful sons of Asclepius (sic) to invent new names of disease, such as dropsies and catarrhs—do you not think this is abominable?"

In terms of attitude toward size and shape, the Greeks were not as stringent as is current American fashion; e.g. Homer[7] described Helen of

Troy as "the well rounded" and "of the beautiful cheeks." The Venus de Milo is a little over 5 feet in height, yet her measurements are 37-27-38, with a 22½ inch thigh and an almost 13-inch upper arm.[8] A woman this shape in American culture would probably be on a reducing diet.

The Greeks developed a great interest in cooking, and professional cooks were highly-respected, well-paid artisans. The Greeks considered a new dish as important as a new poem. In Sybaris, cooks who served the best dish at a banquet were crowned on a dais in front of the guests.[9]

ROMANS

The early Romans were frugal eaters, but later wealthy and powerful Romans developed elaborate and luxurious eating practices. Our word cereal comes from Ceres, the Roman goddess of agriculture and the harvest. Eating to excess was apparently common among wealthy dilettantes. Vomitoria have been described and Seneca wrote "men eat to vomit and vomit to eat."[10] A modern parallel can be seen in the binging-vomiting behavior of anorexia nervosa patients who often come from relatively wealthy families.

In Imperial Rome obesity was apparently rampant. Lucretius wrote in the fifth book of DeRerum Natura that "In the old days lack of food gave languishing limbs to Lethe, contrariwise today surfeit of things stifles us."[11]

The Roman rulers were alarmed by the excessive eating and periodically laws were passed to curb the excesses. Some laws limited the amount that could be spent on food, and others limited the number of guests at a dinner party. In recent times, similar sentiments about obesity have been expressed. For example, in the 1920's, Sweden attempted to levy a tax on obesity: roughly a dollar for every pound over 200 pounds.[12] Recently, Stunkard[13] has suggested tax incentives for maintaining a reasonable weight.

MIDDLE AGES

The Christian religion influenced attitudes toward eating and weight during the Middle Ages. On the one hand, obesity was considered a gift of God (and probably rather uncommon, since food was scarce and plagues rampant), but, on the other hand, gluttony was considered a venial sin. In Dante's Inferno, one of the circles of hell is devoted to gluttons.[14]

Asceticism, the religious doctrine that one can achieve a higher spiritual state by rigorous self-denial and abstinence, was commonly practiced in the Middle Ages and applied to fasting as well as chastity. The belief that devotion to an ideal and self-worth can be measured by the extent of abstinence from hedonistic pleasures, remains a common cultural thread in our society. The caricature of this belief is seen in the emaciated anorexia nervosa patient who considers herself "bad" or "sinful" if she eats a carrot stick. Abstaining from certain foods (e.g., ham or pork by Jews) is still considered evidence of devotion. Fasting is common to all religions. Probably because food was so scarce, giving or abstaining from food was one way of showing respect. In the Islam religion, the religious beliefs are called the Five Pillars of Islam; fasting is the fourth pillar. The Koran promises reward beyond bounds for fasting for God's sake.

The ascetic influence was particularly evident with the Puritans, who believed that any indulgence was sinful. The idea that overindulgence in food or alcohol is sinful is still seen in many weight-reduction groups in modern society. Louderback[15] has said that we are a society still driven by conscience and anxious about salvation, but that these concerns have been secularized into needs for social acceptance and upward mobility. Allon[16] has described the religious connotations of some group-dieting interactions. For example, many group dieters label themselves as good or bad depending on whether they have lost or gained weight. Group dieters often use religious language: sinner, saint, absolution, and diet bible. Some offer testimonials to the "ideal of thinness" and talk about "really living" for the first time in their lives. Like Alcoholics Anonymous, confessions of cheating on diets pervade the meetings. Thus, the ancient ascetic belief that abstinence can purify and cleanse the soul can still be seen, in somewhat altered form, in contemporary group dieting.

Although food was precious throughout the Middle Ages, there were some areas that remained prosperous with abundant food. For example, in the late Middle Ages, Italy was relatively affluent and Italian cooks famous. Catherine de Medici reportedly took her Italian cook with her when she left Italy for France.[17] In 1248 the King of France formed a guild for the men who roasted meats on heavy chains, La Confrerie de la Chaine de Rotisseurs.[18] Today, it remains one of the most prestigious food and wine societies in the world. Thus, gastronomy continued through the Dark Ages, albeit limited to the wealthy and powerful.

AGE OF EXPLORATIONS

The age of explorations from 1420–1620 A.D. was initiated, in part, to find spices to cover the spoiled and unpalatable flavors of meat. Columbus was looking for the Spice Islands when he landed in the new world. Vasco de Gama's spice cargo was worth 60 times what it cost to outfit his 16 ships which sailed around the Cape of Good Hope. Marco Polo told of fortunes to be made in spice trading. Eastern spices such as pepper, cloves, ginger root, nutmeg, mace, and coriander were effective in covering the flavor of spoiled meat, and became as precious as gold. In this vein, it is interesting to note that in 1968 the world's spice trade report stated that the largest user of spices was still the meat industry.[19] Thus, the taste and flavor of food, not just food for survival, has been important to man for centuries.

RENAISSANCE

During this period, Renaissance artists and writers reflected cultural attitudes toward eating and body shape. In Shakespeare's *Merchant of Venice*,[20] Nerissa said that " . . . they are as sick that surfeit with too much as they that starve with nothing." René Dubos[21] cites a story of a man alleged to have died of surfeit in 1635. This man, Thomas Parr, lived in Shropshire, England and was reported to be 152 years old. The Constable of England ordered him to London where he wined and dined with the King and died immediately. William Harvey performed the autopsy and found no abnormalities. It was declared that he died of surfeit. Thus, overeating was considered a hazard to life even in Shakespearean times.

Although overeating was considered dangerous, large women were in vogue. Renaissance artists painted women who were large and buxom. Bathsheba, painted by Rembrandt, is a large, imposing woman. Rubens painted fulsome women. It is said that to pose for Rubens the model had to weigh at least 200 pounds. Certainly by today's standards these models would be considered fat and urged to diet.

NINETEENTH CENTURY

Big women continued to be popular throughout the 19th century. Reichman[22] quotes Alexander Walker (London 1836) who wrote *Beauty Illustrated Chiefly by an Analysis and Classification of Beauty in Women*: "Her face is round . . . her shoulders are softly rounded . . . her bosom, in its luxuriance, seems literally to protrude on the space occupied by her arms; her waist, though sufficiently marked, is, as it were, encroached on by the embonpoint of all the contiguous parts, her haunches are greatly expanded; her thighs are large in proportion . . . the whole figure is soft and voluptuous in the extreme."

AGE OF CORPULENCE

Admiration of large size and voracious appetites continued until the 1920's through what has been called the Age of Corpulence in America. In the early 1900's Lillian Russell, an American actress and singer, vied with "Diamond Jim" Brady in eating contests. "Diamond Jim's" eating capacity is legend. It is said that he once reviewed a lengthy menu and told the waiter that he saw nothing to object to, and was brought and ate everything from the menu. At the turn of the century the French painters Monet, Renoir, and Toulouse-Lautrec depicted women with ample figures.

MODERN CHANGES IN ATTITUDE

After World War I, in America, there was a sudden shift to a "boyish" silhouette and an emphasis on an exaggerated slimness. "Flappers" were admired for nearly shapeless figures. With Mae West and the cinema there was a brief return to admiration of a curvacious figure. However, after World War II the trend to slimness began again. In the 1950's and 1960's extremely thin, almost emaciated models were featured in fashion magazines like *Harper's Bazaar* and *Vogue.* This trend was epitomized by the model aptly nicknamed "Twiggy" in the late 1960's. The last two decades in America have been characterized by a societal preoccupation with thinness. It has been estimated that the American public currently spends $16,000 per minute in an attempt to become fashionably thin.[23] Dieting has become big business. For example, Table 9.1 lists the books available on nutrition and dieting at a typical bookstore in a 1978 survey. Parenthetically, only one of these books was by a well recognized authority in the field of nutrition (*A Diet For Living* by Dr. Jean Mayer[24]). *Zen Macrobiotics,*[25] written by George Ohsawa, and agreed upon by experts to be a highly dangerous regimen was as easily available to the unwary consumer.

There are some recent indications that a backlash to the national obsession with slimness is developing. Isaac Rubin, author of the *Thin Book by a Formerly Fat Psychiatrist*[26] believes that the whole issue of fatness has been exaggerated in the United States. He suggests that in a land of abundant food, the elite are distinguished by extreme slenderness. *Fat and Thin: A Natural History of Obesity,*[27] by Anne Beller emphasizes the historical popularity of an ample figure. Stella Reichman presents a colorful argument against the "Think Thin Trauma" in *Great Big Beautiful Doll.*[8] The National Association to Aid Fat Americans (NAAFA) has eloquently described the rejection and disgrace experienced by many obese persons in American society.[12] Mann[28] has argued that the scientific evidence linking obesity to various serious diseases is for the most part circumstantial. Denigration of

Table 9.1
Diet and Nutrition Books available at a popular bookstore in Tampa, Florida (1978)

The Thin Game Including the Master Plan	Nutrition and Your Mind
The Compulsive Overeater	Stop Dieting! Start Losing!
The Great Nutrition Robbery	Sweet and Dangerous
Banish Those Unsightly Cellulite Bumps Forever	A Diet for Living
I Almost Feel Thin	Sugar Blues
Zen Macrobiotics	Weight Control through Yoga
Lose Pounds the Low Carbohydrate Way	Natural Foods Dieting Book
Doctor Romano's Megatetics Weight Reduction Guide	Fat Destroyer Foods: The Magic Metabolizer Diet
Fat is a Feminist Issue	The Woman Doctor's Diet for Women
From Fat to Skinny	Think Yourself Thin
Eat, Think and Be Thinner: The Weight of Life Way	Mental Health through Nutrition
Jazzercize	Fasting as a Way of Life
	The Last Chance Diet

the obese, particularly the mildly obese, may, therefore, be more on social, moral, and cultural grounds than on sound scientific medical evidence.

ANTHROPOLOGICAL VIEWPOINT

DICHOTOMY BETWEEN "RIGHT" AND "WRONG" FOODS

Anthropological studies have revealed a wide variety of eating practices and attitudes toward obesity. In some societies, young brides-to-be are purposely overfed; huge hips and thighs are particularly valued and have been given a special name, steatopygia.[29] One great advantage of cross-cultural studies is illumination of some of the cultural influences on our own eating practices, some of which may militate against health.

Margaret Mead[30] has said that in America the resistances and acceptances of food are thought of in terms of morality. People think that they ought to eat what is good for them, rather than what is palatable; and conversely, food that makes the body healthy is unpalatable. She notes that this attitude is so ingrained in our culture that it comes as a surprise to learn that many other cultures do not have this dichotomy. In many cultures, the foods believed to make people strong and healthy are the very foods that are regularly eaten and that people like to eat. In the American home both the "right" and "wrong" foods are placed on the table and the child is rewarded with good-tasting "wrong" food, for example, chocolate cake. Children are punished by having the "wrong" food taken away from them. The repetitive message is that what is delicious is an indulgence and what is good for you is unpalatable. In a recent novel attempt to change the status of a "good" food to a delicious and palatable food, one television advertisement emphasized that eating green vegetables is an indulgence. In our society where food choice is a moral decision, people will probably never joyously and unquestioningly eat the best food that nutritional science can provide.

CHILD-REARING PRACTICES

Mead believes that resistance to changing food habits is related to child-rearing practices. If food was intimately associated with warmth and loving, food comes to symbolize affection, and any change in food habits is difficult. In other cultures, food may be a private affair. For example, in some parts of Melanesia and Polynesia the rule is that men and women should never see each other eat.[31] In northern Arabia there is a widespread notion that one should not be seen to eat by anybody.[32] In the United States there are widespread differences in eating practices and attitudes toward obesity. In some ethnic groups large size is synonymous with strength and prowess. Loss of weight to what most physicians would consider normal weight might be considered hazardous to health by such groups. These cultural attitudes are not negligible and must be considered if change is to be effected.

DEFINITION OF FOOD

Even what is defined as food is culturally determined. The Ifugao of the Phillipine Islands regard dragonflies as human food.[33] They eat three species of the dragonfly, as well as locusts which are boiled, dried, powdered, and stored as food. They fry crickets and flying ants in lard. Although milk is considered a nutritious food item in the United States, there are some societies that regard it with disgust as akin to a mucous discharge. In colonial America, wild greens, like dandelion and cowslip were considered animal fodder; some cultural groups consider these green vegetables a delicacy today. Food preparation and serving is also dictated by society. For example, in Peru foods are classified as "hot" or "cold" and hot foods are appropriate only for certain occasions. Wellin[34] describes resistance toward boiling water to prevent infectious disease, because it would change the classification of water from a cold to a hot food.

FOOD TABOOS

Food taboos may be based on realistic dangers or may arise from superstitions, myths, or folk tales. Certain foods may symbolize evil or uncleanliness. Avoidance of food may result in an increased group cohesiveness and improve survival. Rejection of food may be based on fear of disease. For example, for centuries tomatoes were believed to be poisonous. The reason that pork was rejected by the early Jews, Moslems, and Hindus is not known, but may have been related to the fact that the pig was a scavenger and suspected of harboring disease. Although the relationship between uncooked pork and trichinosis is well known today, probably early man did not know of this relationship.

Many of the cultural restrictions on food are connected with sex and reproduction. Among the Zulus, milk cannot be drunk by pregnant, lactating, or menstruating women and preferably not at all after pubescence.[35] The origin of this food taboo is the Zulu belief that the reproductive function of women is somehow dangerous to the welfare of cattle and that cattle might be affected adversely through the medium of milk. In other cultures some foods are taboo for fathers, or prospective fathers, or for boys entering adolescence. Or, only certain members of a society may be permitted to eat a particular food; for example, among the Murngin of Australia, only men who are fathers may eat porcupine, snake eggs, or crayfish.[36]

Whatever the origin of the food taboo, it may have a potent influence on the eating behavior of a culture. In *African Notebook*,[37] Schweitzer describes cases in which individuals unwittingly broke a food taboo and died within a day. Some group dieters in America regard fatty foods as taboo. The anorexia nervosa patient who is terrified of eating anything that contains fat may be but an extention of our cultural obsession with slenderness and the erroneous belief that fat is taboo.

Although some food habits and food taboos may appear strange or irrational, it is usually wise to consider the consequences of any widespread belief about food. For example, centuries ago, burnt sponge was recommended for goiter; only later was it learned that it contained iodine. The English fed limes to sailors suffering from scurvy, and not until centuries later was a deficiency of vitamin C identified as the cause of scurvy.

THEORY OF HUMAN NEEDS (MASLOW)

One method of evaluating the function of food in a society is Maslow's theory of human needs.[38] He classifies human needs into (1) physiological needs, (2) safety or security needs, (3) belongingness and loving needs, (4) esteem or status needs, and (5) self-actualization needs. The idea behind this theory of human motivation is that a minimum satisfaction of one need is necessary before the person can move up to seek satisfaction of the next need in the hierarchy (See Fig. 9.2).

PHYSIOLOGICAL NEED FOR FOOD

Hunger, defined as an urgent need for food, is a crucial physiological need. The need for food dominates a hungry man's entire existence. Maslow has said, "For the man who is extremely and dangerously hungry, no other interest exists except food . . . he dreams about food, he remembers food, he thinks about food, he emotes only about food, he perceives only food, and he wants only food."[39] For the hungry person, culture, politics, family and friends are irrelevant. An interest in the welfare of others is impossible if one is physiologically hungry.

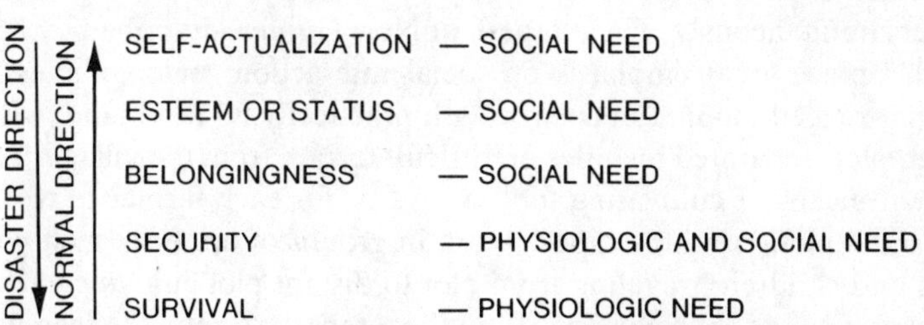

Figure 9.2. Maslow's theory of human needs (adapted from Lowenberg[2]).

SAFETY OR SECURITY NEEDS

The next need in Maslow's hierarchy is the need for safety or security. In terms of food, this means knowing where your next meal is coming from. As the economic situation of the individual improves, he may move upward in the hierarchy to the security level, which represents both a physiological need and a social need.

Individuals can quickly be reduced to survival strategies in searching for food. For example, one woman describes a harrowing escape from starvation during World War II in Nazi Germany. Although she now has an abundant food supply, holds a prestigious position at a university, and often prepares gourmet meals, threats to self-esteem result in a return to the security level and she stockpiles food in cabinets and refrigerators.

In times of disaster, or threatened disaster, man quickly reverts to the security or survival stage. Forecasts of war or nuclear holocausts, such as in the civil defense movement in the 1960's in the United States, resulted in millions storing food in shelters.

BELONGINGNESS NEEDS

After the survival and security needs are met, food is used to meet the needs for belongingness and affection. Food can be used to promote interpersonal acceptance; "breaking bread" with friends has a long cultural history. In fact, inviting friends to visit, but failing to provide food and drink, is considered inhospitable. For centuries, food has been given to signify friendship. Usually such gifts are difficult to prepare or to obtain and range from homemade preserves to exotic elaborate packages. Gifts of food are particularly common at Christmas. Gourmet magazines feature expensive foods that can be ordered and family magazines give detailed instructions for preparation of elaborate foods. Food is important at funerals and may symbolize sympathy for the grieving relatives. The offering of "chicken soup" to someone who is unhappy may be a genuine attempt to console and to include that person in a caring and cohesive group.

In some situations the needs for survival, safety, and belongingness may be met simultaneously. The Arapesh of New Guinea, described by Margaret Mead,[40] place great emphasis on social interaction (belongingness). They live in a rugged mountainous area with practically no level land, with small garden plots separated by miles of difficult terrain from the village. The most efficient means of cultivating food would be for each farmer to work alone on a small plot, but the Arapesh work in groups of up to six men with their wives and children, traveling from plot to distant plot enjoying each other's company and the sharing of work. In the Arapesh society, the men will carry coconut saplings miles to plant them on the house sites of others and will hunt only to give their kill away, since the lowest form of humanity is the person who eats his own kill. Thus, everything that is eaten is the product of social interaction.

Another similar example is found among the Hopi Indians in the Southwestern United States and Mexico.[41] Corn functions as food, but is also an integral part of the entire religious cycle of ceremonies that is bound to the growing cycle of the corn. To be considered a member of the Hopi tribe, a baby must have corn during the first hazardous 20 days of life. Corn (maize), then, is a symbol of love, affection, and belongingness.

ESTEEM OR STATUS NEEDS

The fourth level in the hierarchy is the need for esteem or status. Certain foods may be visible evidence of rank or high status. Foods that are expensive, difficult to obtain or prepare are the ones most likely to be used in obtaining status. For example, in the United States, steak or lobster tail is expensive and may be the dinner of choice when improvement in social status is sought. Gifts of food or invitations to meals may be used to promote esteem or increase status. Food may symbolize a family's wealth. For example, in Ruanda, the Urundi reportedly keep cattle not for meat or milk, but as a bank account.

Status needs may predominate over wise nutritional practices. For example, whole wheat bread has always been considered more nutritious, but during the Middle Ages and the Renaissance in England, white bread was scarce and more expensive, and was preferred. There is even an old saying: "the whiter the bread, the sooner you're dead." Nevertheless, white bread continued to be prestigious until recently, when dark bread has become more expensive and sometimes difficult to obtain and consequently often more prized.

Feasts and festivals may meet both the needs for belongingness and esteem or status. Tiberius Caesar, one of the late Roman emperors, wrote a cookbook in which he discussed 17 ways to cook suckling pig and reportedly he committed suicide after spending 100 million sesterces on food and had only 10 million left.[42] In America, the Northwest Coast Indians feasted frequently. The potlatch was a huge feast to which a chief invited both friends and enemies to demonstrate how powerful he and his tribe were. These feasts became very competitive as rival tribes strove to attain superior status. Today, cooking contests and gourmet clubs may serve to increase the esteem of the cooks as well as meet self-actualization needs, the fifth level described by Maslow. An exotic, expensive meal requiring hours of preparation may increase the esteem and status of a gourmet club member as well as express his or her creativity.

Classification of Foods Reflect Status

Even the classification of edible materials is intricately associated with status considerations. The Committee on Food Habits of the National Research Council[43] noted that food is classified as inedible; edible by animals; edible by people, but not my kind of people; edible by people like me; and edible by myself. For example, clay is considered inedible by most people, but believed to be a required nutrient by some pregnant women in the Southeastern United States. Powdered dragonflies may seem unappetizing to us, yet are a staple food item for the Ifugao. Bacon and eggs for breakfast is perfectly acceptable for many Americans, but anathema to traditional Jews and consumption would result in a rapid decline in status and esteem.

Political Power of Food

Food is also used to influence the behavior of others, i.e., to meet power needs. Increasing power is one way of increasing status and esteem. Perhaps the most common example is the use of food to control the behavior, emotions, or attitudes of children. Food, especially sweets, may be used to reward good behavior or may be withheld to punish unacceptable behavior. Special dinner parties may be given to influence the decisions of someone in power. "Wining and dining" is a well known ploy to influence others.

A more dramatic example is withholding of food or destruction of crops to attain political ends. For example, in Biafra in the late 1960's, hundreds of thousands died during a famine created by the Nigerian blockade aimed at weakening the Biafran military resistance. In China in 1943 in the Honan province, a country's own troops emptied the countryside of food to prevent the enemy from benefiting from available foods. The resulting famine caused the deaths of millions of people, including large numbers of children. The United States destroyed crops in South Vietnam with herbicides in the 1960's as a strategic weapon. The underlying theory is that crop destruction will eliminate rations for the troops. As Mayer[44] has noted, however, it is invariably the children who suffer and die first.

In the United States in the 1960's, farmers were paid by the government to let fields lie fallow, so that the grain supplies would not be a glut on the international market and decrease profits from grain sales. Meanwhile, about one-seventh of the world's population was starving or severely undernourished. In the Civil War, during Sherman's notorious March to the Sea, his troops burned crops to weaken Southern resistance. Thus, the need for power may influence food policies that have widespread effects.

The political power of food is enormous. The intimate relationship between food distribution and politics does much to explain the seemingly anomalous position of the Nutrition Committee in the United States Department of Agriculture. It has been argued that this committee should be in the Department of Health, Education and Welfare, where problems of overnutrition and undernutrition could best be studied. However, in the overall world view of nutrition problems, the Department of Agriculture may be the correct organization.

SELF-ACTUALIZATION NEEDS

The fifth level in Maslow's hierarchy refers to self-actualization needs. In terms of food, at this stage the person may devise a new recipe or serve exotic food or attempt to prepare dishes which require complex procedures and equipment. The gourmet cook may be meeting his needs for self-actualization. Of course, if high-calorie meals are prepared and eaten very often, obesity may result. Historically, both the Greeks and the Romans used cooking to express creativity. During the time of Pericles in the Greek Golden Age about 20 cookbooks were produced. Archestratus produced *Gastrology* in 350 B.C., which included recipes he had collected in his travels; some of the recipes are still in use today.[45] Also, in the old Greek plays, cooks gave out recipes over the footlights. Cooking was considered an art then, as now. Modern bookstores have entire sections devoted to cookbooks that range from preparation of simple, nutritious meals to the creation of elaborate banquets. Chefs may become famous television personalities, such as James Beard or Julia Child. The creative use of food to meet self-actualization needs, however, requires that physiological need for food as well as the need for security, belongingness, and status be met first or simultaneously.

SYMBOLIC MEANING OF FOOD

LANGUAGE

The close association between eating and the development of various aspects of our culture is symbolized in language, folklore, fairy tales and children's stories. As Cameron[46] has noted, humans regularly use the techniques they develop for satisfying physiological needs to meet biosocial needs that are only indirectly, or symbolically, related to the physiological need. In *The Psychology of Behavior Disorders* he says:

> "Our language is full of ambiguous illusions to social acceptance and rejection, to verbal assaults, to gastric need for food and to the spiritual need for sustenance. Thus, we eat our words and swallow our wrath, the Lord spews us forth, we sink our teeth into a problem, drink in a message, find an explanation indigestible, and reject with biting comments. When the human being, with all his verbal ambiguities and his behavior, becomes confused, he often acts out as social operations what was intended to be only verbal metaphors."

In American slang, even people are classified according to food. Thus, a "hot tomato" is a sexy woman, the "apple of my eye" is a preferred (usually young) person; "fruit cake" is a person with bizarre or unusual behavior; and a "vegetable" is an incompetent, often comatose, person. Our feelings or attitudes about a person may be expressed in cooking terms: a person may be "boiling mad" or "burned up" (with anger) or may have opinions that are "half-baked." Our verbal repertoire includes similies comparing physical or personality attributes to food: a person may have a "peaches and cream" skin, a "face as red as a beet," "a mouth like cherries," or "may look good enough to eat." Some proverbs use food or eating symbolically. For example, "don't cry over spilt milk" means: don't worry about what can't be changed. The symbolic use of food terms may be used for political ends. For example, in an editorial castigating bureaucratic waste, the *Washington Post* said:[47] "Of course, there is still a food problem—an enormous one. Some people in this country and many around the world are hungry, and some federal programs have gotten so rich as to be indigestible."

NURSERY RHYMES

Fairytales, children's stories, and nursery rhymes are replete with references to food, eating, and weight. A 19th century German poem (see Fig. 9.3) describes a boy who refused to eat and died.[48] This rhyme clearly communicates a direct message—one must eat to live—but also symbolizes another societal injunction, that one must partake of what is offered in life to be truly alive and aware. The negativism in the rhyme is reminiscent of anorexia nervosa patients whose need for emotional control overrides even the physiological need for food.

In the nursery rhyme "Little Jack Horner,"[49] eating is associated with morality:

Little Jack Horner
Sat in a corner
Eating a Christmas pie;
He put in his thumb
and pulled out a plum
and said, "What a good boy am I" (p 53).[49]

Some children even learn their alphabet through the medium of food, as in the nursery rhyme, "A as an apple pie." The origin of the "clean plate club" in which children are encouraged to finish every bite, may be from the nursery rhyme, "Jack Sprat":

Jack Sprat could eat no fat
His wife could eat no lean
And so between them both you see,
They licked the platter clean (p 66).[49]

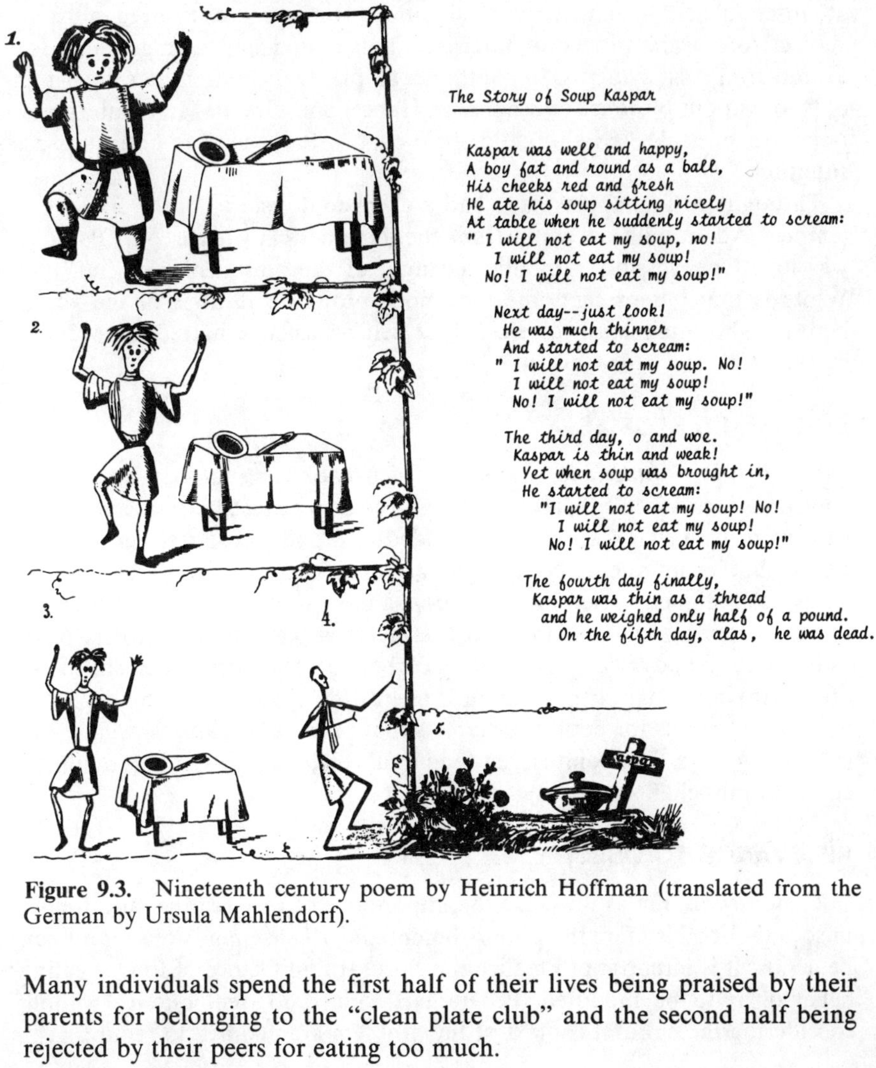
1.
2.
3.
4.
5.
The Story of Soup Kaspar
Kaspar was well and happy,
A boy fat and round as a ball,
His cheeks red and fresh
He ate his soup sitting nicely
At table when he suddenly started to scream:
" I will not eat my soup, no!
I will not eat my soup!
No! I will not eat my soup!"
Next day--just look!
He was much thinner
And started to scream:
" I will not eat my soup. No!
I will not eat my soup!
No! I will not eat my soup!"
The third day, o and woe.
Kaspar is thin and weak!
Yet when soup was brought in,
He started to scream:
"I will not eat my soup! No!
I will not eat my soup!
No! I will not eat my soup!"
The fourth day finally,
Kaspar was thin as a thread
and he weighed only half of a pound.
On the fifth day, alas, he was dead.
Kaspar

Figure 9.3. Nineteenth century poem by Heinrich Hoffman (translated from the German by Ursula Mahlendorf).

Many individuals spend the first half of their lives being praised by their parents for belonging to the "clean plate club" and the second half being rejected by their peers for eating too much.

FAIRY TALES

There are numerous references to food and eating in fairy tales. For example, the wicked stepmother gives Snow White a poisoned apple, an action rich in symbolic meaning. Bettelheim[50] suggests that the symbolism in fairy tales is interpreted differently by children as a means of resolving current emotional conflicts. He believes that the reason fairy tales have survived for centuries is because they speak directly to the unconscious problems faced in childhood. Since children have a wide variety of conflicts at different ages and in varying situations, the symbolism used must be subject to a wide variety of interpretations. Food and eating are classic examples of such symbols. In another example, two children literally eat an old woman out of house and home in Hansel and Gretel. Many interpretations are possible and the child may choose the one that best suits his situation.

Throughout time apples have had a checkered history. In the Bible, Eve tempted Adam with an apple from the Tree of Knowledge, and Paradise was lost. One possible symbolic meaning of the poisoned apple in Snow White is that it represents the venomous projected feelings of the young heroine who must learn to reject these self-destructive hatreds in order to mature.

CHILDREN'S STORIES

In *Alice in Wonderland*,[51] one bite of a cookie resulted in an instant, enormous increase in size, and drinking from a vial caused instant shrinkage. This work by Lewis Carroll was intended as a political satire. Perhaps one reason that it continues to be so popular a century later, is that the symbolism lends itself to such varied interpretation. For example, the sudden increase in size is reminiscent of many anorexia nervosa patients who grossly overestimate their body width after eating carbohydrates. The sudden shrinkage after drinking a vial of fluid reminds one of the wishful thinking exploited by advertisements for potions or tablets that promise a dramatic weight loss in hours or days. The point is that food and weight can be symbols of almost any cultural belief.

RELEVANCE TO OBESITY

These few examples illustrate the importance of food, eating, and weight in society. Food is more than nourishment and affects many areas of human behavior. It is important to realize the cultural significance of food if eating behavior is to be modified. Programs designed to treat obesity without considering the cultural context of the problem are doomed to failure.

INFLUENCE OF ADVERTISING

INACTIVITY AND TELEVISION

Television is a potent means of communicating information and influencing attitudes and behavior. In the area of developing food preferences and eating habits, television has had a profound effect and medical science is only now beginning to consider the consequences. Mayer[24] has repeatedly stressed that we are progressively becoming a more sedentary society. He believes that inactivity is the most important factor explaining the increase in frequency of obesity in modern society.

Television has been described as the national sport. Children probably spend at least 3 or 4 hours a day sitting in front of the television set. This obviously decreases the time a child might spend in physical activity, thus increasing the tendency toward obesity.

Television is only one of the many technological advances that result in decreased caloric expenditure. Jeffrey and Katz have given several prosaic but interesting examples.[52] For example, a secretary who uses an electric rather than a manual typewriter uses 12 fewer calories per hour (90 as opposed to 102). Over the course of a year, if she types 20 hours a week, this equals about 12,000 calories, or a gain of 3.4 pounds per year. In 10 years this would result in a 34-pound weight gain. Another everyday example is the telephone extension which reduces walking by an average of about 70 miles per year, or 6,160 calories less are expended per year. Thus, if everything else remains the same, and a telephone extension were installed at age 20, a person could gain 40 to 50 pounds by age 50, simply by not using as much energy to walk to the phone. These examples, however, are probably minor compared to the calorie excess accumulated during television watching (See Fig. 9.4). Furthermore, snacking while watching television is notorious for increasing the total daily calories ingested.

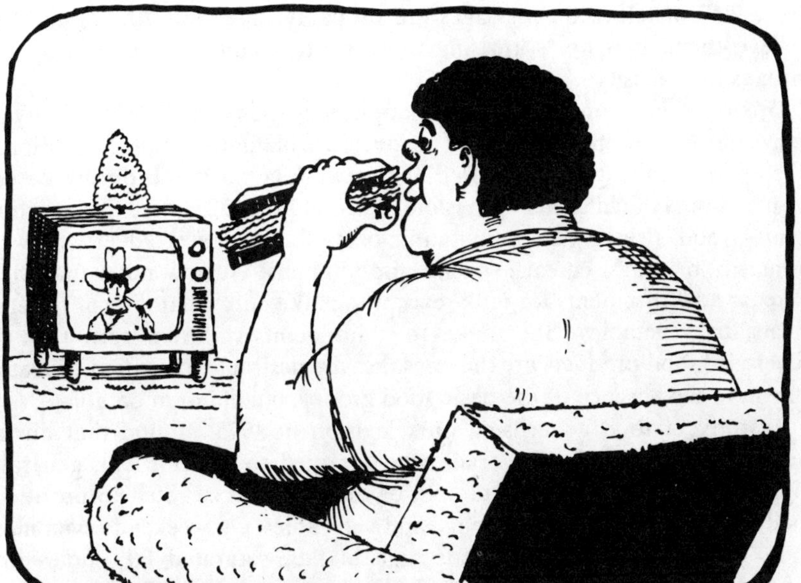

Figure 9.4. Inactivity contributes to obesity.

NUTRITIONAL VALIDITY OF TELEVISION ADVERTISEMENTS

The advent of television advertising has had a tremendous impact on the eating habits of everyone, but has probably had the most influence on the food preferences of children. Smith and colleagues[53] evaluated health information presented during a week of television and found that 70% of all health messages viewed were judged by a panel of experts to be inaccurate or misleading or both. Lewis and Lewis[54] asked two groups of fifth and sixth graders to watch "messages" on television concerned with health and illness. The children were asked to describe the messages and report their conclusions. If the message was a commercial they were asked if they or their parents had ever tried the product. More than 85% of the messages viewed were advertisements. These investigators found that about 70% of these messages were believed by the children, even though a high proportion of the messages was probably incorrect. There was a positive correlation between parental use of a product and credibility of the advertisement. Thus, if a parent used the product, the child was more likely to use the product and to believe the message. The modeling behavior of the parents seemed to be of more importance than the child's own experience with the advertised product. The actual content of the advertisement was compared to the intended message, and 90% of the students made the inferences intended by the sponsors. The implication is clear: television can and does influence behavior and attitudes of children, particularly if parents use the product. Since 70% of television messages are probably false, and 70% of children believe them, it is not surprising that nutrition education is making few inroads into obesity.

Gussow[55] has concluded from her investigations that the majority of television advertisements for food products are blatantly counter-nutritional. She and her colleagues monitored 388 network commercials during a week with 19 hours of childrens' television and found that 82% were for ingestible items—food, drink, gum, or vitamin pills. The products advertised were primarily breakfast cereals, snacks, and vitamins. Gussow notes that there were no advertisements for milk (except to make milk palatable) or for eggs, meats, or vegetables. She makes a valid point: children learn that the advertised food products are the ones that are desirable. Nutrition educators may note the absence of the basic food groups, but children do not.

A study of food advertising on television in 1975[56] found that during weekdays almost 70% of the ads were devoted to low-nutrient, generally high-calorie foods. Only about 15% of the time was devoted to nutritious food such as bread, seafood, fruits, and vegetables. On weekends even more time, 85%, was devoted to foods high in fats, saturated fat, cholesterol, refined and processed sugar, and salt. During the weekend, for example, no advertising was devoted to fruits or vegetables.

Recently we[57] surveyed 12 hours of children's television programs on Saturday morning from three different television stations and found no improvement from Gussow's 1972 report. More than 90% of the advertisements were for edible products. Again, breakfast foods and snacks accounted for the majority of advertisements. The overwhelming majority of advertisements were for sweet, chocolate, high-calorie food products.

Advertisers decide what to advertise, when, and to whom on the basis of anticipated profit. Nutritional considerations are rarely taken into account and then usually only when required by government regulation. In their own defense, businesses have claimed that children left to their own devices can choose a nutritious diet, and an early study is misused to prove this contention. Davis[58] offered three newly weaned infants a self-selected diet of simple natural foods. Their growth and development over the next year was judged normal. However, as Gussow[55] notes, at no time were these infants offered snack food, soda, or colored sugar breakfast cereals. Fruit Loops, Pop Tarts, and Cookie Crisps were not part of their diet. Thus, from groups of nutritious foods, these youngsters did select nutritious diets. Therefore, it cannot be concluded from this report that children will routinely choose nutritious foods from all products currently available. Furthermore, although this was an interesting well-documented study, only three children were studied.

TASTE PREFERENCES EASILY INFLUENCED

Taste preferences are established early in life and are susceptible to a variety of influences. In a 1938 study,[59] nursery school children were given a choice between a pleasant-flavored chocolate solution and a very sweet sugar solution with a medicinal flavor. Initially, the children preferred the chocolate taste. They were then read a 5-minute story in which the chocolate taste was portrayed as tasting very bad, but the overly sweet taste was preferred by the story's hero. After the story and for the next few days, the children preferred the medicinal overly sweet taste they originally disliked. Clearly, children's taste preferences can be easily influenced, particularly when the taste in question is imbued with a positive meaning. Television bombards children with nutritional messages that are not only inaccurate, but guide their taste preferences toward sweet chocolate food products. An exclusive preference for sweet-tasting high-calorie non-nutritious foods undoubtedly predisposes to obesity in childhood that may persist through adult life.

FAST FOOD RESTAURANTS

Other avenues of advertising also encourage increasing consumption of high calorie atherogenetic diets. Slogans like "Big Mac Attack" broadcasted over radio and television effectively convey the message that McDonald's hamburgers are irrestible, delicious, and addicting. Certainly several billion of these hamburgers have been consumed at a caloric cost of 1300 calories with french fries and a chocolate milk shake. McDonald's and other quick food restaurants also exploit the use of food to meet the social needs for affection and belongingness. For example, recently a McDonald's contest awarded family dinners at McDonald's, including air fare, to transport members of the group to the winner's city. The enterprise was entitled "Family Reunion." One can even register to vote at McDonald's! Clearly, these restaurants are a potent cultural force in our society.

It is possible, of course, that marketing decisions could be nutritionally wise and also be profitable. Since large numbers of people eat in restaurants, even small changes in the menus could have a dramatic effect on eating habits. Stunkard,[60] for example, has reported that a small chain in Houston, Texas has begun to list the calorie content of a few items on its menu which were selected for their limited fat content and prepared with polyunsaturated oils. There was sufficient increase in consumption of these products to induce the company to expand the number of such items available.

The ways food or food products are promoted also influence eating habits. For example, the arrangement of foods in a cafeteria line is known to influence selection. If sweet desserts are placed first in line, or at a point where the consumer must wait before paying the bill, these foods will be chosen more often. Simple reordering of the available food will result in a more nutritious selection.

VENDING MACHINES

In a mobile society that emphasizes speed and achievement, it is not surprising that fast food restaurants and vending machines are popular. Although there is nothing necessarily wrong with convenience foods, or with selling foods from vending machines, much of what is sold is sweet, high-calorie, and non-nutritious. For example, in the medical school complex at the University of South Florida, there are two vending machines. On the day of this writing, 18 of 20 offerings were sweet; the two exceptions were peanut butter crackers and "bacon smackers." Six varieties of sweet sodas were available, four types of gum, five varieties of candy, and three kinds of cookies. Three of the choices were low-calorie, but sweet: sugarless Mr. Pibb, Carefree Gum, and Tab. It is apparent that the available selections are non-nutritious and even the low-calorie selections reinforce cravings for sweets.

Some educational institutions are beginning to examine the influence of vending machines on student eating habits, along with their role in increasing the intake of high-calorie, rich foods. The Dallas School Board passed a regulation in 1975[61] that vending machines offer nutritious foods or drinks without a highly concentrated sugar base. Although this is a laudable change, the idea has not been widely implemented.

RISE IN CONSUMPTION OF SUGAR

The rise in sugar consumption exemplifies current trends in America. In the past century, the U.S. consumption of sugar has increased dramatically, while the consumption of high fiber foods has decreased substantially. In 1875, the average consumption of sugar was 40 pounds per year per capita, and in 1975 there was an increase to 120 pounds per person per year.[62] These figures give some credence to the notion that we are becoming a "nation of carboholics." Advertising that is focused almost exclusively on sweet food products promotes this tendency.

HUGE PROFITS FROM FOOD PRODUCTS

Food and beverage companies are big businesses in the United States. Advertisements alone cost 1.15 billion in 1975.[63] Profits from sales of non-nutritious foods are phenomenal. Many books are available on how to entice the customers to buy a product, whether or not he needs it, or even wants it. Only in a society characterized by abundance could the following statement be made:

> "The economy is marked not by a scarcity of goods, but by a scarcity of markets. The major problem of most firms is to find sufficient customers for their output."[64]

Creating a need or a desire for a food product is the goal and requires elaborate planning and strategic maneuvering. The selection of a brand name may be the result of chance or inspiration, but more often is the subject of intense marketing research. One group of marketing analysts note that:

> "as products, services, even companies become more alike in function and appearance, the name has assumed new significance. Often it is the sole tangible, differentiating element between one brand and another."[65]

These authors even list the principles for selecting a name that will ensure a specific, unique brand identity. For example, a name must have both sound and sight appeal. Not only must the name look good on packages and ads, but the sound of the words must convey the desired message.

Packaging products in ways that promote sales has also been carefully studied. In an article entitled "The Package as a Communication" Gardner[66] notes that a package arouses a complex set of reactions in the potential consumer. The material used, the form and shape, the colors used, and the label all influence this reaction. That emotional feelings can be evoked by colors or materials is well known. Big businesses are developing ever more sophisticated techniques for exploiting these emotional factors in order to increase profits.

PHYSICIANS UNAWARE OF POTENT INFLUENCE OF ADVERTISING

Underlying these analyses of marketing methods is the belief that a continuous increase in consumption is good for the nation as well as the individual. Not only is this belief probably fallacious, but in a nation of abundance, it is dangerous to health. Of great importance is the fact that businessmen have a much greater understanding of the cultural influences on eating habits than do physicians. Their marketing acumen often rests on solid scientific data that far outstrips the information available to a practicing physician. It is little wonder that more Americans are eating "junk food" and that physicians have little success in treating obesity.

DEHUMANIZATION

An increasingly mechanized approach to the provision of food may have profound psychological and cultural influences. For example, changes in the food service practices at the Montgomery County Detention Service in Maryland have been reported.[67] For 5 or 6 years inmates had been fed TV dinners in aluminum foil pans. During this time they regularly threw their trays against the wall in anger. When a change was made to fresh foods prepared by an inmate chef, complaints about food decreased precipitously. It was hypothesized that the taste and nutritional value of TV dinners were less important than the fact that the feeding process had become dehumanized and was, therefore, dehumanizing. The report notes that the morale improved immediately after the switch.

Bruno Bettelheim, a well known psychologist with broad experience in the care of institutionalized children, believes that the circumstances surrounding eating can profoundly influence all aspects of behavior. He says: "Eating experiences condition our entire attitude toward the world, not so much because of how nutritious is the food we are given, but because of the feelings and attitudes with which it is given."[68] In his book, *A Home for the Heart*,[69] he describes in detail the way in which food is selected, prepared and served at an institution with very severely emotionally disturbed children. The interpersonal transactions between the children and staff concerning the food are considered an integral part of the therapeutic process. For example, whereas many institutions use plastic dinnerware to avoid breakage, Bettelheim's group selected china dinnerware with the youngsters and noticed that there was less breakage. The children felt that the decision about the dinnerware was partly theirs and, therefore, the china was valuable to them as well as to the staff. The attitude that this was a home in which food was served lovingly, rather than mechanically, was part of their treatment program. Also, the entire staff, including the top of the hierarchy, take their meals together. Bettelheim remarks that the entire social climate changes when everyone eats together. Violent outbreaks are less frequent and the interpersonal relationships improve between all members of the group, therapists and patients alike. Nothing is more divisive than when people eat a different fare, in different rooms. In this vein, it is worth noting that some of the worst race riots have evolved around who can eat where. Thus, the attitudes toward food and eating permeate our entire lives and are intimately associated with our deepest feelings. The nutritional need for food is only part of the importance of food, or in Bettelheim's words "the distinction between physical and emotional need, between body and intellect, is in reality a false one."[68]

HOLISTIC VIEWPOINT

The preceding discussion highlights numerous factors that influence nutritional practices. Technological changes, business, political decisions, religious practices, scientific and medical knowledge, and history all influence eating habits. The socialization process initiated by the family has tremendous psychological impact on the individual's food consumption. Figure 9.5 illustrates the major influences that determine what, when, and how a person eats. Furthermore, all these factors influence one another. For example, in the late 1960's and early 1970's during the "Green Revolution" (a technological advance in agriculture) new wheat varieties had taken hold in Mexico and northwestern India and new varieties of rice in the Phillipines promised a high yield crop for the people of Southeast Asia. Worldwide production of wheat was rising. The harvest from the seas was continuing to increase. There was a growing optimism that the worldwide need for food could be met. Then, in 1972, unfavorable weather changes (a climate effect) resulted in two sudden, short-term simultaneous crop failures in several areas. This gave rise to massive purchases of grain by Russia which eliminated American reserves and caused international prices of wheat, corn, and rice to rise sharply (an economic effect with political consequences). Thus, a change in climate had dramatic economic and political consequences. Changes in any of the factors influencing nutrition may affect other aspects often in unforeseen and unpredictable ways. Therefore, a holistic understanding of obesity is more likely to result in planning that will effectively combat the problem.

A corollary of the holistic view of obesity and the other eating disorders is that the problem cannot be solved without the involvement and contribution of all fields, including medicine, social work, psychiatry, sociology, business, politics, education, and research. This is a concept that is often

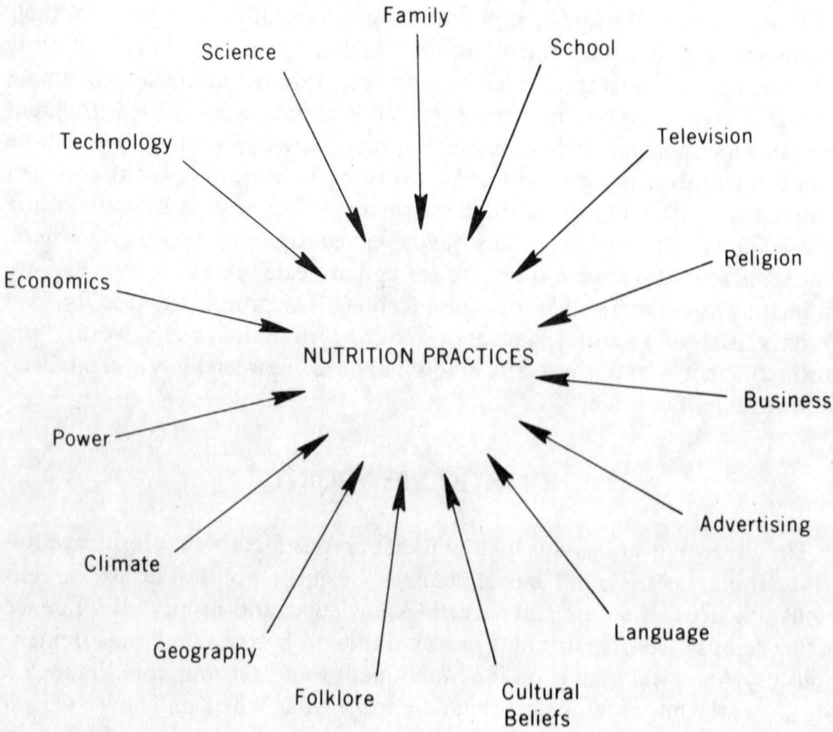

Figure 9.5. Multiplicity of factors influencing eating practices (adapted from Lowenberg[2]).

ignored by the medical profession. The social consequences of various scientific discoveries and medical treatment methods have been largely ignored. As Dubos notes in *Mirage of Health*, "This happy phase of social irresponsibility is over and the scientist will be called to account for the long-term consequences of his act."[70]

An example of a scientific advancement that has widespread deleterious consequences is formula feedings. Although initially intended for babies whose mothers could not breast-feed, these formulas have mushroomed into a million dollar business, with incalculable effects on health, notably obesity and known associated conditions, e.g., diabetes and hypertension. The change in the mother-child relationship with bottle-feeding rather than breast-feeding may prove to have cultural effects even more devastating than the rise in obesity. The medical scientist will need to continuously investigate the consequences of any new discovery or treatment method. The ability to do this effectively will require the interdisciplinary cooperation of many fields.

WORLD FOOD SUPPLY PROBLEM

A related consideration is the world's food supply. Although it is popular to consider only the needs of one's own family, neighborhood, state, or country, this isolationist attitude may be hazardous. It is well known that wars have been fought to obtain food; thus, ignoring the fact that one seventh of the world is starving is unwise. Furthermore, it is ironic and sad that many deaths in the United States are secondary to an overabundance of food when huge numbers of people die from starvation. Surely some plan could be devised to assure more healthy distribution of food and thereby reduce the mortality and morbidity from both obesity and starvation. This is, of course, not a new idea and is one that has explosive political potential. Nonetheless, consideration of the problem of obesity in the context of world food supplies may facilitate plans that are beneficial to all.

An example of a strategy that would benefit both groups (i.e., the overnourished and the undernourished) is provided by Lappe in "*Diet for a Small Planet.*"[71] She advocates a shift to vegetable sources of protein from the usual meat protein sources. The cost of the legumes and grains needed to provide the daily protein requirement is generally less than the cost of meats to provide equivalent protein (less than $1.00 compared to more than $1.00). Furthermore, grains and vegetables have no cholesterol and polyunsaturated fats as do meats, and therefore, are less atherogenic. Also, in terms of the world food supply, production of beef requires large amounts of grain which could supply protein to a greater number of people. Thus, even a small shift in eating habits with an increased consumption of grain and legumes, and a decrease in meat consumption, would be less expensive and more nutritious for Americans, and would permit continued export of grains to other countries with deficient supplies. Such a change might meet with great resistance for a variety of reasons, but is feasible with the cooperation of all groups in society.

CULTURAL ATTITUDE TOWARD SIZE

One of the prevailing notions about health is that a big baby is a healthy baby and the larger and the faster the baby grows, the better. It is also widely believed that an overweight child will outgrow his "baby fat." Despite the evidence that fewer than 20% of such babies do outgrow their fat, the idea of rapid growth is a widely accepted criterion of health. The main advantage of this criterion is that weight and height can be easily measured and are convenient, objective characteristics on which to agree, and in a society with abundant food, can generally be readily achieved. However, there is little proof that rapid achievement of large size portends future health or happiness or even an individual's ability to cope in society. Size and weight are not in themselves desirable. Dubos[72] describes an assay by Boycott entitled "On the Size of Things or the Advantages of Being Rather Small" in which he concludes that an animal about the size of a medium dog has the optimal size. Nonetheless, many people, including some physicians, continue to believe that big babies are necessarily beautiful, healthy, and happy.

However, the cultural attitude toward large size is reversed in later childhood, adolescence, and adulthood, at least in the United States. The fat child is often teased and called nicknames like "fatso," "baby elephant," "tubby," etc. These taunts, although painful in childhood, are even more difficult to tolerate during puberty and may result in permanent self-deprecatory attitudes toward one's body. In adolescence, any deviation from the accepted cultural norm for size and shape may result in criticism from peers. More important in terms of enduring attitudes toward one's body, however, is the family's reaction. An obese youngster whose family accepts him and offers support, and not criticism, is less likely to develop a disturbance in body image.

In the United States there is tremendous cultural pressure, particularly for women, to conform to a relatively narrow range of size and shape. This societal pressure increases as one rises in socioeconomic status. For example, a current fashion model, Tatiana Kalatschova, is 5 feet 7 inches tall and weighs 117 pounds, and is described as the perfect size 8.[73] She is reportedly the toast of the garment industry who see her as the standard for middle America. While her size and shape may be fine for her, there is no reason why everyone should be her size. The concept that there is *one* ideal size is fallacious. There is undoubtedly a range of sizes and shapes that does not pose a risk to health.

STIGMATIZATION OF THE OBESE

PSYCHODYNAMICS

The stigmatization of obese individuals is particularly apparent in middle and upper socioeconomic groups and pervades all areas of social interaction. Stigmatization involves the rejection and disgrace of persons with a condition viewed either as a physical deformity or a behavioral abnormality. The psychodynamics of stigmatization of people with unusual behavior or physical deformities have been studied by a variety of workers, notably Bettelheim.[69] The initial rejection of a person who is different is usually based on fear. The rejecting person often fears the same thing may happen to him, e.g., that he may become fat. Rejection of the obese person increases the emotional distance between the obese person and the non-obese person, facilitating the sense of security and superiority of the slim individual. The fear that one may become fat, i.e., physically deformed or behaviorally deviant, is thereby submerged. This process of rejection compounds the initial problem in a variety of ways.

EXAMPLES OF STIGMATIZATION

In a series of studies, Richardson and colleagues[74, 75] found that both children and adults devalue overweight children even more than children with other physical disabilities. The subjects were shown drawings of a normal child, a child with a brace, a child in a wheelchair, a child with a left hand missing, a child with a facial disfigurement, and a grossly obese child. The grossly obese child was consistently ranked less likable than the other children. Allon[16] reports his preliminary work which suggests that the obese adult is devalued even more than the obese child. Not surprisingly, such disparagement may be internalized in the obese person, resulting in a decrease in self-esteem, and a vicious cycle may be set up. This decrease in self-esteem may result in decreased social involvement, hence a decrease in physical activity. Solace may be sought by eating and even greater obesity may result.

Obese people, particularly women, are subject to criticism in a variety of other ways. The fashion industry, for example, designs clothes for very slim women. Louderback[76] notes that some wedding dresses are not made beyond size 10. Perhaps the implication is that women over this size are so unattractive that they will never get married. Advertisements for clothes often range from size 6 to 12, or 14, and women requiring larger sizes may have a very narrow choice of clothing available. Shopping can be a humiliating experience for a woman who is obese or simply larger than the cultural standard. Salesladies may scorn a woman who is unable to wear a certain size. Sometimes the shopper is told outright that she should lose weight (as if deciding to lose weight is all it takes) or more frequently told her size is not available. There are chain stores specializing in clothes in larger sizes, but frequently these clothes have drab colors, lack style, and fit like tents. For obese persons who have an associated body image disturbance, the experience of shopping may be so painful that they would rather wear outdated unflattering clothes.

Obesity decreases chances of admission to college. Canning and Mayer[77] found that the obese had less chance of admission even with comparable grades, IQ scores, and attendance records. Since education, occupation, and income are strongly interrelated social class variables, such discrimination against the obese may prevent them from rising in socioeconomic levels. They conclude that obesity may be one cause of downward social mobility. Thus, a girl may be in a lower socieconomic class because she is obese rather than obese because she is in a lower socioeconomic class.

ATTITUDES OF PHYSICIANS

Physicians often have negative attitudes toward obese individuals. In one study,[78] the physicians polled were found to dislike obese patients and preferred not to treat them. Treatment was expected to fail. These physicians believed obesity was unattractive and indicative of a lack of control. The severely overweight person was described as "weak willed," "ugly," and "awkward." The physicians evaluated the obese individuals even more harshly that the obese judge themselves. This negative stereotyping results in part from prevailing cultural attitudes. The "disease" concept of obesity, based on the narrow view that obesity has one cause and one treatment, also hinders the ability of physicians to empathize with the wide variety of problems experienced by an obese patient. The fatalistic view that obesity cannot be treated may well set up a self-fulfilling prophecy. Obesity may be difficult to treat, but, then, so is leukemia. It is the attitude that obesity could be controlled, if only the patient tried, that prevents the physician from intervening as effectively as possible. Recently, even the advances in understanding the development of adipose tissue have been taken as confirmation of the idea that obesity is untreatable. Thus, it is argued, if fat cell number is determined early in life, and loss of weight only decreases fat cell size, not fat cell number, treatment attempts are doomed to failure. Such sweeping generalizations are not justified.

FAT POWER

A group has been formed called the National Association to Aid Fat Americans, Inc. (NAAFA). This association includes fat and thin people who are aware of the stigma and social discrimination faced by obese persons. Grosswirth,[79] one of the leading spokesmen for this group, vividly describes the stigmatization that is all too frequently experienced:

> "You are a glutton. Your physician has probably told you so. Or you have read a magazine article by some "expert" who demolished all those "myths" concerning frame size, metabolism and heredity. About the only thing your physician or expert is willing to concede is that there are some psychological factors involved: you lack willpower, i.e. strength or character. You are a weakling. You are also, in the bargain, antisocial at best, suicidal at worst. You are an emotional mess as manifested by the fact that you are a physical slob" (p 29).[79]

He goes on to advocate "Fat Power" and advises fat people to take pride in shopping and to aggressively seek out stores that carry their size and welcome their business. Reichman, who weighs 199 pounds and is proud of it, describes an incident in which she went to a store to try an article of clothing advertised as "one size fits all." When scorned by the saleslady, she demanded the manager and said she was a spokesman for 20 million American women over size 14.[80]

Some proponents of the "fat can be beautiful" concept suggest that the obese might march en masse to certain clothing stores and demand a clothing section for fat women. This group prefers the word "fat" to its many euphemisms, as they take pride in their non-thinness. The NAAFA has engaged attorneys to investigate possible discrimination against obese students who apply for college admission. Although a certain size and shape are rarely listed requirements for employment, large or obese persons probably do have less chance of securing certain jobs than their thin peers. It has been suggested that anti-discrimination laws are needed to protect obese people.

Although the concept of "fat power" seems to be an over-reaction, since obesity *is* hazardous to health, the idea that there is a broad range of sizes and shapes that are healthy and attractive is valid. Furthermore, indiscriminate recommendation of weight loss to individuals who are significantly overweight is unwise before the meaning of their obesity is clearly understood.

CHANGING FOOD HABITS

Changing the food habits of a given cultural group is an arduous undertaking fraught with unexpected difficulties. To change fundamental food habits an entire culture must change. To affect large numbers of obese individuals significantly, changes that will affect many different segments of society must be instituted. Several steps are necessary to deliberately bring about a change in food habits.[81] Those who possess knowledge about a desirable change in food habits must want to communicate this information. The group whose practices require modification must be aware of this fact and motivated to make the change. And, the food required to make the change must be available.

IDENTIFICATION OF HARMFUL FOOD PRACTICES

To possess the knowledge that certain food habits need change requires careful analysis of all the food practices in a cultural group. Jelliffe and Bennett[82] propose the following classification of nutritional practices:

1. Beneficial practices which should be supported and encouraged; for example, breast feeding.
2. Neutral practices which have neither beneficial nor harmful effects should be left alone; for example, moderate intake of Vitamin C to prevent colds.
3. Unclassifiable practices which may or may not be deleterious should be investigated further; for example, use of certain food additives.
4. Harmful practices should be identified; for example, accelerating consumption of cholesterol and saturated fats.

Once the harmful practices have been identified, the most dangerous should be the focus for change.

GROUP DECISION METHOD

The next step requires that the group be aware of the needed changes and motivated to make them. Many worthy projects flounder at this step. Lewin[83] compared two methods of changing food habits. In the first method, called the *Group Decision Method*, the group decided for itself whether it wanted to change and to what extent it would change. In the second method, called the *Request Method*, a group was asked to make a change in food habits and goals were set by people outside the group. The goal of the nutritional change was to increase the consumption of whole wheat bread compared to that of white bread. At the time of this experiment, in 1942, white bread was not enriched and contained fewer nutrients than whole wheat bread. Lewin found that the Group Decision Method resulted in a greater consumption of whole wheat bread than did the Request Method, and that the change was longer-lasting. Others have confirmed these findings in experiments designed to change other food habits.[84] Lewin has discussed the possible reason for the greater effectiveness of the Group Decision Method compared to the Request Method. Resistance to change is based in part on fear of social rejection; in the Group Decision Method the decision to change receives social reinforcement.

TOWN MEETING MODEL

In the United States some of the major nutritional practices that result in obesity and related conditions have been identified and are agreed upon. The next step is to facilitate cultural change of target eating habits. Methods incorporating the Group Decision Method are most likely to be effective. For example, group participation in formulating the goals, enumerating the resistances, and devising appropriate strategies for achieving the goals might use the "Town Meeting Model" devised by The Institute of Cultural Affairs.[85] The method involves a four-step process:

1. Voicing future hopes; for example, a decrease in obesity-related conditions.
2. Determining the challenges; for example, promotion of high-calorie, high-cholesterol foods on television.
3. Articulating the underlying contradictions; for example, freedom of producers to advertise versus hazards to the consumers.
4. Finally, discovering a workable group of responses; for example, inviting a producer of "junk foods" to a seminar at an obesity clinic.

The value of such a method is that it can represent the conjoint effort of a large group of people and, therefore, has the greatest potential for success.

FOOD ADDITIVES

Controversy over food additives is increasing, particularly over artificial sweeteners used to decrease caloric content of certain foods. The hapless consumer is daily bombarded with reports of cancer in laboratory animals caused by intake of commonly used additives, as well as with promises of improved health and vigor through the use of "natural" and "organic" foods. Loss of energy and frequent colds are widely believed to result from subclinical deficiencies of various vitamins. Vitamins are routinely added to various foods, particularly breads and breakfast foods. The increasing number of reports of the hazards of various additives is bewildering, even to the expert. For example, in one review of substances "generally recognized as safe" (GRAS) there were more than 20,000 references to vitamin A and glutamic acid.[86] It is not surprising that many people are confused about which foods are safe.

VALUE OF ADDITIVES

An additive is a minor ingredient added to food to achieve a specific effect. Of the 1500 pounds of foodstuffs consumed per capita, 139 pounds are additives.[87] Additives are used as preservatives, to improve flavor, texture, and appearance, and to aid health and nutrition. Historically, additives have been used as preservatives for centuries. It was learned that the addition of salt and vinegar would permit longer storage and a wider distribution of foods. Spices have been used since ancient times to improve the flavor and taste of foods, particularly meats. Fifty years ago, pellagra caused the deaths of 7,000 people in the United States each year. In the southwestern states, niacin was added to the traditional diet of cornmeal, and this deficiency disease was virtually eliminated.[87] As the prevalence of obesity has continued to rise, there has been an increasing demand for low-calorie foods, many of which are prepared with artificial sweeteners, notably cyclamates and saccharin. Cyclamates were banned in 1969 after ingestion of large quantities was found to cause cancer in laboratory animals. Saccharin is still sold but contains a label indicating that it has caused cancer in laboratory animals.

The food industry has made tremendous technological advances, including use of various additives, and there is now a wide selection of foods available to greater numbers of people. For example, in 1928, the average grocery offered 867 food items; in 1950 the number was 3750; today it is more than 11,000 items.[88] The ability of additives to prolong shelf life of food items is in large part responsible for this greater choice.

QUESTIONABLE SAFETY OF ADDITIVES

Despite the increase in palatable foods available, debate continues as to the safety of the additives. Miller[89] has enumerated several reasons for this growing national concern. First, there has been rapid addition of many new additives in the past decade. In the past, introduction of a new additive took centuries and society had extensive experience with each new additive or technique. Thus, people had ample opportunity to observe any hazardous effects of the change. Furthermore, because of slow communication, even an acutely toxic additive harmed only a few people before it could be removed. In contemporary society, mass advertising, coupled with rapid distribution of food products, increases the hazards of new additives.

The second major reason for the increasing concern over additives is the dramatic rise in numbers and types of food additives. Probably fewer than 50 additives were in common usage until this century, whereas today, there are more than 2000. Furthermore, several additives may be used in the same product and interactions among them may be important. The many uses of these agents also makes evaluation difficult.

The concept of safety and toxicity is the third factor contributing to the controversy about additives. The food industry and the public both tend to view toxicity in terms of pharmacology: i.e., does the additive adversely affect health? Much of the laboratory testing is on animals, and it is well known that what is hazardous for humans may not be hazardous to rats and vice versa. (For example, thalidomide did not cause teratogenesis in rats, but did in humans.[90]) Also, acute toxicity is the easiest to detect, but is only part of a total toxicological evaluation of an additive. For example, the effects of chronic usage on the individual and his children as well as the potential for mutogenesis, teratogenesis, and carcinogenesis must be considered. Because of the rapid introduction of many new additives, research is scanty and incomplete. For example, information was deficient on fetal exposure for four fifths of the substances reviewed by the Select Committee on GRAS substances.[86] For most people, establishing that an additive poses no acute hazard is not sufficient. The consumer not only wants to live to be a healthy and hale centenarian, but expects his children and grandchildren to have the same opportunity. Thus, unproven additives are regarded with suspicion.

DELANEY AMENDMENT

The misconception that an additive is either safe or hazardous pervades reports on additives. The Delaney Amendment to the Food and Drug laws in effect declares illegal any compound or chemical which causes cancer. In the biological sciences, there is probably no absolutely safe drug or additive. The relative risk weighed against the potential benefit is what must be considered. For example, cyclamate is an artificial sweetener that was used extensively in low calorie beverages and dietetic fruits. As part of a balanced diet, such foods have great potential in weight reduction programs. However, cyclamates were banned in the United States when some laboratory animals developed cancer after ingesting large amounts of a mixture of cyclamate and saccharin.[91] Canada, The Netherlands, Belgium, Switzerland, West Germany, and Spain followed a more moderate course and permitted the use of cyclamates up to a maximum recommended intake of 3.5 g per day.

Recently, the Food and Drug Administration has been more cautious in handling reports of cancer in laboratory animals. The potential benefit of artificial sweeteners in weight reduction programs must be weighed against the risk of cancer extrapolated from animal studies. The question of carcinogenesis is a very emotional one and the first reaction to laboratory studies suggesting that an additive may produce cancer is the banning of that substance. However, it is very likely that any substance, including food itself, can produce cancer if ingested in large enough quantities or if embedded in certain organs.

DISTRUST OF FOOD INDUSTRY

The growth of marketing techniques which focus almost exclusively on how to sell a product, rather than on the nutritional content, has fostered consumer criticism. Miller[89] notes that the credibility of the food industry has plummeted. Many people now routinely question the claims made for any food additive. This distrust and lack of confidence has resulted in vociferous criticism, militant consumer groups, and some over-reactions. The increasing popularity of health food stores, "organic" foods, "natural" foods, and unprocessed foods stems in part from distrust of the food industry.

FOOD FALLACIES

"ORGANIC" AND "NATURAL" FOODS

Many health food stores advertise "organic" foods, but in fact, all foods are organic in that they contain carbon. Many people mistakenly believe that all "organic foods" are produced without pesticides and artificial fertilizers and are free of additives. However, there are no legal standards for "organic" foods and they may be no different from foods purchased elsewhere, except that they are more expensive. Another misconception is that "pure" foods are free of chemicals. All foods are chemicals. In fact, all animal and plant life is chemical. A "natural" food is one with little or no processing and usually grown without chemical fertilizers or pesticides. Thus, some health food stores still sell certified raw milk, which has not been pasteurized and thus could potentially contain pathogenic organisms.

HEALTH FOOD STORES

Although a number of misconceptions are promulgated by "health food stores," in at least two important areas there is substance to the claims. First, refined sugar is overused and overpromoted in our society, and probably has contributed significantly to the rise of obesity-related diseases. Youngsters are conditioned to prefer sweets, and sugar-containing foods are readily available. However, the "raw" sugar and "natural" sugar sold as substitutes are also concentrated carbohydrates, high in calories and low in nutritional content. The second claim which has some validity is that "processed" foods can be hazardous to health. Some food processing, such as pasteurization, promotes health, but some does not. For example, most of the food products advertised on children's programs are the result of several processing steps and contain excessive calories for their nutritional worth. However, to categorically condemn *all* food processing does not promote health. The emotional ambiance of "health food stores" is also misleading. Storekeepers often wear white coats and make extravagant claims for various products, especially certain vitamins, and bolster their claims with pseudoscientific literature on nutrition. Adelle Davis' book, *Let's Eat Right to Keep Fit*,[92] is widely available and has been estimated to contain at least one error per page.[93]

The prevalence and popularity of "health food stores," however, is related in part to the apathy of the medical profession toward nutrition and preventive medicine. If our zeal for "curing" disease were matched with an interest in preventing disease, there might be fewer misconceptions about nutrition and its relationship to health.

MISCONCEPTIONS ABOUT CURATIVE VALUES OF FOODS

Misconceptions about the nutritional and curative values of food are not new. Even Hippocrates had some mistaken notions about food. For example, he thought that one should starve a fever, that fruit should be restricted in diarrhea, and that garlic was a good purgative and diuretic. In our scientific era, one might expect such erroneous ideas to be rare. However, many common food fallacies persist.[94] For example, many people believe that citrus fruits are too acid to be handled by the body. In fact, after absorption, the organic acids in fruits are oxidized to carbon dioxide and water and the inorganic residue remaining is basic in reaction. Another common misconception is that honey is not fattening. Actually, a tablespoon of strained honey contains 65 calories whereas a tablespoon of white sugar contains only 45 calories.

NATURAL TOXINS

Few people are aware that many nutritious, safe foods contain natural toxins.[87, 89] Cyanide, for example, is a poison found in apricot pits and lima beans. Nitrates and nitrites, which are used to cure meats, have a relationship to nitrosamine, a substance that has been shown to cause cancer in laboratory animals. However, in the public outcry against using these additives, it has been generally overlooked that nitrates are present in spinach, beets, lettuce, eggplant, celery, and turnip greens and that people often consume more nitrates from these vegetables than from cured meats. Other naturally occurring toxins include caffeine, a stimulant found in coffee and tea. A wide variety of toxins occur in seafood. Cheese and pineapple juice contain pressor amines and Valencia oranges contain a cholinesterase inhibitor. These are but a few examples of naturally occurring toxins which, if consumed in large quantities, would be dangerous. However, small amounts are not dangerous. Diets that include a wide variety of foods are the safest. Perhaps a reasonable goal for the food industry regarding additives is to attain a level of safety that is commensurate with the safety of naturally occurring foods.

FOOD FADDISM

Obese individuals are particularly at risk for food faddism. Our society places a high premium on slenderness, yet actively encourages overconsumption of food. Since weight loss is so difficult to achieve, and even more difficult to maintain, many obese people follow a variety of food fads that promise quick and permanent weight loss. Often no apparent damage results from following these fads because the enthusiasm wanes quickly when the initial weight loss does not continue. However, the disappointment and sense of failure, which often follow termination of a fad diet, cause much misery to many obese subjects who already may suffer from low self-esteem.

A fad is a style or custom that is enthusiastically endorsed by many people for a short time. Some of the recent reducing fads have included the grapefruit diet, the "Last Chance Diet" (the notorious liquid protein diet), the "Calories Don't Count Diet," and the "Zen Macrobiotic Diet." There are many reasons why such nutritionally dangerous diets flourish, but a major factor is the failure of the medical profession to treat obesity adequately. This relates in part to the nature of obesity itself. Even in carefully designed treatment programs, the majority of patients do not maintain significant weight losses. However, physicians generally fail to appreciate the complex nature of obesity and may arrogantly recommend that the patient "simply push himself away from the table". Such attitudes damage both the physician and the patient, and increase the patient's vulnerability to food fads and quackery.

TYPES OF FOOD FADDISTS

Food fads may serve a variety of conscious or unconscious needs. Beal[95] has attempted to classify food faddists into groups on the basis of the need met by the fad. Probably many reducing diets become popular for the same reasons. The *miracle-seeker* tries to regain health or energy by following a certain diet. For example, an obese individual with emotional problems and with an associated body image disturbance may erroneously believe that weight loss alone will improve his self-concept and alleviate all problems. He may choose to follow any of many diets guaranteed to result in quick weight loss, and even if significant amounts of weight are lost, he may regain the weight when he finds he still suffers from low self-esteem. Perhaps this sequence of events accounts for the tendency of reduced subjects to regain even more weight than was initially lost. The "miracle-seeker" may be easy prey to any of the "get thin quick" remedies that are widely available. Anti-obesity drugs are very popular with patients and physicians, despite the fact that none has been shown to be effective in the long run and many are known to be dangerous. The miracle-seeker, be he physician or patient, is susceptible to the claims made for these drugs.

Another group of food faddists *distrust* the *medical profession.* Beal posits that these individuals need to establish control over their destiny and not be dependent on unknown others. Most obese people have not maintained significant weight loss by following physicians' recommendations and this may contribute to distrust of pronouncements made by medical groups. However, often more important is that the reducing diet may be promoted by individuals who are personable, persuasive, and willing or able to spend more time with the patient. Obese individuals who distrust the medical profession or do not have a positive relationship with their physician often do not check on claims by promoters of various dietary nostrums.

A third group identified by Beal are called *fashion followers.* The psychological need is to gain approval and acceptance from others. Probably few patients attempt to lose weight in order to prevent or ameliorate the obesity-related diseases such as diabetes or hypertension. The tremendous cultural pressure to be thin is often the major reason that people follow diets. The need for acceptance and approval (belongingness) may result in selection of a popular, but dangerous, reducing diet. On the positive side, however, the belongingness need may motivate a person to join a group such as TOPS (Take Off Pounds Sensibly) or Weight Watchers, which generally recommend sensible reducing diets, and cooperate with the medical profession.

The food faddist described as an *authority seeker* meets his need for recognition of self-competency by apparent knowledge about food. Sometimes this results in an improved nutritional status. However, since the covert purpose is to establish competency rather than attain a healthy weight, such individuals may accept only those nutritional ideas that bolster self-esteem.

The other types of food faddists include the *anti-establishmentarian*, whose goal is self-realization and the *super health seeker* who needs to forestall awareness of aging. Faddists described as *truth seekers* and those *concerned about* the *uncertainties of life* may be reacting to an unstructured environment. These individuals may be looking for stability in a rapidly changing society. Valid nutritional facts which do not fit their pre-existing pattern may be ignored or discarded because they are threatening. These attitudes impair the ability to evaluate new food products critically and may lead to enthusiastic endorsement of some non-nutritious foods.

GROUPS AT RISK

The groups particularly at risk for food fads are adolescents, the elderly, the chronically ill, and the mentally ill. The emotional upheaval of adolescence renders teenagers vulnerable to peer pressure and many may enthusiastically adhere to a fad diet for a short period. Fortunately, most of these fads are short-lived and neither overnutrition nor undernutrition develops. Obese adolescents, however, are particularly prone to faddish reducing diets and to the discouragement that generally ensues when weight loss does not continue. Many chronically mentally ill patients are obese, secondary either to inactivity, or the side effects of various psychotropic drugs. Many such patients hope for a more complete relief of their symptoms without the side effects of drugs and may follow food fads or use vitamins in an attempt to relieve their symptoms.

EXAMPLES OF DANGEROUS DIETS

The *Zen Macrobiotic Diet* is a dangerous collection of food fallacies which offers a cure for obesity, schizophrenia, syphilis, and meningitis, to name just a few. This diet is a series of 10 stages which progressively eliminates various foods until only unpolished rice is consumed. Although in the early stages animal foods, fruits, and vegetables are permitted, a minimum intake of water is advised. Also white sugar and all of the foods containing sugar are to be avoided. The final diet, consisting exclusively of rice, is extremely dangerous, and the American Medical Association has cited cases of scurvy, anemia, hypoproteinemia, hypocalcemia, emaciation, and kidney failure.[96] The macrobiotic food cult has also recommended that macrobiotic foods be used instead of milk for infants. A mixture called kokoh has been used and consists of sesame seeds, brown rice, aduki beans, wheat, oats, and soya beans mixed with water. Robson[97] found that the mixture contained proteins of good quality but was too dilute to provide adequate intake energy for infants.

The *liquid protein diet*[98, 99] recently became notorious when several people died while following these diets, sometimes under medical surveillance. The diet initially devised was a 600-calorie per day reducing diet. The protein was given to prevent breakdown of body protein and it was alleged that the liquid protein was more effective than conventional equicalorie diets. However, conventional protein-containing foods contain better quality proteins than the liquid protein, and are at least as effective in preventing negative nitrogen balance. Furthermore, diets consisting exclusively of protein are dangerous, since the body also requires other nutrients.

Certain cultural factors have contributed to the popularity of this diet. The title "Last Chance Diet" was appealing to large groups of obese people who have tried and failed to maintain weight losses. Also, the prevalent cultural belief that "fat is bad" obscures the fact that certain dietary fats are essential for survival. Protein is considered to be a "good" dietetic food, and it is generally not realized that excess energy intake in any form—protein, carbohydrate, or fat—will be stored as fat. Thus, a "Last Chance," liquid protein diet would be expected to have wide appeal.

SUMMARY

The cultural and social factors that impinge on obesity have been largely ignored by the medical profession. Means of preventing illness are rarely taught in medical school and only recently are nutrition courses being added to the curriculum. In practice, the physician is often overwhelmed trying to treat patients who suffer the consequences of obesity. However, it is difficult to overestimate the importance of these factors which include historical, political, economic, and religious influences. Effective treatment programs will require consideration of all these factors.

References

1. Eppright ES: Factors influencing food acceptance. J Am Diet Assoc 23: 579–587, 1947.
2. Lowenberg ME, Todhunter EN, Wilson ED, et al: Food and Man. Ed 2. New York, John Wiley and Sons, 1974, p 8.
3. Lowenberg ME, Todhunter EN, Wilson ED, et al: Food and Man. Ed 2. New York, John Wiley and Sons, 1974, p 10.
4. Hippocrates, cited by Dubos R: Mirage of Health. Perennial Edition. New York, Harper and Row Publ Inc, 1971, pp 134–143.
5. Young N: Our national diet survey. Glamour, July 1978, pp 162–165.
6. Plato: Republic, cited by Dubos R: Mirage of Health. Perennial Edition. New York, Harper and Row Publ Inc, 1971, p 143.
7. Homer, cited by Reichman SJ: Great Big Beautiful Doll. New York, The Great American Library Inc, 1977, p 20.
8. Reichman SJ: Great Big Beautiful Doll. New York, The Great American Library Inc, 1977.
9. Lowenberg ME, Todhunter EN, Wilson ED, et al: Food and Man. Ed 2. New York, John Wiley and Sons, 1974, p 34.
10. Seneca, cited in Lowenberg ME, Todhunter EN, Wilson ED, et al: Food and Man. Ed 2. New York, John Wiley and Sons, 1974, p 45.
11. Lucretius, cited in Lowenberg ME, Todhunter EN, Wilson ED, et al: Food and Man. Ed 2. New York, John Wiley and Sons, 1974, p 45.
12. Louderback L: Fat Power: Whatever You Weigh is Right. New York, Hawthorn Books Inc, 1970, p 39.

13. Stunkard AJ: Obesity and the social environment: current status, future prospects. NY Acad Sci 300: 315, 1977.
14. Dante A: Divine Comedy. New York, Columbia Univ Press, 1951.
15. Louderback L: Fat Power: Whatever You Weigh is Right. New York, Hawthorn Books Inc, 1970, p 25.
16. Allon N: The stigma of overweight in everyday life. In: Obesity in Perspective. Fogarty International Center Series on Preventive Medicine. Vol 2, Part 2. National Institutes of Health. Bethesda, Md, Oct 1–3, 1973.
17. Wason B: Cooks, Gluttons and Gourmets. New York, Doubleday, 1962.
18. McDuffie A: Culinary craft and artful eating. The Tampa Tribune: June 29, 1978.
19. Lowenberg ME, Todhunter EN, Wilson ED, et al: Food and Man. Ed 2. New York, John Wiley and Sons, 1974, p 58.
20. Shakespeare W: Merchant of Venice. Stirling B (ed). New York, Penguin, 1960.
21. Dubos R: Mirage of Health. Perennial Edition. New York, Harper and Row Publ Inc, 1971, p 201.
22. Reichman SJ: Great Big Beautiful Doll. New York, The Great American Library Inc, 1977, p 23.
23. Jeffrey DB, Katz RC: Take It Off and Keep It Off: A Behavioral Program for Weight Loss. Englewood Cliffs, NJ, Prentice-Hall Inc, 1977, p. 12.
24. Mayer J: A Diet for Living. New York, Pocket Books, 1977.
25. Ohsawa G: Zen Macrobiotics: The Art of Rejuvenation and Longevity. Oles L, Suehle SO (eds). New York, Japan Publs, 1977.
26. Rubin T: Thin Book by a Formerly Fat Psychiatrist. New York, Pinnacle Bks, 1975.
27. Beller AS: Fat and Thin: A Natural History of Obesity. New York, Farrar, Straus & Giroux, Inc, 1977.
28. Mann GV: The influence of obesity on health. N Engl J Med 291: 226–232, 1974.
29. Rudofsky B: The Unfashionable Human Body. New York, Doubleday and Co Inc, 1971.
30. Mead M: Dietary patterns and food habits. J Am Diet Assoc 19: 1–5, 1943.
31. Lowenberg ME, Todhunter EN, Wilson ED, et al: Food and Man. Ed 2. New York, John Wiley and Sons, 1974, p 135.
32. Sumner WG: Folkways. New York, Mentor Books, 1960.
33. Goldman I: The Ifugao of the Philippine Islands. In: Cooperation and Competition Among Primitive Peoples. Mead M (ed). New York, McGraw-Hill Co, 1937, pp 153–179.
34. Wellin E: Water boiling in a Peruvian town. In: Health, Culture and the Community. Paul BD (ed). New York, Russell Sage Foundation, 1955.
35. Lee DL: Cultural factors in dietary choice. In: Nutrition. Brennan R (ed). Dubuque, Iowa, Wm C Brown Co, 1967, pp 22–29.
36. Warner W: Black Civilization, A Social Study of an Australian Tribe, Rev Ed. Magnolia, Mass, Peter Smith Pub Inc, 1937.
37. Schweitzer A: African Notebook. New York, Henry Holt & Co, 1939.
38. Maslow AH: Motivation and Personality. New York, Harper and Row Publ Inc, 1970.
39. Maslow AH, cited by Lowenberg ME, Todhunter EN, Wilson ED, et al: Food and Man. Ed 2. New York, John Wiley and Sons, 1974, p 149.
40. Mead M: The Mountain Arapesh. II. Socio-Economic Life. Anthr Pap American Museum Natural History 49: Pt 3, 1947.
41. Simmons L: Sun Chief. New Haven, Yale University Press, 1942.
42. Lowenberg ME, Todhunter EN, Wilson ED, et al: Food and Man. Ed 2. New York, John Wiley and Sons, 1974, p 43.
43. Committee on Food Habits. Manual for the Study of Food Habits. National Research Council Bull III. National Academy of Science, Washington DC, 1945.
44. Mayer J: Crop destruction in Vietnam. Science 152: 291, 1966.
45. Lowenberg ME, Todhunter EN, Wilson ED, et al: Food and Man. Ed 2. New York, John Wiley and Sons, 1974, p 34.
46. Cameron N: The Psychology of Behavior Disorders, A Biosocial Interpretation. Boston, Houghton Mifflin Co, 1947.
47. Washington Post editorial January 31, 1977.

48. Hoffman H: Struwwelpeter. New York, Warne, Frederick & Co, 1844.
49. Best Loved Nursery Rhymes and Songs. Baker A (ed). New York, Parents Magazine Enterprises Inc for Playmore Inc, 1974.
50. Bettelheim B: The Uses of Enchantment: The Meaning and Importance of Fairy Tales. New York, Alfred A Knopf, 1976.
51. Carroll L: Alice's Adventures in Wonderland. New York, Penguin, 1950.
52. Jeffrey DB, Katz RC: Take It Off and Keep It Off: A Behavioral Program for Weight Loss and Healthy Living. Englewood Cliffs, NJ, Prentice-Hall Inc, 1977, pp 16–17.
53. Smith FA, Trivax G, Zuehlke DA, et al: Health information during a week of television. N Engl J Med 286: 516–520, 1972.
54. Lewis CE, Lewis MA: The impact of television commercials on health-related beliefs and behaviors of children. Pediatrics 53: 431–435, 1974.
55. Gussow J: "It Makes Even Milk a Dessert." A Report on the counternutritional messages of children's television advertising. Clin Pediatr 12: 68–71, 1973.
56. Masover L, Stamler J: Presentation to the 1976 Convention of the American Public Health Assoc, reported in Dietary Goals for the United States. Ed 2. Prepared by Select Committee on Nutrition and Human Needs. United States Senate, Dec 1977, p 59.
57. Powers PS, Younger D, Fernandez R: Television advertising and childrens food preferences. Submitted to 2nd Regional Congress of American Association of Social Psychiatry, Louisville, Ky, 1979.
58. Davis C: Self-selection of diet by newly weaned infants. Am J Dis Child 36: 651–679, 1928.
59. Duncker K: Experimental modification of children's food preferences through social suggestion. J Abnorm Soc Psychol 33: 489, 1938.
60. Stunkard AJ: Obesity and the social environment: current status, future prospects. Ann NY Acad Sci 300: 298–320, 1977.
61. Jeffrey DB, Katz RC: Take It Off and Keep It Off: A Behavioral Program for Weight Loss and Healthy Living. Englewood Cliffs, NJ, Prentice-Hall Inc, 1977.
62. Dietary Goals for the United States. Ed 2. Prepared by Select Committee on Nutrition and Human Needs. United States Senate, Dec 1977, p 28.
63. Dietary Goals for the United States. Ed 2. Prepared by Select Committee on Nutrition and Human Needs. United States Senate, Dec 1977, p 59.
64. Kotler P: Marketing Management Analysis, Planning and Control. Englewood Cliffs, NJ, Prentice-Hall Inc, 1967.
65. Lippincott and Margulies Inc: The name's the thing. Design Sense 24, cited by Lowenberg ME, Todhunter EN, Wilson ED, et al: Food and Man. Ed 2. New York, John Wiley and Sons, 1974, p 241.
66. Gardner B: The package as a communication. In: Marketing for Tomorrow . . . Today. Moyer MS, Vosburgh RF (eds). 1967 Conference Proceedings. American Marketing Assoc, Chicago, 1967.
67. Dietary Goals for the United States. Ed 2. Prepared by Select Committee on Nutrition and Human Needs. United States Senate, Dec 1977, p 52.
68. Bettelheim B: Food to nurture the mind. School Review, May 1975, cited in Dietary Goals for the United States. Ed 2. Prepared by Select Committee on Nutrition and Human Needs. United States Senate, Dec 1977, p 53.
69. Bettelheim B: A Home for the Heart. New York, Alfred A. Knopf, 1973.
70. Dubos R: Mirage of Health. Perennial Edition. New York, Harper and Row Publ Inc, 1971, p 271.
71. Lappe FM: Diet for a Small Planet. Revised Edition. Westminster, Md, Ballantine, 1975.
72. Dubos R: Mirage of Health. Perennial Edition. New York, Harper and Row Publ Inc, 1971, p 262.
73. Scott M: Nobody's perfect—except Tatiana. The Tampa Tribune and the Tampa Times, Parade Magazine: July 2, 1978, p 12.
74. Richardon SA, Hastorf AH, Goodman N, Dornbusch SM: Cultural uniformity in reaction to physical disabilities. Am Sociol Rev 26: 241–247, 1961.
75. Goodman N, Richardson SA, Dornbusch SM, Hastorf AH: Variant reactions to physical disabilities. Am Sociol Rev 28: 429–435, 1963.

76. Louderback L: Fat Power: Whatever You Weigh is Right. New York, Hawthorn Books Inc, 1970, p 62.
77. Canning H, Mayer J: Obesity—its possible effect on college acceptance. N Engl J Med 275: 1172–1174, 1966.
78. Maddox GL, Liederman V: Overweight as a social disability with medical implications. J Med Educ 44: 214–220, 1969.
79. Grosswirth M: Fat Pride: A Survival Handbook. New York, Jarrow Press Inc, 1971.
80. Reichman SJ: Great Big Beautiful Doll. New York, The Great American Library Inc, 1977, p 123–124.
81. Lowenberg ME, Todhunter EN, Wilson ED, et al: Food and Man. Ed 2. New York, John Wiley and Sons, 1974, p 127.
82. Jelliffe DB, Bennett FJ: Cultural and anthropological factors in infant and maternal nutrition. Fed Proc 18: 185, 1961.
83. Lewin K: Forces behind food habits and methods of changes. In: The Problem of Changing Food Habits. Committee on Food Habits. National Research Council Bull 108, 1943, pp 35–65.
84. Radke M, Caso EK: Lecture and discussion as method of influencing food habits. J Am Diet Assoc 24: 23–31, 1948.
85. Institute of Cultural Affairs, Chicago, IL 60640.
86. Select Committee on GRAS Substances. 1977. Evaluation of health aspects of food additives: lessons learned and questions unanswered, cited by Miller SA: Additives in our food supply. Ann NY Acad Sci 300: 397–405, 1977.
87. Chou M: National myopia: food additives. Research Memorandum #48. Hudson Institute. HI-2718/4-P. Feb 1978.
88. Grinnell G: Trends in Grocery Retailing. USDA Economic Statistics and Cooperatives Services. National Food Review, 1978, p 17.
89. Miller SA: Additives in our food supply. Ann NY Acad Sci 300: 397–405, 1977.
90. Rementeria JL: Drug Abuse in Pregnancy and Neonatal Effects. St Louis, CV Mosby Co, 1977, p 185.
91. Goldblith SA: The use and abuse of food technology in the quality of our food supply. Ann NY Acad Sci 300: 161–166, 1977.
92. Davis A: Let's Eat Right to Keep Fit. New York, Harcourt Brace Jovanovich, 1970.
93. Mann G, cited in Rynearson EH: Americans love hogwash. Nutr Rev Suppl: 1–14, 1974.
94. Wilson ED, Fisher KH, Fuqua ME: Principles of Nutrition. New York, John Wiley and Sons, 1967.
95. Beal VA: Food faddism and organic and natural foods. Presentation at National Dairy Council Food Writers' Conference, Newport, RI, May 1972, cited in Schafer R, Yetley EA: Social psychology of food faddism. J Am Diet Assoc 66: 129–133, 1975.
96. Council on Foods and Nutrition, Zen Macrobiotic Diets. JAMA 218: 397, 1971.
97. Robson JRK: Food faddism. Pediatr Clin North Am 24: 189–201, 1977.
98. Wolfe S: The new drop dead diets. Mother Jones, June 1978, pp 13–14.
99. Liquid protein and sudden cardiac deaths—an update. FDA Drug Bulletin, May–July 1978, pp 18–19.

CHAPTER

10

Other Eating Disorders

Throughout history, eating, food and weight have been tremendously important, both in terms of survival and interpersonal relationships. Although less time and societal effort are now required to ensure adequate nutrition for survival, the importance of food symbolically and interpersonally is difficult to overestimate. It is not surprising, therefore, that there are a myriad of other eating disorders including anorexia nervosa, bulimia, pica, and rumination. Eating dysfunctions are also associated with some of the hypersomnias. Anorexia or megaphagia may occur with systemic disease, e.g., disseminated carcinoma or hypothyroidism.

ANOREXIA NERVOSA

Anorexia nervosa is an uncommon condition that has fascinated physicians for more than a century. It was initially recognized as a separate entity by Morton[1] in 1689 who named it phthisis nervosa. Sir William Gull[2] rediscovered it in 1868 naming the disease anorexia nervosa and Lasèque[3] spoke of anorexic hysterique in 1873. Morton's initial vivid description is still clinically accurate. He describes an 18-year-old woman as follows:

> "In the month of July she fell into a total suppression of her Monthly Courses from a multitude of Cares and Passions of her Mind. . . . From which time her Appetite began to abate and her Digestion to be bad; her flesh also began to be flacid and loose, and her looks pale . . . . She was wont by her studying at Night, and continual pouring upon Books, to expose herself both Day and Night to the injuries of the Air. . . . I do not remember that I did ever in all my practice see one, that was conversant with the living, so much wasted with the greatest degree of a Consumption (like a Skeleton only clad with Skin) yet there was no Fever but on

the contrary a coldness of the whole Body . . . only her Appetite was diminished, and her Digestion uneasy with Fainting Fits, which did frequently return upon her."

Morton's patient refused the medication offered and died 3 months later.

EPIDEMIOLOGY OF ANOREXIA NERVOSA

Prevalence

In the century following Gull's rediscovery of anorexia nervosa, there has been a plethora of clinical reports and investigations. Most estimates of prevalence range from 1.3 to 2.4 per 100,000 of the general population in the United States. Some investigators, however, believe that usual prevalence rates are spuriously low because patients with mild forms of the condition recover spontaneously or are successfully treated at home. Some estimate prevalence at 1 in 250 in female Caucasians between 12 and 18.[4]

Sex Distribution

Although an occasional investigator has defined anorexia nervosa as occurring only in females, most agree that 90–95% of the patients are females and 5–10% are male. The reason for the female preponderance is not clear but two major explanations have been proposed. The first theory is that adolescent girls, in developed countries, are subjected to more intense pressure to maintain a svelte figure and, consequently, psychopathology is more likely to be expressed by an eating disorder, namely anorexia nervosa or obesity. This explanation does not, of course, account for the much higher prevalence of obesity than anorexia nervosa among adolescent girls. The second theory is that anorexia nervosa is a neuropsychiatric disorder that includes primary hypothalamic-pituitary malfunction and that the control system for the hypothalamic-pituitary axis is more complex in females than males; consequently malfunction is more likely in females.

Age of Onset

Anorexia nervosa usually begins in adolescence after menarche in females, and incidence is highest between 12 and 18 years of age. Rarely, it may begin prepubertally or in the early 30's. The diagnosis is often missed in the occasional prepubertal girl with anorexia nervosa because she never had menarche and consequently secondary amenorrhea does not occur. Furthermore, a prepubertal child may not lose much body weight but may grow in height such that she is emaciated; the diagnosis may be missed because she did not lose weight, but, rather, failed to gain weight commensurate with her height. Since anorexia nervosa may have a chronic course, older patients may present with the disease, but a careful history will usually reveal that the condition started in adolescence or early adult life. One patient with anorexia nervosa came for treatment at age 54 but initially lost more than 25% of her body weight at age 21.

Socioeconomic Class

Most patients in the United States and England are from the upper or upper middle socioeconomic classes; those few from the lower socioeconomic classes are from families with an abundance of food readily available. Anorexia nervosa is rarely reported in the underdeveloped countries.

Nearly all patients described are Caucasian, and only one black patient has been reported.[5] A variety of explanations may account for these epidemiological findings, but the most likely is that self-starvation as an interpersonal tool is ineffective in the absence of adequate food. The black patient reported is from a family with abundant food. In her case the diagnosis was initially missed because of marked cultural differences between this black patient and her Caucasian physicians. The patient never revealed to her physician her preoccupation with food and weight. Only after several weeks in the hospital did she confide to the black janitorial staff her obsession about food and her intense fear of becoming fat; and it was a black kitchen worker who witnessed her bulimic episodes.

PRIMARY ANOREXIA NERVOSA (BRUCH)

Hilde Bruch,[6] who has contributed the most to our understanding of the psychological characteristics of anorexia nervosa has noted that, paradoxically, with increasing observation and investigation the clinical picture has become less distinct than in the initial description by Morton. For example, by 1960 Bliss and Branch[7] had defined anorexia nervosa as present if there had been a weight loss of 25 pounds attributable to psychological causes.

At present there are three major classifications of anorexia nervosa, which are used, with some minor variations, by most investigators in the English-speaking countries (See Table 10.1). Although most of the patients would be identified using any of these three systems, Bruch's diagnostic scheme for primary anorexia nervosa, which includes important psychological criteria, might exclude some patients diagnosed by the other methods.[8, 9]

Bruch postulates that in primary anorexia nervosa, food is refused to achieve control and maintain a sense of self through bizarre control of the body and its functions. She identifies three major areas of psychological disturbance: a disturbed body image that may be of delusional proportions, decreased internal awareness, and a paralyzing sense of ineffectiveness.

Body Image Disturbance

Body image is a concept that includes one's view of himself psychologically, physically, and interpersonally. Various attempts have been made to

Table 10.1
Anorexia nervosa classification systems.

Bruch	Feighner et al	Russell (Britain)
Primary Anorexia Nervosa	1. Onset before 25	1. Pattern of behavior aimed at weight loss
1. Body image disturbance	2. Loss of 25% body weight	2. Persistent pursuit of excessive thinness
2. Decreased internal awareness	3. Distorted attitude toward eating, food or weight	3. Emaciation to 80% of standard
3. Sense of ineffectiveness	4. No other medical illness	4. Amenorrhea · 3 months
Secondary Anorexia Nervosa	5. No other psychiatric illness	5. Absence of other physical or psychiatric condition
	6. Two of following	
	• lanugo • bulimia	
	• bradycardia • vomiting	
	• over activity • amenorrhea	

elucidate the nature and extent of body image disturbances in anorexia nervosa including the "Draw-A-Person" test which is thought to reflect the person's own perception of himself. Estimation of various body widths permits an operational definition of the perceptual disturbance of body image. One study[10] found that anorexia nervosa patients report body widths (face, chest, waist, and hips) to be 24–50% greater than is actually the case; however, the patients were accurate in estimating the widths of other objects. This study did not, however, evaluate the patients' estimates of the widths of significant people in their lives and inaccuracies might have occurred in these estimates.

In another study of anorexics,[11] a reduction in body size estimate was associated with a good outcome. This finding is consonant with Bruch's belief that recovery requires a more accurate body image.

Although these studies of the perceptual disorder in anorexia nervosa are preliminary and inconclusive, they are fascinating and unique in providing an operational method of elucidating the complex psychophysiological concept of body image.

Decreased Internal Awareness

The second major psychological criterion for anorexia nervosa described by Bruch is a decreased internal awareness of both bodily sensations and emotional feelings. Awareness of hunger, in the normal sense, seems to be absent. The anorectic patient may have episodes of compulsive overeating (bulimic episodes) unassociated with any awareness of hunger sensations. The pathogenesis of this deficient awareness of internal cues is postulated to be as follows. From birth there is behavior that originates in the infant and behavior in the infant in response to stimuli. The family producing the disturbed patient does not respond appropriately to cues coming from the infant because of their preoccupation with their own needs. Instead, the child is bombarded with expectations and demands and learns to respond to her parents' needs and is confused about her own feelings, thoughts, and wishes. Characteristically there is a strong symbiotic tie between the mother and daughter and the anorectic patient may come to believe that she is really the puppet of someone else's feelings (usually her mother). Much of the negativistic behavior seen in anorectics is a desperate attempt to avoid control by others. Yet the anorectic is deficient in her own sense of separateness and cannot function independently. The father in this situation is usually ineffective and does not intervene in the mother-daughter symbiosis. Fig. 10.1 was drawn by a friend of a family with a daughter with anorexia nervosa.

The overactivity observed in a severely cachectic anorexia nervosa patient may also reflect a deficient awareness of internal body cues and a denial of fatigue. The absence of sexual feelings may also reflect this decreased internal awareness.

Most of the patients are unaware of their own emotional states and may

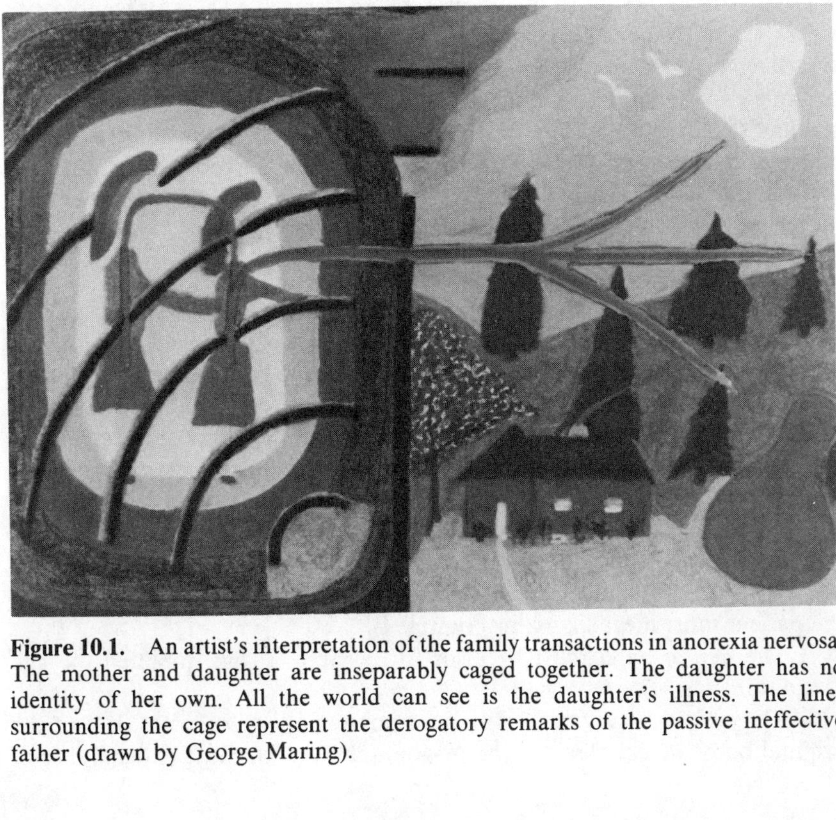

Figure 10.1. An artist's interpretation of the family transactions in anorexia nervosa. The mother and daughter are inseparably caged together. The daughter has no identity of her own. All the world can see is the daughter's illness. The lines surrounding the cage represent the derogatory remarks of the passive ineffective father (drawn by George Maring).

proclaim themselves happy even in the face of dramatic evidence to the contrary. In this area, anorexia nervosa patients are similar to some patients with obesity. Stunkard's work[12] relating gastric motility to reports of hunger in obese and normal weight individuals showed that the normal weight subject reported hunger coincident with stomach contractions whereas in the obese, self-reports of hunger were significantly less often correlated with gastric contractions. That is, in both anorexia nervosa patients and the obese subjects studied by Stunkard, the internal sense of hunger is apparently deficient and unrelated to the physiological state of the subject.

Sense of Ineffectiveness

The third major psychological disturbance in primary anorexia nervosa is a paralyzing sense of ineffectiveness which pervades all thinking and activities. Despite the apparent stubborness and negativism seen in many of these young women, particularly vis-à-vis eating, there is an underlying sense of helplessness affecting all areas of functioning. Bruch's theory is that these patients gain a sense of mastery by effectively controlling their weight, which accounts for their willingness to resort to vomiting or purging.

Using Bruch's criteria, other cases of anorexia which are secondary to schizophrenic or neurotic needs are classified as secondary anorexia nervosa. Her theory of anorexia nervosa has the great advantage of describing a possible etiology and providing a rational basis for the re-educative psychotherapy she prescribes. The patient is assisted in becoming more aware of her own feelings and bodily sensations as a means of recognizing her own separateness and identity. Therapy focuses on her right to satisfy her own basic needs in healthy ways.

OTHER CRITERIA FOR ANOREXIA NERVOSA (FEIGHNER)

Another major classification system in vogue was described by Feighner and colleagues[8] and has been used with minor modifications by many investigators, notably those studying possible endocrine abnormalities in anorexia nervosa. It does not attempt to explain the etiology of the condition and probably some cases classified as secondary anorexia nervosa by Bruch would be included in this scheme. The one advantage of this system is that its use requires a less detailed and sophisticated psychological evaluation, and consequently a more homogeneous group of patients may be identified.

To qualify for the diagnosis of anorexia nervosa using Feighner's criteria, the patient must meet six major criteria.

1. The *age of onset* must be prior to 25 (Spitzer[4] has qualified the age range from 10–30).

2. There must be anorexia with accompanying *weight loss of 25%* of the original body weight. Many experts would argue that most patients do not

have true anorexia, i.e., a loss of appetite, but rather are hungry and stringently ration their food.

3. The patient must demonstrate a *distorted implacable attitude* toward eating, food, or weight that overrides hunger, admonition, reassurances and threats. Examples of this distorted attitude are denial of illness with a failure to recognize nutritional needs, or apparent enjoyment in losing weight with overt manifestation that food refusal is a pleasurable indulgence, or unusual hoarding or handling of food. An example of the latter would be one patient who collected dozens of recipes; she was a gourmet cook who spent hours daily preparing meals for her husband, but refused to eat anything but carrot sticks and celery.

4. *No known medical illness* accounts for the anorexia and weight loss.

5. *No known psychiatric illness* accounts for the condition. Anorexia and weight loss are common findings in the affective disorders, particularly depression, and the loss of appetite may be explained by self-derogatory remarks such as, "I don't deserve to eat, I'm such a bad person." Rarely, however, is the weight loss a driving force in the patient's life. Also the later age of onset of depression and other associated symptoms help to distinguish this condition. Schizophrenia may initially present as anorexia nervosa and some investigators consider the core problem of anorexia nervosa and schizophrenia to be the same, namely, a lack of a sense of separateness with a consequent loss of ego boundaries. However, usually the patient with anorexia nervosa has an appropriate affect and no evidence of a formal thought disorder (e.g. loose associations). The anorexia nervosa patient may have a disturbance in the content of thought amounting to a delusion in her belief that she is fat even when actually emaciated, but this alone does not justify the diagnosis of schizophrenia. Obsessive compulsive neurosis and phobic neurosis must also be considered in the differential diagnosis but there is rarely as dramatic a weight loss in either of these conditions.

6. The patient must demonstrate at least two of the following manifestations: (a) amenorrhea, (b) lanugo (fine body hair on arms and legs), (c) bradycardia (persistent resting pulse of 60 or less), (d) periods of overactivity, (e) episodes of bulimia, (f) vomiting (may be self-induced).

These criteria are often used in the United States and a similar less complex scheme is used by Russell[9] and most investigators in Great Britain. Russell's criteria are itemized in Table 10.1.

PERSONALITY TYPES IN ANOREXIA NERVOSA

No One Personality Type Identified

Although there is broad general agreement that there are psychological factors that account for part of the syndrome of anorexia nervosa, experts disagree about possible predisposing personality types or the existence of precipitating psychological factors. Classically, the young girl who develops anorexia nervosa has been described as perfectionistic, compulsive, and above average in intelligence. The patient has often been an outstanding student, compliant with expectations of her family and teachers. Typically as the patient's weight loss progresses she becomes obsessed with thoughts of food, repetitive in handling or hoarding food, and frequently these adolescents begin to work harder in their studies and begin to deny themselves every pleasure. Eating, food, and the control of weight become the prime focus of the patient's life.

Obsessive-compulsive personality style was long believed to be an essential feature of the disease but systematic studies using any of the three schemes described earlier, have failed to confirm this belief. Parenthetically, observations of war victims suffering from starvation suggest that some of the signs and symptoms, including obsessions about food, compulsive behavior, and infantile regression, may be secondary to the starvation.

One large study[13] distinguished three major personality types: "obsessional," "hysterical," and "mixed." In a group of 30 patients, Crisp[14] thought hysterical or obsessional symptoms developed as the patient lost weight. In another study[15] of 13 patients, three personality trends were observed: passive-aggressive, obsessive-compulsive and passive-dependent.

Precipitating Factors

Evaluation of possible precipitating factors has also yielded conflicting results. Traditionally a sexual conflict, either in reality or fantasy, was thought to trigger the initial weight loss, but systematic attempts to elucidate this factor have not been convincing. Commonly, however, these adolescents have been mildly to moderately overweight prior to the onset of the disease and the patients often state that teasing by family or peers was the motivating factor to start a diet. A number of possible precipitating factors have been identified[16] including disturbance within the family, concern about personal experience, and teasing about weight.

Anorexia nervosa is probably a complex neuroendocrine psychiatric condition that may occur in patients with a wide variety of personality types under certain psychosocial stresses. The relative importance of the physiological, social, and psychological factors must be assessed for each individual patient and the unique constellation of stresses for that person identified.

ENDOCRINE FINDINGS IN ANOREXIA NERVOSA

Weight Loss and Amenorrhea

Amenorrhea is the one finding in anorexia nervosa that may not be functional and it has been the impetus for many detailed endocrine studies.

Menses cease before any significant weight loss has occurred in one third to one half of the patients.[17] Furthermore, although menses are notoriously sensitive to emotional turmoil, amenorrhea does not regularly occur in any other psychiatric disorder.

As discussed in Chapter 3, there is a relationship between body weight and puberty. Frisch[18] found that the mean body weight of girls at menarche was 48 kg even though the age and height of the girls varied considerably. She theorized that with the attainment of a mean critical body weight there is a change in metabolic rate to a level at which the hypothalamus becomes increasingly sensitive to gonadal signals, resulting in a decreased inhibition of gonadal hormones and puberty ensues. One of the reasons anorexia nervosa patients have been so exhaustively studied is that as anorectics regain weight, there is a unique opportunity to study the relationship of body weight to endocrine function. If the regulation of body weight can be understood in this relatively homogeneous small group of patients, perhaps this will facilitate an understanding of obesity, which is both more prevalent than anorexia nervosa and includes a more disparate group of patients in terms of psychopathology and endocrine abnormalities.

As these anorectic patients achieve a normal weight and dietary intake, investigation should lead to a better understanding of the evolution of gonadotropin activity which may depend on weight and nutrition-related feedback mechanisms. For example, it is known that there are low plasma[17, 19] and urinary[20] gonadotropins and an absent response to clomiphene citrate[21] during the acute phase of the disease. Several studies[22, 23] have documented the normal release of luteinizing hormone (LH) and follicle-stimulating hormone (FSH) after administration of gonadotropin-releasing hormone (GnRH), thus suggesting a disturbance in the hypothalamus rather than in pituitary gonadotropin synthesis and release.

Immaturity of LH Pattern

Boyar and co-workers[24] have described an "immaturity" of the 24-hour luteinizing hormone secretory pattern in anorexia nervosa. In the normal prepubertal girl there are low levels of LH secretion of the same magnitude during sleeping and waking. In the early pubertal premenarchal girl there are increased levels of LH secreted during sleep. In the late post-menarchal girl there is normally a marked increase of LH secretion during sleep and also an episodic secretion of LH during waking. In the normal adult pattern there is normally episodic secretion of LH of equal magnitude during sleeping and waking. In their study of nine patients with anorexia nervosa they found an arrest (in those patients with primary amenorrhea) or a regression (in patients with secondary amenorrhea) to the prepubertal, early, or late pubertal pattern of LH secretion that was inappropriate for their age

(See Fig. 10.2). One 22-year-old patient who was studied during an acute phase and during remission showed a pre-pubertal pattern of LH secretion at 40.2 kg and a normal adult pattern at 50.7 kg. This provides some evidence that body weight is one of the determinants of the functional integrity of the hypothalamic pituitary gonadal axis and indirect evidence for Frisch's critical weight theory.

Boyar and colleagues postulate that any mechanism that leads to a critical increase or decrease in body weight may result in corresponding initiation or regression of the pubertal LH secretory pattern. Although these studies are very interesting, the results must still be regarded as tentative since a relatively small number of patients have been studied. One clinical observation of patients with anorexia nervosa is that often menses do not commence in these young women as they regain weight in excess of the postulated critical 48 kg; the reason for this is not clear.

Although there are less data available on male patients, male anorectics have been shown to have low levels of urinary testosterone and low total gonadotrophic activity in the urine.[25]

Low Tri-Iodothyronine Syndrome

Many patients with anorexia nervosa have symptoms suggestive of deficient thyroid activity including bradycardia, dry skin, low basal metabolic rate, elevated serum cholesterol and elevated carotene levels. Moshang et al[26] have shown significantly low tri-iodothyronine (T_3) levels in anorexia nervosa but a normal mean basal thyroid-stimulating hormone (TSH) concentration and normal mean maximum increase in TSH after thyroid releasing hormone, and normal thyroxine (T_4) levels. The current theory is that there is a "low tri-iodothyronine syndrome" that occurs in chronic and severe illness or acute starvation due to *diminished peripheral deiodinization of T_4 to T_3*. It is estimated that 60–80% of the daily production of T_3 is secondary to extrathyroidal conversion of T_4 to T_3. Wilcox[27] studied 10 obese women following jejunoileal bypass who had a dramatic decrease in their calorie intake but little change in weight and found significantly lower T_3 in these patients than in normal weight control subjects. This finding supports the idea that body weight *per se* does not determine T_3 levels but calorie deprivation does. At both extremes of body weight, anorexia nervosa and obesity, the pituitary-thyroid axis is normal, but in anorexia nervosa and calorie-deprived obese T_3 is low.

Boyar and colleagues[28] have also studied cortisol secretion and metabolism in anorexia nervosa. They noted that the 10 patients studied had significantly elevated 24-hour mean plasma cortisol levels, with preservation of the normal circadian variation of cortisol secretory levels. These patients also had a significant decrease in the metabolic clearance rate of cortisol and an

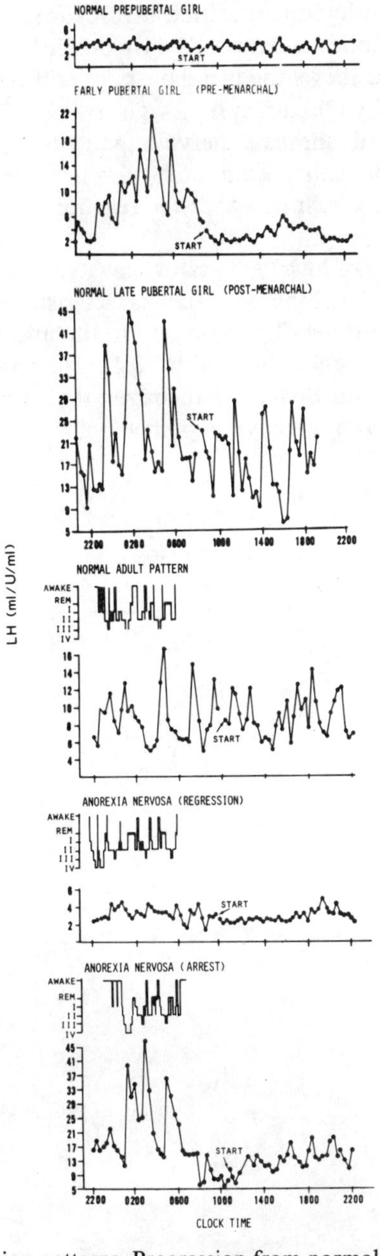

Figure 10.2. LH secretion patterns. Progression from normal prepubertal pattern to normal adult pattern. In one anorexia nervosa patient there was "regression" to the prepubertal pattern and in another anorexia nervosa patient the LH pattern was "arrested" at the early pubertal stage (adapted from Boyar et al[24]).

elevation of the tetrahydrocortisol-tetrahydrocortisone ratio. This *elevated THF/THE ratio* implies a decreased 11-oxidation of cortisol to cortisone (See Fig. 10.3 which shows the metabolism of cortisol and cortisone by the liver and excretion by the kidney).

Another study[29] of anorexia nervosa patients has shown a *decreased androsterone:etiocholanolone ratio,* both of which are metabolites of testosterone. 5α reductase which catalyzes the reaction of testosterone to androsterone is decreased.

The three findings of low T_3/T_4 ratio, elevated THF/THE ratio, and low androsterone:etiocholanolone ratio are characteristic of the "low tri-iodothyronine syndrome" and may be secondary to the undernutrition in anorexia nervosa or chronic illnesses (See Table 10.2). The enzymes involved are all present in the liver, and Boyar has theorized that these thyroid and steroid findings may serve a "protective hypometabolic" function in the face of a catabolic state.

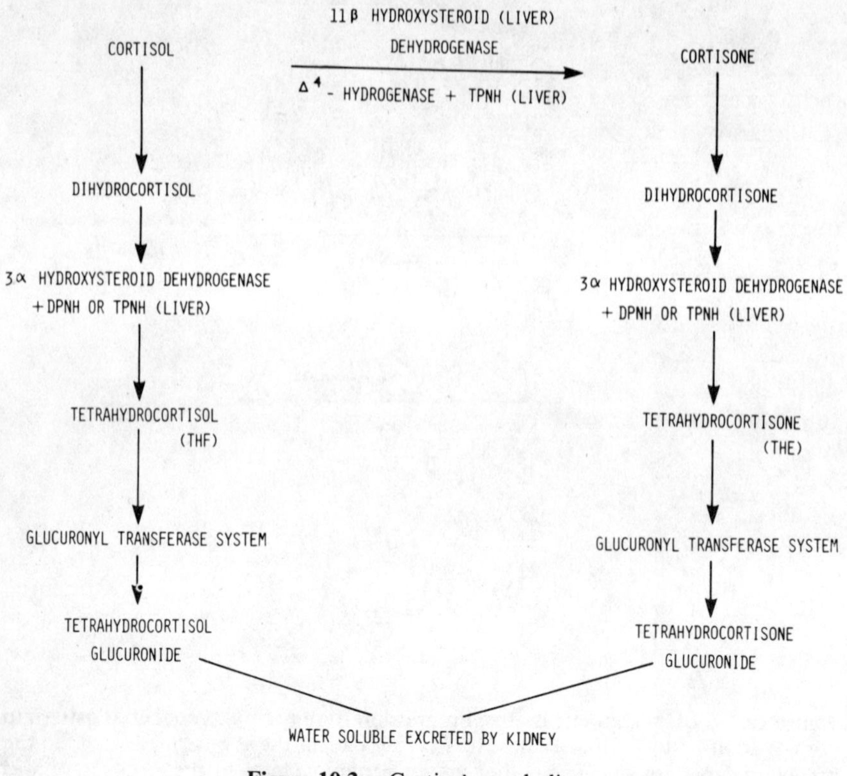

Figure 10.3. Cortisol metabolism.

Table 10.2
Low tri-iodothyronine syndrome.

Occurs in some chronic diseases, starvation, and perhaps in anorexia nervosa
1. Elevated THF:THE (tetrahydrocortisol:tetrahydrocortisone) ratio
2. Low T_3:T_4 (tri-iodothyronine:thyroxine) ratio
3. Low androsterone: etiocholanolone ratio

Evidence for Hypothalamic Dysfunction

Mecklenburg and associates[23] studied five anorexia nervosa patients, four of whom had an abnormal increase in urine osmolality after administration of exogenous anti-diuretic hormone (ADH). They concluded that these patients had partial diabetes insipidus, although noting that a number of factors can interfere with the method used. They hypothesize that an abnormality of the hypothalamus near the supraoptic nucleus accounts for the partial diabetes insipidus. These same five patients were studied under cold stress at a temperature of 50° F (10° C) and all failed to shiver, had an abnormal decrease in core temperature and did not stabilize their temperature. Furthermore, four of the five patients had decreased compensatory responses to heat stress. The authors note that the primary motor center for shivering is thought to be in the posterior hypothalamus under inhibition from the anterior hypothalamic thermosensitive cells. Although they conclude that their findings are positive evidence of hypothalamic dysfunction, the number of subjects studied was small. Table 10.3 lists the endocrine and metabolic abnormalities in anorexia nervosa.

Prolactin Levels

Thyroid-releasing hormone is known to be a highly potent prolactin releaser. Patients with abnormalities in prolactin levels would be interesting theoretically since a decrease in central dopaminergic activity is thought to increase prolactin output from the anterior pituitary. An increase in dopamine may also inhibit feelings of hunger. Amphetamines, which at least temporarily inhibit appetite in some people, are thought to increase central dopaminergic activity (See Fig. 10.4). Chlorpromazine, a dopamine antagonist, is a known potent stimulus of prolactin secretion, and administration

Table 10.3
Metabolic and endocrine abnormalities in anorexia nervosa.

- Low Plasma and Urinary LH and FSH (gonadotrophins) but normal release after GnRH
- Regression or "arrest" of LH secretory pattern
- Low tri-iodothyronine syndrome
- Thermoregulatory abnormalities
- Questionable partial diabetes insipidus
- Elevated GH
- Low insulin levels

often results in increased hunger and weight gain. However, Wilcox[27] noted that obese calorie-deprived patients (ostensibly hungry) had high normal prolactin levels.

PROGNOSIS OF ANOREXIA NERVOSA

The course of anorexia nervosa is variable. It may be chronic with remissions and exacerbations or it may progress to death or there may be but one episode. The mortality rate has been estimated to be between 10 and 20%. One study suggests that the mortality rate is higher in male patients.[30] Starvation is the usual listed cause of death but the actual terminal event is often not known.

Evaluation of studies investigating morbidity in patients who have regained to normal weight is difficult because of the wide variety of criteria used to assess "morbidity." However, a large proportion of these patients have significant residual psychopathology even if their weight is normal.

Beumont and associates[16] have evaluated a group of 31 patients divided into "dieters" (those who have lost weight by dieting, food refusal, and strenuous exercising) and "vomiters and purgers" (those who have induced vomiting or abused laxatives or diuretics). The "dieters" were generally obsessive and socially withdrawn individuals whose anorectic behavior started in response to psychological stress and these patients were more likely to have a full recovery. The "vomiters and purgers" were more outgoing in personality and most had previously been obese; these patients had a poor prognosis both in terms of weight and anorectic behavior. Another study[31] found that onset at an early age and employment in professional and skilled occupations were associated with a good outcome. Factors associated with poor prognosis included vomiting, laxative abuse, psychosomatic complaints, and moderate to severe depression and obsessive-compulsive manifestations.

TREATMENT OF ANOREXIA NERVOSA

Treatment of anorexia nervosa is still largely a matter of controversy. Most agree that hospitalization in the acute phase is necessary. Metabolic imbalances, intercurrent infections, or other acute problems must be treated medically.

At present the most effective therapy appears to be a combination of re-educative psychotherapy and behavior modification.

Re-educative psychotherapy, rather than intensive insight psychotherapy, is more likely to be effective. Bruch[6] encourages patients to focus on stimuli arising within themselves including feelings and physical sensations. Transactional analysis[15] has also been used with emphasis on the patients' own thoughts and feelings. Whatever method is used, treatment is often difficult, requiring close coordination and communication among all members of the treatment staff. Usually the patient must be hospitalized for several months.

The behavior modification method that has been commonly used is an operant conditioning program individually designed for each patient with positive reinforcement of social activity, increased physical activity, and visiting privileges contingent on weight gain. For example, in a study by Halmi and co-workers,[32] the patient was expected to gain 0.5 kg/5-day period. If she gained the required weight, she was given an additional hour out of her room daily and an additional hour with a visitor. If the patient did not gain weight at the end of 5 days, she earned no additional privileges. If she lost weight, she was tube fed until she attained the weight she was at the beginning of the 5-day period. The patients were started on formula feedings, Sustacal (1 cal/ml) in a total 24-hour feeding of 125% of basal requirements.

Although there has been great interest in the behavior therapies in the treatment of anorexia nervosa, it must be remembered that most of the studies have relatively brief follow-up periods, usually less than a year. It is well known that follow-up is necessary since weight gain at discharge does not ensure against relapse. In fact, one collaborative study[33] of behavior therapy for anorexia nervosa in 81 patients showed no significant improvement in the more seriously ill patients with behavior modification. Most likely, behavior modification techniques will eventually prove to be effective tools as part of a holistic treatment plan for certain patients with anorexia nervosa.

IMPORTANCE OF ANOREXIA NERVOSA RESEARCH FOR OBESITY

Although a relatively rare condition, elucidation of the endocrine, metabolic, and psychological abnormalities of anorexia nervosa might permit a better understanding of obesity, which in Western countries, at least, is fast approaching epidemic proportions. Part of the difficulty in studying obesity is that the problem is so common with such a wide variety of associated findings, that even identifying a group to be studied is a gigantic undertaking. Anorexia nervosa, on the other hand, is relatively easy to diagnose, the study group can be easily delimited, and the patient group has a number of clinical features in common. Furthermore, the paradox of voluntarily starving to death, in the face of plenty, provokes curiosity.

Disturbances of Body Image and Eating Patterns

A significant proportion of anorectics was initially at least mildly obese and a small but definite percentage of "recovered" anorectics become obese. Body image disturbances are found in most anorexia nervosa patients and some obese patients. Studies of the perceptual aspect of body image in anorexia nervosa patients has been the impetus to the study of analogous problems in the obese.

Both obesity and anorexia nervosa involve disturbances in eating patterns. An understanding of the bulimic episodes of anorexia nervosa might help us understand the binges that occur in obese patients, particularly those with the binge-eating syndrome. The megaphagia (increased eating) seen in Kleine-Levin syndrome (a hypersomnia that occurs in adolescent males) and in Parkinson's disease may be a variant of bulimia. Marijuana users regularly report increased appetite and overeating (the "munchies").

Metabolic and Endocrine Findings

Some of the anorexia nervosa patients do have anorexia, i.e., a true loss of the sense of hunger; however, many are hungry but control their eating. The hypothalamus is thought to be an important center in the control of eating. The ventromedial nucleus is designated the "satiety" center and ostensibly exerts inhibitory control over the ventrolateral nucleus of the hypothalamus designated the "feeding" center. Most of the conditions that have bulimia or megaphagia are postulated to have abnormalities of the hypothalamus or its neural connections. Many of the studies of anorexia nervosa are focusing on abnormalities of the hypothalamus, but it remains unclear whether these abnormalities are primary or secondary to malnutrition. Likewise the endocrine and metabolic abnormalities of obesity may be secondary to overnutrition. It is possible that in both disorders of extreme weight change, the abnormalities serve to perpetuate the weight disturbance, even if these abnormalities were not causal.

Dopaminergic Theory of Anorexia Nervosa

Study of various conditions with abnormalities of appetite may result in an understanding of the control of appetite and hence the regulation of weight. For example, Barry and Klawans,[34] theorize that unmodulated dopaminergic activity may account for the principle findings of anorexia nervosa.

They cite the following in support of this theory. Amphetamine is an indirect catecholamine agonist that releases dopamine and norepinephrine (the major catecholamines) from their respective nerve terminals and inhibits re-uptake of catecholamines. Also, to a lesser extent, amphetamine inhibits monoamine oxidase.[35] It is hypothesized that the catecholamines act on the ventromedial and ventrolateral hypothalamic centers to induce anorexia. Apomorphine, which probably acts as a direct dopamine agonist, with no effect on norepinephrine receptors, results in a decreased food intake in rats.[36] This action is blocked by pimozide, a dopamine receptor antagonist. Also, megaphagia has been noted in some patients with Parkinson's disease,[37] a condition in which central dopamine is depleted. Conversely, patients with Parkinson's disease taking L-dopa lose weight, initially secondary to nausea and vomiting but later weight losses may be due to increased dopamine activity.[38] Furthermore, prolonged administration of chlorpromazine, a dopamine blocking agent, is well known to cause weight gain. Therefore, unmodulated dopamine activity, of unknown cause, may account for the

SUBSTANCE	DOPAMINE EFFECT	EFFECT ON APPETITE
Amphetamine	↑	↓
Apomorphine	↑	↓
Pimozide	↓	↑
Parkinson's Disease (untreated)	↓ (block receptor)	↑ (?)
Parkinson's Disease (treatment with L-Dopa)	↑	↓
Chlorpromazine	↓	↑

Figure 10.4. Dopamine and anorexia. Summary of evidence for the theory that unmodulated dopamine activity results in anorexia.

anorexia in anorexia nervosa (See Table 10.4). One problem with this aspect of the theory is that many patients claim not to be anorexic, but rather to rigidly control their intake.

Furthermore, the hyperactivity of the anorectic patient might also be related to the catecholamines. Amphetamine induces hyperactivity through the noradrenergic system.[39] Although there are many dissimilarities between amphetamine psychosis and anorexia nervosa, in both there are distortions of body image and perception, hyperactivity and obsessive-compulsive manifestations. The behavior of some anorexic patients appears stereotypic, particularly vis-à-vis food. The stereotyped behavior seen in animals intoxicated on amphetamines has been shown[36, 40] to be due to release of dopamine which is densely distributed in the nigrostriatal area.

Amphetamine users describe gross distortions of body image[41] including feelings of transparency and invisibility. The body image disturbance in anorexia nervosa is usually a misperception of actual size. Amphetamine abusers also report visual distortions. This effect of amphetamine is thought to be mediated by dopamine.[42]

Finally, animal studies suggest that substances that stimulate dopamine receptors inhibit LH-releasing hormone (GnRH) and stimulate prolactin release. Therefore, unmodulated dopamine activity could account for the amenorrhea and the occasional finding of galactorrhea[23] in anorexia nervosa.

This theory does not account for why dopamine is unmodulated, and it may prove to be oversimplified or incorrect, but it does suggest ways of studying the control of appetite and weight which may eventually lead to a better understanding of both obesity and anorexia nervosa.

Sensitivity to External Cues

At both extremes of weight, some patients in each group are more sensitive to external cues than to the sensations arising within themselves. Although

Table 10.4
Increased catecholamine theory of anorexia nervosa (adapted from Barry and Klawans[34]).

Effects of Dopamine	Effects of Norepinephrine
• Anorexia	• hyperactivity
• Amenorrhea (inhibition Gn RH)	
• Body image distortion	
• Ritualistic stereotyped behavior	

the evidence is contradictory, there appears to be at least a subset of the obese population who are more sensitive to external cues.[43] Anorexia nervosa patients who claim not to be hungry, tired, or emotional may actually be more attuned to external cues than to their own internal body signals. This idea fits well with Bruch's theory of faulty parental transactions resulting in decreased internal awareness in the child.

Complicated Problems

Both anorexia nervosa and obesity are conditions that are complex and bridge several fields of medicine including internal medicine, pediatrics, family practice, and psychiatry. A clear understanding of either disease will require the collaboration of investigators in all these areas. Even though there is much experimental work underway in both animals and humans, this work is for the most part tentative and often has not been practical for the clinical management of these patients, whose numbers are rapidly increasing.

EATING DISORDERS WITHOUT WEIGHT ABNORMALITIES

Abnormalities of eating may occur without a change in weight. Bulimia and pica are the two most distinct conditions which have thus far been identified. Eating disturbances may occur in conjunction with psychiatric conditions, such as schizophrenia or phobic disorders.

In schizophrenia a delusion may involve food:

> Jennifer, a patient with hebephrenic schizophrenia had a thought disorder and inappropriate affect. She was also delusional and believed that her family was plotting to hurt her and that her mother had poisoned her food. Therefore she refused to eat.

In certain drug ingestions, abnormalities of eating may occur. With LSD, the patient may "taste in color"; that is, after eating he may experience a colorful visual hallucination (synesthesia); depending on the person's subjective reaction to this experience he may increase or decrease eating. With amphetamine ingestion there is initially a marked decrease in appetite and with marijuana, megaphagia (the "munchies") is prominent.

Various neurological conditions also involve eating abnormalities. In patients with bilateral temporal lobe destruction, a Kluver-Bucy-like syndrome may occur with insatiable appetite, placidity, sexual exhibitionism, and visual agnosia (vision is intact physically but there is an inability to discriminate objects meaningfully). As noted earlier, untreated Parkinson's disease may be associated with megaphagia. Kleine-Levin syndrome, a periodic hypersomnia, may be associated with megaphagia.

BULIMIA

Bulimia as a separate syndrome has only recently been popularized[4] and is distinct from the symptom of bulimia (episodes of overeating) that is seen in a wide variety of conditions. Bulimia is an episodic pattern of binge eating that occurs primarily in female adolescents and young women, which is often associated with little or no weight change. In striking contrast to anorexia nervosa patients, these young women are aware of their disordered eating patterns and often seek psychiatric assistance. There is no amenorrhea or significant weight loss. The patients often fear they will be unable to stop eating voluntarily. They are very concerned about their weights and try to control their weight with diet, self-induced vomiting, or cathartics. During a binge, food is eaten as inconspicuously as possible with minimal chewing and food often has a high calorie content with a sweet taste. Once a binge has started, other foods may be sought to continue the binge. The binge is terminated with abdominal pain, sleep, self-induced vomiting, or social interruption. Even though the patient may describe the binge as pleasurable, it is followed with self-condemnation and, often, a very rigid diet. In severe cases, there may be no period of normal eating and the patient may alternate between fasts and binges.

Prevalence is unknown and there are no known precipitating factors. Some patients have a history of intermittent drug abuse, particularly barbiturates, amphetamines, or alcohol. The course is usually chronic with occasional remissions. Bulimia has some similarities to the binge-eating syndrome and may be the same condition but without weight gain.

The following case history illustrates some of the findings typical of bulimia:

> Annette is a 20-year-old college senior who complained, "I think about food constantly and I'm afraid I will lose control and not be able to stop eating." Two years prior to the initial evaluation she weighed 150 pounds and was 5 feet 4 inches tall; she decided to diet by following a non-carbohydrate diet of 300 calories. After losing 10 pounds her menstrual periods stopped. She continued to diet over the next 6 months until she weighed 85 pounds. She felt she was a good person for losing weight but still "felt fat" and thought she would look even better at 80 pounds. However, she realized, intellectually, that she actually needed to gain weight. She was with friends who were her constant companions on a tour of Italy and she decided to gauge her food intake to theirs rather than judging by whether she felt fat. She regained to 130 pounds. Her menses started when she weighed 112 pounds.
>
> However, during the last 8 months, she has continued to think incessantly about food and dream about food. She has binges of overeating in which she will consume large quantities of a current favorite food in less than 15 minutes. A recent favorite was cookies. She also chews about 30 packs of sugarless gum per day. The binge is terminated when she develops abdominal pain, or when all the food in the refrigerator is gone, or when she is interrupted. Her weight fluctuates between 125 and 130 pounds. Her menses are normal and she is very aware of the

abnormal eating pattern. Following a binge, she is guilt-ridden for days and considers herself a bad person. Between binges she tries not to eat at all, but sometimes will allow herself a small helping of a very low calorie food, for example, string beans.

She notes that binges are more likely when she is emotionally upset and comments that she has made food the most important thing in her life because it is the only area of her functioning over which she has some control. She adds that she knows intellectually that she is not fat and knows that fasting does not prove that one is a good person, but knowing this does not alter her feelings. She receives outstanding marks in college, although she did not want to go to school. She performs well on her job, but dislikes secretarial work. She is an attractive woman who dresses well but since breaking up with a boyfriend 2 years ago has dated only infrequently. She lives with her parents and was in constant and bitter conflict with them until she began obsessing about food.

This young woman probably would have been diagnosed as having anorexia nervosa early in her history but currently the diagnosis of bulimia is more appropriate since she has primarily an eating disturbance without a weight abnormality. She feels helpless to control many areas of her life and thinks most decisions have been made for her rather than by her, and food intake is the only area of her life that she controls. The psychodynamics of a pervasive sense of helplessness and disturbed body image are the same in this patient as in primary anorexia nervosa as described by Bruch.

PICA

Pica is the persistent eating of non-nutritional substances and is usually not associated with weight changes. It occurs most frequently in children or pregnant women. A variety of non-food substances may be ingested ranging from starch, clay, ashes, and paint to hair. The childhood form usually begins in the second year but may also start somewhat earlier. It is more common in retarded children, and in these youngsters may start later. It usually remits spontaneously.

There is dispute as to whether pica causes certain deficiency states or is the consequence of a deficiency state. For example, a group of 38 iron-deficient patients had excessive ice consumption and with iron therapy two thirds lost their craving for ice.[44] Furthermore, Lanzkowsky[45] studied 12 children who chronically ingested sand, soil, and clay, and had iron-deficiency anemia. Treatment with intramuscular iron injections reversed the habit. Others postulate that iron deficiency anemia can be caused by various ingested substances that prevent iron absorption.

Gastrointestinal malaise may also be an important etiological factor in pica. Geophagia (consumption of clay or soil) was reported to relieve nausea and vomiting by the early Greeks and Arabs. Even animals have been suspected of relieving gastrointestinal malaise by pica. Virtually every dog owner has observed his pet eating soil or grass during illness.

The propensity of pregnant women for this condition has been noted since the middle ages. In some cultures, pica is extremely common during pregnancy. O'Rourke et al[46] studied 200 obstetric patients in Augusta, Georgia, and found that 55% of them ate clay or starch. The majority had pica only during pregnancy. Typically, the women with pica during pregnancy believed ingestion of the various substances would relieve nausea and vomiting or headaches and ensure beautiful children. Frustration of a craving was believed to cause a birthmark on the fetus. There also is a relationship between eating dirt as a child and pica during pregnancy. In the study by Keith et al,[47] for example, 27% of pregnant women with pica also ate dirt in childhood.

Prolonged ingestion of non-nutritive material can lead to general malnutrition by compromising the absorption of nutrients or a specific deficiency state from eating materials with a high affinity for certain trace elements such as zinc or iron. Parasitic infections can occur from eating contaminated soil. Ingestion of substances containing a high concentration of lead or other heavy metals can result in systemic poisoning. Furthermore, in pregnant women the incidence of toxemia has been reported to be twice as great in those who have pica as in those who do not.[46]

RUMINATION

Rumination is an eating disorder that starts in infancy between 3 to 12 months; it is usually associated with weight loss or failure to thrive. It rarely occurs in adults but if it does is called merycism. Typically, a rumination episode is as follows.[48] Food is regurgitated into the mouth without nausea, retching, or disgust, and is ejected, chewed, or reswallowed. Concomitantly the back is arched, sucking movements of the tongue occur, and the activity appears pleasurable to the infant. Between rumination episodes the infant is usually hungry and irritable.[49] There is no associated gastrointestinal disease.

Characteristically the diagnosis is missed during an extensive and costly work-up in which the child is studied and restudied with a tube in every orifice. Observation of the infant during and after feeding will clarify the situation. The various diagnostic tests may actually be associated with an increased incidence of rumination episodes. It is critical that the clinician closely observe the infant to determine whether the regurgitation is voluntary.

It is probably a relatively rare condition, although closer observation might reveal that many "vomiting" infants who fail to thrive actually are ruminating. The cáuse of the condition is thought to be a poor mother-baby relationship.

Flanagan[49] recommends a mother substitute initially as a role model. Individual psychotherapy for the mother may also be needed, although spontaneous remissions have been reported. The disorder is potentially fatal and mortality may be as high as 25%.[50] If the consequent failure to thrive is untreated, developmental delays may occur in all spheres. After rumination has ceased, it is not known whether there are subsequent feeding difficulties or personality abnormalities.

RELATIONSHIP BETWEEN EATING AND SLEEPING DISORDERS

The Kleine-Levin syndrome and the Pickwickian syndrome are two sleep disorders that are associated with abnormalities of eating.

KLEINE-LEVIN SYNDROME

The Kleine-Levin syndrome is a periodic hypersomnia often associated with megaphagia that occurs predominantly in adolescent males. Striking behavioral symptoms may preceed, follow, or coincide with the sleeping episode; these include motor restlessness, truculence, and uninhibited sexuality. Other reported psychiatric symptoms include alterations in sensorium, amnesia, affective symptoms, delusions, and hallucinations. The sleeping episodes characteristically start gradually, last several days, recur at intervals of several months, and cease completely by the third decade. The patient typically is completely normal between episodes. Patients are often amnesic for the hypersomnia and bizarre behavior. EEG abnormalities of a diffuse generalized type may occur during the episodes. Treatment with cerebral stimulants may abort an episode. Megaphagia or bulimia occurs in perhaps half the patients during the sleepy periods but usually does not result in weight gain since the total episode is only a few days every several months. For a review see Powers and Gunderman.[51]

This is a rare condition; fewer than 50 cases have been reported in the literature. It is even less common in females than in males. Billiard and colleagues[52] report one adolescent girl who had the typical sleeping episodes which regularly occurred close to the end of her menstrual cycle. A therapeutic trial of premarin prevented the hypersomnia. This patient also had an abnormal increase of 5-hydroxyindolacetic acid (5-HIAA) in the cerebral spinal fluid after the probenecid test, suggesting an increased turnover of 5-hydroxytryptamine during the periodic hypersomnia.

PICKWICKIAN SYNDROME

The Pickwickian syndrome is a hypersomnia associated with obesity. The condition was named after Joe, the fat boy in Dicken's *Pickwick Papers*. These grossly obese patients are typically sleepy, short of breath, and cyanotic. One study of 22 patients[53] revealed a marked reduction in pO_2 and an increase in pCO_2. Secondary polycythemia and right ventricular hypertrophy with signs of cor pulmonale and right ventricular failure were frequent. Nearly one third of these patients died and the remainder were likely to have serious morbidity including pulmonary emboli and severe papilledema. It was initially thought that the increase in fat resulted in mechanical difficulty in breathing and hence decreased perfusion of the lungs, but probably the situation is much more complex.

NEUROENDOCRINE CORRELATES OF SLEEP AND EATING DISORDERS

SEROTONIN AND CATECHOLAMINES IMPLICATED

The Kleine-Levin syndrome and the Pickwickian syndrome which involve disorders of both eating or weight and sleeping are interesting since animal studies suggest that certain areas of the brain are concerned with both eating and sleeping. The hypothalamus, classically thought to mediate eating, has many neural interconnections to the reticular activating system which is involved in modulating sleep. The raphe nuclei containing serotonin neurons are located in the lower midbrain and upper pons and are part of the reticular activating system. The axons of these nuclei ascend via the medial forebrain bundle (MFB) to terminate primarily, but not exclusively, in the hypothalamus.

Animal studies implicate serotonin as responsible for slow wave sleep because lesions in the median raphe abolish slow wave sleep.[54] The increase of 5-HIAA, a metabolite of serotonin in a somnolent patient with Kleine-Levin syndrome, is consistent with this theory.[52] However, Dement studied cats treated with p-chlorphenyalanine (which inhibits serotonin synthesis) and they still slept.[55]

Jouvet[54] also proposes that connections from the medial raphe to the norepinephrine-rich nucleus ceruleus trigger rapid eye movement (REM) sleep. The dorsal norepinephrine pathway originates in the nucleus ceruleus and terminates in the hippocampus and cerebral cortex. The hippocampus, located in the temporal lobe, has neural interconnections via the fornix to the mammillary nuclei (part of the hypothalamus). The ventral norepinephrine pathway originates from nuclei in the brainstem and ascends via the medial-forebrain bundle to the hypothalamus.

RITUALISTIC COMPULSIVE BEHAVIOR

Obsessive compulsive characteristics have been noted in several of the eating disorders. Many anorexia nervosa patients obsess about food and are ritualistic in their handling of food. Obese patients with the binge-eating syndrome may eat in a compulsive manner when emotionally upset. In the

Kleine-Levin syndrome the bulimic episodes may be ritualistic and some of the bizarre behaviors have been described as "irresistable urges."[51] The cingulate gyrus which is part of the limbic system is thought to mediate some aspects of ritualistic compulsive behavior. Kelly et al[56] treated patients with intractable obsessions and compulsions with lesions in the anterior cingulate gyrus. Apparently some of these patients responded to treatment. The amygdala, also part of the limbic system, is known to influence eating and sexual behavior, at least in animals with the Kluver-Bucy syndrome. There are many complex neural interconnections between amygdala and hypothalamus.

LIMBIC SYSTEM

The limbic system includes Papez's circuit of emotion, and an understanding of the eating and sleeping disorders will require elucidation of the complex relationship between the limbic system, the reticular activating system, and the hypothalamus. That mind and body are not separate is perhaps nowhere clearer than in the eating and sleeping disorders which have a wide variety of psychological and physiological abnormalities. Knowledge of the limbic system, reticular activating system and hypothalamus may eventually permit a holistic theory of these disorders and thereby permit more realistic treatment plans.

HYPOTHALAMUS AND PITUITARY HORMONES

The hypothalamus is also well known to be crucial in the neuroendocrine system. Sleep research laboratories have noted that several hypothalamic and pituitary hormones are closely related to the 24-hour sleep-waking cycle.[57] For example, growth hormone is secreted during the first 2 hours of sleep and it is postulated that there is a relationship to stage III and IV sleep. Urinary and plasma corticosteriod levels also peak during the last part of the night. As the eating and sleeping disorders are studied in more detail, abnormalities in the neuroendocrine system will probably be documented.

SUMMARY

There is a wide variety of eating disorders which may be associated with weight gain, stable weight, or weight loss. Although obesity is by far the most common, research on the other conditions, particularly anorexia nervosa, may provide valuable information about the regulation of weight. The sleep disorders are currently the focus of much interest and also may be associated with eating dysfunctions Although many psychiatric disorders may have associated eating problems, depression is usually accompanied by anorexia and weight loss. Systemic disease, notably carcinoma, is associated with weight loss and anorexia.

References

1. Morton RR: Phtisiologia-or a Treatise of Consumption. London, Smith, 1689.
2. Gull WW: Address in medicine delivered before Annual Meeting of the British Medical Association at Oxford. Lancet 2: 171, 1868.
3. Lasèque EC: De l'anorexie hystérique. Arch Gen Med 21: 385, 1873.
4. Spitzer RL: Eating disorders. In: Diagnostic and Statistical Manual III. Draft presented to the American Psychiatric Association, May 1977, Toronto, Canada.
5. Powers PS: Art work: another dimension in the treatment of psychiatric patients. Art Psychotherapy 5:71–79, 1978.
6. Bruch H: Eating Disorders: Obesity, Anorexia Nervosa and the Person Within. New York, Basic Books, 1973.
7. Bliss EL, Branch CHH: Anorexia Nervosa. New York, Hoeber, 1960.
8. Feighner JP, Robins E, Guze SB, et al: Diagnostic criteria for use in psychiatric research. Arch Gen Psychiatry 26: 57–63, 1972.
9. Russell GFM: Anorexia nervosa: its identity as an illness and its treatment. In: Modern Trends in Psychological Medicine. Price JH (ed). London, Butterworths, 1970, pp 131–164.
10. Slade PD, Russell GFM: Awareness of body dimensions in anorexia nervosa: cross-sectional and longitudinal studies. Psychol Med 3: 188–199, 1973.
11. Crisp AH, Kalucy RS: Aspects of the perceptual disorder in anorexia nervosa. Br J Med Psychol 47: 349-361, 1974.
12. Stunkard AJ, Fox S: The relationship of gastric motility and hunger. Psychosom Med 33: 123–134, 1971.
13. Dally PJ: Anorexia Nervosa. London, Heinemann, 1969.
14. Crisp AH: Clinical and therapeutic aspects of anorexia nervosa: a study of 30 cases. J Psychosom Res 9: 67–78, 1965.
15. Powers PS, Powers HP: Combined therapy in anorexia nervosa: behavior modification and transactional analysis, in preparation 1979.
16. Beumont PJV, George GCW, Smart DE: "Dieters" and "vomiters and purgers" in anorexia nervosa. Psychol Med: 6: 617–622, 1976.
17. Warren MP, Vande Wiele RL: Clinical and metabolic features of anorexia nervosa. Am J Obstet Gynecol 117: 435–449, 1973.
18. Frisch RE: Critical weight at menarche and the initiation of the adolescent growth spurt and control of puberty. In: Control of the Onset of Puberty. Grumbach M, Grave G, Mayer F (eds). New York, John Wiley and Sons, 1974, pp 403–423.
19. Beumont PJV, Carr PJ, Gelder MG: Plasma levels of luteinizing hormone and of immunoreactive oestrogens (oestradiol) in anorexia nervosa: response to clomiphene citrate. Psychol Med 3: 495–501, 1973.
20. Russell GFM, Loraine JA, Bell ET, et al: Gonadotrophin and oestrogen excretion in patients with anorexia nervosa. J Psychosom Res 9: 79–85, 1965.
21. Marshall JC, Fraser TR: Amenorrhea in anorexia nervosa: assessment and treatment with clomiphene citrate. Br Med J 4: 590–592, 1971.
22. Wiegelmann W, Solbach HG: Effects of LH-RF on plasma levels of LH and FSH in anorexia nervosa. Horm Metab Res 4: 404, 1972.
23. Mecklenburg RS, Loriaux DL, Thompson RH, et al: Hypothalamic dysfunction in patients with anorexia nervosa. Medicine (Baltimore)53: 147–159, 1974.
24. Boyar RM, Katz J, Finkelstein JW, et al: Anorexia nervosa: immaturity of the 24-hour luteinizing hormone secretory pattern. N Engl J Med 291: 861–865, 1974.
25. Beumont PJV: Anorexia nervosa in male subjects. Psychother Psychosom 18: 365–371, 1970.
26. Moshang T, Parks JS, Baker L, et al: Low serum triiodothyronine in patients with anorexia nervosa. J Clin Endocrinol Metab 40: 470–473, 1975.
27. Wilcox RG: Triiodothyronone, TSH and prolactin in obese women. Lancet 1: 1027–1029, 1977.
28. Boyar RM, Hellman LD, Roffwarg H, et al: Cortisol secretion and metabolism in anorexia nervosa. N Engl J Med 296: 190–193, 1977.
29. Bradlow HL, Boyar RM, O'Connor J, et al: Hypothyroid-like alterations in testosterone metabolism in anorexia nervosa. J Clin Endocrinol Metab 43: 571–574, 1976.

30. Powers PS, Powers HP: Anorexia nervosa in males, in preparation 1979.
31. Halmi KA, Brodland G, Loney J: Prognosis in anorexia nervosa. Ann Intern Med 78: 907–909, 1973.
32. Halmi KA, Powers PS, Cunningham S: Treatment of anorexia nervosa with behavior modification: effectiveness of formula feedings and isolation. Arch Gen Psychiatry 32: 93–96, 1975.
33. Eckert ED, Goldberg SC, Halmi KA, et al: Behavior therapy in anorexia nervosa. Presentation at Annual Meeting of American Psychiatric Association. Toronto, Canada, 1977.
34. Barry VC, Klawans HL: On the role of dopamine in the pathophysiology of anorexia nervosa. J Neural Transmission 38: 107–122, 1976.
35. Baldessarini RJ: Pharmacology of the amphetamines. Pediatrics 49: 694–700, 1972.
36. Ernst AM: Mode of action of apomorphine and dextroamphetamine on gnawing compulsion in rats. Psychopharmacologia 10: 316–323, 1967.
37. Rosenberg P, Herishanu Y, Beilin B: Increased appetite (bulimia) in Parkinson's disease. J Am Geriatr Soc 25: 277–278, 1977.
38. Barbeau A, Mars H, Gillo-Joffroy L: Adverse clinical side effects of levodopa therapy. In: Recent Advances in Parkinson's Disease. Barbeau A, McDowell FH (eds). Philadelphia, FA Davis, 1971.
39. Ellinwood EHJ, Sudilovsky A, Nelson LM: Evolving behavior in the clinical and experimental amphetamine (model) psychosis. Am J Psychiatry 130: 1088–1093, 1973.
40. Fog RL, Randrup A, Pakkenberg H: Aminergic mechanisms in corpus striatum and amphetamine-induced stereotyped behavior. Psychopharmacologia 11: 179–183, 1967.
41. Ellinwood EHJ: Amphetamine psychosis: a multi-dimensional process. Semin Psychiatry 1: 208–226, 1969.
42. Klawans HL, Margolin DI: Amphetamine-induced hypersensitivity in guinea pigs (implications in psychosis and human movement disorders). Arch Gen Psychiatry 32: 725–732, 1975.
43. Schachter S: Some extraordinary facts about obese humans and rats. Am Psychol 26: 129–144, 1971.
44. Reynolds RD, Binder HJ, Miller MB, et al: Pagophagia and iron deficiency anemia. Ann Intern Med 69: 435–440, 1968.
45. Lanzkowsky P: Investigation into the etiology and treatment of pica. Arch Dis Child 34: 140–148, 1959.
46. O'Rourke DE, Quinn JG, Nicholson JO, Gibson HH: Geophagia during pregnancy. Obstet Gynecol 29: 581–584, 1967.
47. Keith L, Brown ER, Rosenberg C: Pica: the unfinished story. Background correlations with anemia and pregnancy. Perspect Biol Med 13: 626–632, 1970.
48. Cameron HC: Forms of vomiting in infancy. Br Med J 1: 872–876, 1925.
49. Flanagan CH: Rumination in infancy-past and present. J Am Acad Child Psychiatry 16: 140–149, 1977.
50. Menking M, Wagnitz JG, Burton JJ, et al: Rumination—a near fatal psychiatric disease of infancy. N Engl J Med 280: 802–804, 1969.
51. Powers PS, Gunderman R: Kleine-Levin syndrome associated with fire setting. Am J Dis Child 132: 786–789, 1978.
52. Billiard M, Guilleminault C, Dement W: A menstruation-linked periodic hypersomnia: Kleine-Levin syndrome or a new clinical entity? Neurology 25: 436–443, 1975.
53. MacGregor MI, Block AJ, Ball WC Jr: Topics in clinical medicine: serious complications and sudden death in the Pickwickian syndrome. Bull Johns Hopkins Hosp 126: 279–295, 1970.
54. Jouvet M: The role of monoamines and acetylcholine-containing neurons in the regulation of the sleep waking cycle. Ergeb Physiol 64: 166–307, 1972.
55. Dement W cited by Freedman AM, Kaplan HI, Sadock BJ: Comprehensive Textbook of Psychiatry. Ed 2. Baltimore, Williams & Wilkins Co, 1975, p 116.
56. Kelly D, Richardson A, Mitchell-Heggs N, et al: Stereotactic limbic leucotomy: a preliminary report on 40 patients. Br J Psychiatry 123: 141–148, 1973.
57. Rubin RT, Kales A, Adler R, et al: Gonadotropin secretion during sleep in normal adult men. Science 175: 196–198, 1972.

CHAPTER 11

Treatment of Obesity: Evaluation, Diet, and Exercise

The treatment of obesity has included a broad range of interventions ranging from calorie-restricted diets, short- and long-term fasts, and bypass surgery to behavior modification techniques. In terms of weight loss, the surgical procedures have produced the most dramatic and long-lasting benefit, but the side effects of the surgery have resulted in significant morbidity and mortality. With the plethora of treatment options available, the physician must carefully evaluate each individual patient and select that combination of techniques most likely to be successful. Collaborative efforts on the part of the physician, nutritionist, psychologist, and social worker are essential.

INITIAL EVALUATION

Once the diagnosis of obesity has been made, preferably confirmed using triceps skinfold calipers, a complete history of the onset and course of the obesity is needed. Agras and colleagues[1] have designed a questionnaire for the Eating Disorders Clinic at Stanford (See Appendix 1). The age of onset of obesity and weights at various ages are determined. Several questions are designed to elucidate the attitude of the family toward the patient's obesity and his attempts to reduce. The patient is asked to describe various methods he has used to lose weight and their effectiveness. A brief social history elicits the patient's occupation, family relationships, and early attitudes toward eating. At Stanford, the patient is not accepted into the clinic until this form is completed. However, in the private practitioner's office, the questionnaire could be used to help the physician obtain a complete history from those patients he has identified as obese.

After the history is obtained, a physical examination will usually identify those patients with an organic or endocrine cause of their obesity as well as identifying obese patients who have already developed medical consequences of their obesity. It is estimated[2] that organic etiologies can be documented in less than 5% of obese patients. In adults, the major conditions that may cause obesity include Cushing's syndrome, hypothyroidism, hypothalamic or hypopituitary syndromes, virilization syndromes, and gonadal deficiency diseases.

UNUSUAL CAUSES OF OBESITY

Patients with Cushing's syndrome have the classical findings of glucocorticoid excess, including truncal obesity, "moon facies," "buffalo hump," plethora, and hypertension. Accurate measurement of blood pressure in any obese subject is critical, since hypertension may be a consequence of obesity and indicates an urgent need for treatment. A normotensive, mildly obese patient with lethargy, cold intolerance, coarse dry skin, or slow speech should be evaluated for hypothyroidism. An obese patient with headaches or visual symptoms should be evaluated for hypothalamic or hypopituitary syndromes with a visual field examination and skull x-rays. Visual field defects are common in pituitary tumors, because as the tumor presses upward from the bony confines of the sella turcica, the optic nerves and optic chiasm are displaced upward until prevented by the anterior arterial arc of the circle of Willis. Tumors usually protrude between the two arms of the optic nerves and exert pressure on the interior medial aspects of the nerves. Initially, therefore, there is usually a superior temporal quadrant defect in one or both eyes which progresses to the bi-temporal hemianopsia classically identified with pituitary tumors. Hypothalamic syndromes may be secondary to craniopharyngiomas, trauma, infection, or leukemic infiltration. Headaches and visual symptoms are characteristically present.

Finally, hirsute or amenorrheic obese females should be evaluated for the virilization syndromes. The differential diagnosis is between ovarian and adrenal etiologies. Adrenal tumors usually secrete a weak androgen and hirsutism results from elevated levels of androgens in the circulation with a consequent rise in the metabolites of androgens (the 17-ketosteroids). Ovarian tumors, on the other hand, excrete potent androgens. Therefore, elevated plasma testosterone in females with normal urinary ketosteroids indicates an ovarian neoplasm.

Bray and colleagues[3] have devised an algorithm for evaluating an obese patient (Fig. 11.1) following essentially the steps outlined above. In addition,

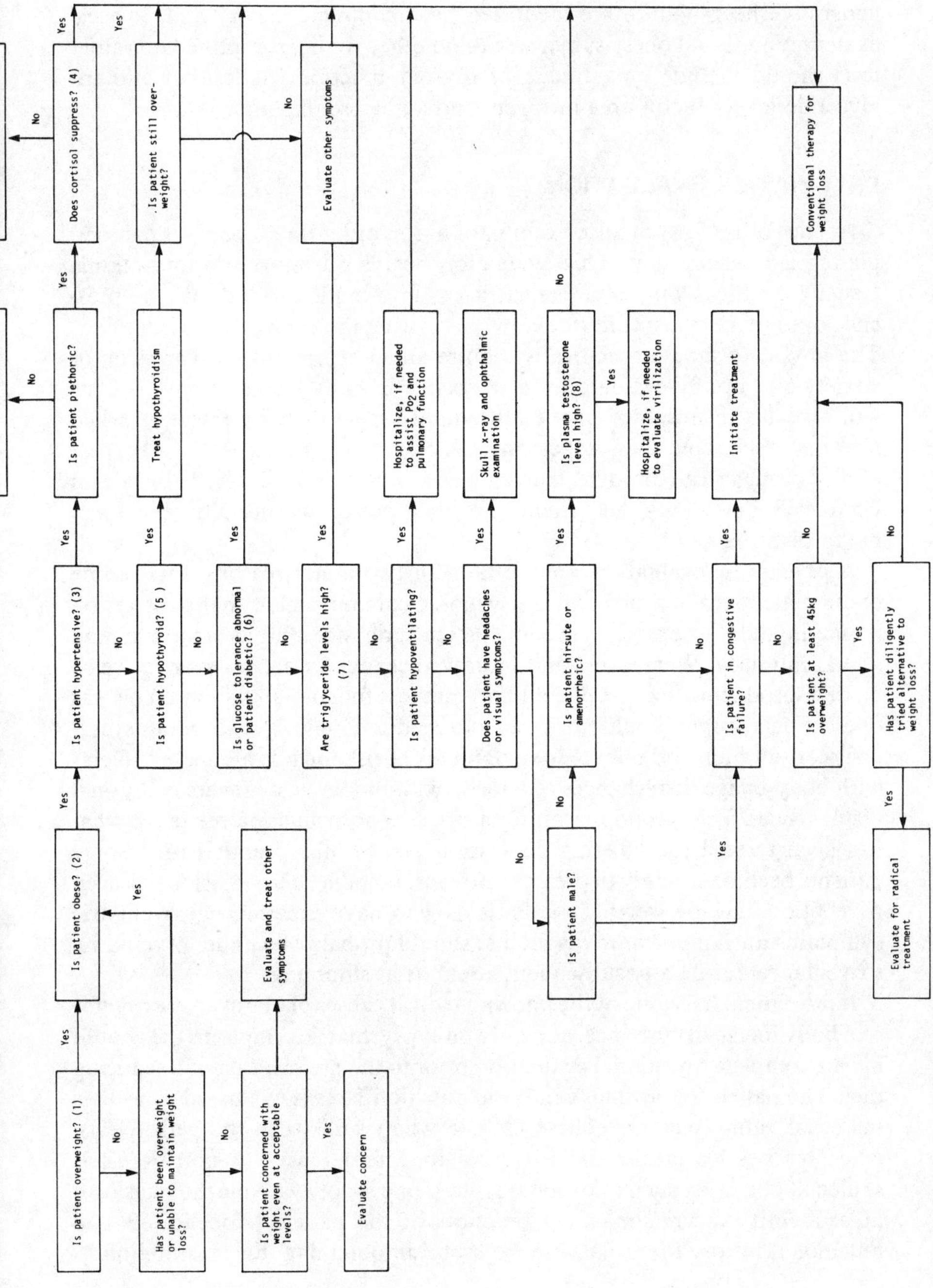

Figure 11.1. Algorithm for evaluating the obese patient. (Reprinted with permission from G. A. Bray, H. A. Jordan, and E. A. H. Sims: JAMA 235: 1488, 1976.)

patients with hypertension, diabetes or the Pickwickian syndrome and congestive heart failure are identified by a complete history and physical examination. In all obese subjects with no other findings, routine laboratory tests should include an estimate of thyroid function, cholesterol and triglyceride levels, blood urea nitrogen, and a glucose tolerance test.

PSYCHIATRIC EVALUATION

At least a brief psychiatric examination is in order for all patients contemplating a reducing diet. This evaluation begins during the history-taking. Usually a patient will volunteer sufficient information to indicate the presence or absence of psychiatric symptoms during the course of the interview. The physician should specifically inquire about symptoms of depression or anxiety and briefly evaluate for disturbance in body image. Many patients will reveal a disturbance in the attitudinal aspect of body image if asked how they feel about their appearance. A distortion in the perceptual aspect of body image can be detected with any of the procedures described in Chapter 8, but asking the patient to draw a person will usually reveal any major disturbances.

A psychiatric evaluation is important for two major reasons. First, some obese patients have a precarious psychological adjustment that depends on remaining fat. For example, in some patients, obesity inhibits emotional and sexual intimacy. Weight loss and improved sexual attractiveness may be so anxiety-producing that the patient becomes less functional than when he was obese. Such people should not be encouraged to lose weight without psychiatric consultation and intervention. Patients at risk include all obese subjects with body image disturbances and those with moderate or severe emotional disturbances. The second reason for a psychiatric evaluation relates to what has been termed the "dieting depression" by Stunkard and Rush.[4] Some patients become severely depressed, anxious, irritable, and occasionally even psychotic following weight loss. Patients who have experienced psychiatric symptoms during previous weight loss should probably be under psychiatric surveillance during any subsequent attempts at slimming.

If the patient has none of the known medical causes of obesity, no evidence of a body image disturbance, and only mild psychiatric symptoms, he should have a complete nutritional evaluation prior to the prescription of a reducing diet. The patient's knowledge of basic nutrition facts is evaluated as well as his usual eating patterns. These include where and when the person eats, who prepares his meals, and his usual food preferences. A nutritionist is skilled at obtaining such information, but if one is not available the physician must identify the major eating practices of the patient. Appendix 2 is a nutritional history form that may be useful in obtaining this information.[5]

EVALUATION OF OUTCOME

DIFFERENT SELECTION CRITERIA

Evaluating the effectiveness of any treatment program for obesity is difficult, partly because different investigators have selected subjects by widely differing criteria. For example, patients selected for bypass surgery are usually referred by internists and often have one or more of the consequences of obesity. By contrast, early studies on behavior modification techniques were usually done with mildly obese subjects who were self-referred, otherwise healthy, female college students. Comparing results of treatment on two such disparate groups is inappropriate. In addition, there are a number of other issues that are important in comparing the outcome of treatment in obese patients.

ATTRITION RATE

Attrition from various treatment programs is a major problem in obesity research. Dropout rates during treatment and at follow-up both merit consideration. Stunkard and McLaren-Hume[6] reported that with conventional out-patient treatment (diet, nutritional instruction, or medication), dropouts ranged from 25% to as high as 75%. With behavior programs, the dropout rates during treatment have been reported to average 10% or less.[7] Various techniques including earning back of deposits or contingency contracting have contributed to the decrement in the dropout rate during treatment.

However, the attrition rate from various behavioral research programs at follow-up is another issue. Although only 4% of the survivors were lost to follow-up in one recent well-documented study,[8] in another study,[9] 60% of the initial group were lost to later follow-up. The average lost to follow-up has been estimated at approximately 20%.[10] It may be that patients who are lost to follow-up do continue to follow new eating patterns, but it is more likely that they have reverted to old patterns and regained weight. Follow-up data is of crucial importance because weight loss is usually not maintained, even by those patients who succeed in losing weight during treatment.

Several solutions to the dropout problem at follow-up have been suggested which may be applicable to any of the various modes of treatment. Deposits, or portions of deposits, may be refunded at follow-up. Sobell and Sobell[11] recommend the following steps. First, at the beginning of the program, the details and importance of follow-up are stressed. Second, follow-up is more likely to be successful if it is frequent and involves personal contact from the therapist. Third, the names of friends and relatives of the subject can be obtained and these people can be contacted during the follow-up period to locate the subject. However, these steps are time-consuming and may fail.

SYMPTOM SUBSTITUTION

Another aspect of treatment outcome is the possibility of symptom substitution. Theorists who believe that obesity is but a symptom of an underlying emotional conflict contend that elimination of the obesity may result in the emergence of another, possibly more serious, symptom. Some behaviorists, on the other hand, think that obesity is a learned pattern of behavior that can be unlearned without risk of symptom substitution. Extreme viewpoints on this issue can be found in the literature. Bookbinder[12] believes that symptom substitution always occurs and Yates[13] claims that it never occurs. Probably symptom substitution can occur in predisposed individuals and careful follow-up to detect such occurrences is needed. Perhaps patients whose obesity has rich symbolic meaning for them are more at risk for symptom substitution. For example, one patient in our clinic believed that his large girth symbolized strength and, as he lost weight on a reducing diet, he became increasingly arrogant and occasionally inappropriately aggressive. It is possible that subtle personality or behavior changes may represent symptom substitution, yet be missed during follow-up evaluation unless a careful pre-treatment psychological assessment has been done. In any case, this is an issue which has yet to be resolved.

REPORTING RESULTS

COMPARISON OF TREATMENT RESULTS

Various investigators have reported their findings in very different ways, often preventing comparison with other treatment modalities. As Stunkard[14] has noted, group summary statistics are often quite misleading. Means and standard deviations provide little basis for evaluating the range of effects of that treatment. A few extreme results in either direction may affect the mean dramatically. If one or two subjects lose a considerable amount of weight, it might appear that the treatment was effective for all the subjects and prevent investigation of the parameters that predicted success in a few subjects. Feinstein[15] has recommended that a *weight reduction index* (RI) be calculated for each subject and reported. This index takes into account weight, height, amount overweight, goal, and pounds lost:

$$RI = [W_l/W_s)\ (W_i/W_t)]\ 100 = \text{excess weight loss} \times \text{relative initial obesity}$$

where W_l = weight loss, W_s = surplus weight, W_i = initial weight, and W_t = target weight. Calculation of this index results in a value between 0 and 200. The value is zero if there has been no weight loss and 200 if there is a very large weight loss. Although simple to calculate, thus far this index has not been widely used.

Jolliffe and Alpert[16] have calculated a *performance index* which can be used for individuals or groups. The method is as follows. Using the food nomogram of Boothby and Berkson[17] (Fig. 11.2), the estimated caloric expenditure rate at pre-treatment weight is calculated. The "calorie deficit" on a reducing regimen is calculated and the time in weeks to lose 25 pounds is determined. Then the individual performance index is calculated using the following formula:

$$\frac{\text{observed weight loss}}{\text{predicted weight loss}} \times 100 = \text{performance index}$$

The average of the individual performance indices gives the group performance index. Although very successful or unsuccessful patient response may skew the results, this method provides a method for comparing treatments of obese patients who vary widely in their degree of obesity.

CLINICAL SIGNIFICANCE

It is important that treatment results in clinically significant changes. For example, it has been reported[18] that both positive covert reinforcement and negative covert sensitization were more effective than the minimal treatment control group, but there was only a 4- to 5-pound difference, which is statistically significant but not clinically relevant. In terms of effectiveness, what is needed is a treatment that significantly reduces the incidence of obesity-related diseases of diabetes, hypertension, and coronary artery disease. A procedure that does not decrease morbidity or mortality or significantly improve body image or alleviate serious psychological problems, is of little value to medicine.

FOLLOW-UP

Follow-up reports have often documented only a brief interval and the method of reporting has been inconsistent. Probably a 6-month follow-up is minimally necessary to evaluate adequately the potency of any treatment in maintaining significant weight loss. The editorial policy of at least one well-known journal now requires a minimum 6-month follow-up before accepting a report.

Stunkard[19] recently proposed a graphic method for reporting results of follow-up studies (Fig. 11.3 illustrates a modified version of this proposal). Weight lost from the beginning of treatment to the end of treatment is plotted on the ordinate, and weight lost from the beginning of treatment to the follow-up is plotted on the abscissa. If weight loss were maintained until follow-up, the result would appear on the diagonal line and if more weight were lost by follow-up than at the end of the treatment, the result would be

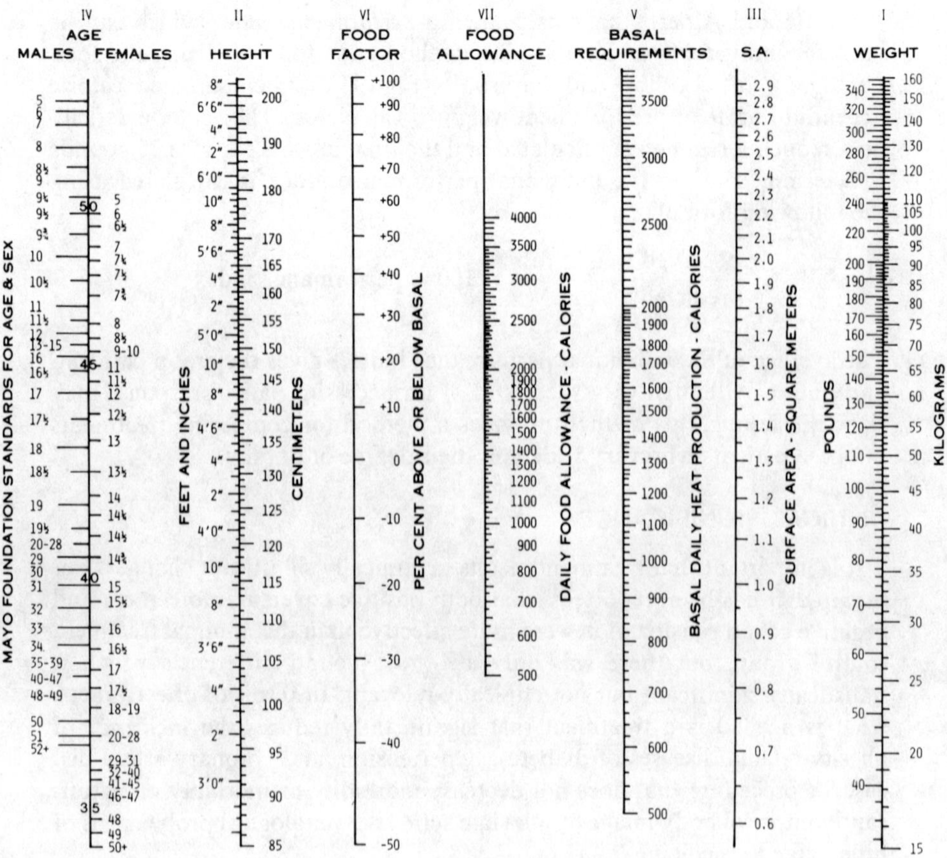

Figure 11.2. Food nomogram. Directions: the standards for age are arranged on the basis of the common method of expressing age as of the last birthday. To determine the desired calorie allowance, proceed as follows: (1) Locate the weight on scale I by means of a pin stuck through the eraser of a lead pencil. (2) Place the edge of the ruler against the pin and swing the other end of ruler to the patient's height on scale II. (3) Transfer the pin to the point where the ruler crosses scale III which gives the surface area in square meters (this value need not be read). (4) Holding the ruler against the pin on the surface area scale, swing the left-hand end of the ruler to the patient's standard for age and sex given on scale IV. (5) Transfer the pin to where the ruler now crosses scale V which gives the basal heat production of the patient for 24 hours and represents the calories of food required by the fasting patient when resting in bed (basal calories). The calories needed for activity bear a relationship to those demanded for the resting condition. The so-called "white collar worker" when at work will need about 50% more than his basal calories. When activity is restricted, as in the hospital, the extra calories necessary will range from 10–30% of the basal calories. Therefore (6) estimate the percent of calories above the basal and locate this point on scale VI. With the ruler connect this point with the point located previously on scale V, and where the ruler now crosses scale VII read the amount of food calories to be provided by the diet. (Reprinted from E. H. Rynearson and C. P. Gastineau: Obesity. Springfield, Charles C Thomas, 1949.)

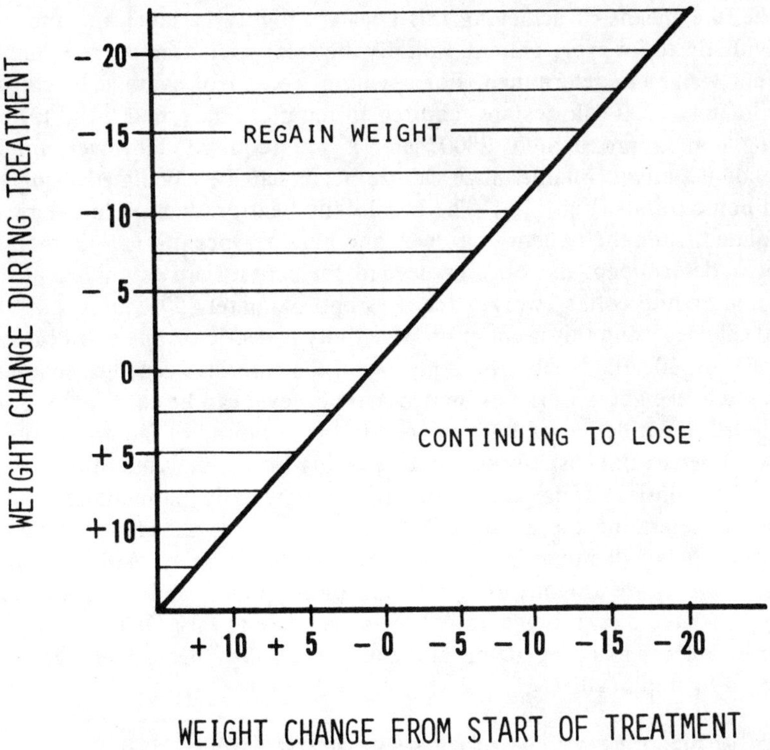

Figure 11.3. Method for reporting follow-up results. If patient maintains the weight lost during treatment, the result will be plotted on the diagonal line. If additional weight is lost, the result will be below the diagonal line. If weight is regained, the result will appear above diagonal line (adapted from Stunkard[19]).

plotted below the diagonal line. If the subject regained weight lost during treatment, the result would be plotted above the diagonal line; e.g., if 20 pounds were lost during treatment and maintained at follow-up, the result would appear on the diagonal; if 10 pounds were regained, the result would be above the diagonal line. This method of reporting follow-up results is easy to visualize and interpret, although it gives no information about the percentage of surplus weight lost, which may be more important medically.

DIET

CALCULATION OF CALORIE NEEDS

Once all the relevant data have been collected, an individual treatment plan is devised. At the core of any regimen is a reducing diet. Although it is agreed that for weight loss to occur, caloric expenditure must exceed caloric intake, the means of achieving this goal are highly variable and must be individualized for every patient. Initially the caloric requirement to maintain current weight is determined. For a young woman of average height approximately 2200 calories are required to maintain a normal weight; for a young man approximately 2800 calories are required. However, for an individual patient, maintenance caloric needs can be calculated using the food nomogram[17] (Fig. 11.2). The basal daily heat production in calories is calculated using the patient's age, sex, and height. Once this caloric requirement is determined, the calories needed for activity are estimated (Table 11.1). A "white collar" worker requires approximately 50% more than his basal calories using this nomogram. If activity is restricted, the extra calories range from 10–30%. Using the nomogram, the calories needed to maintain the current weight with the estimated activity level can be calculated. Since it requires a net deficit of 3500 calories to lose 1 pound of fat, and a loss of 1 pound per week is usually optimal, resulting in minimal loss of lean body mass, 500 calories per day are subtracted from the daily maintenance caloric needs to determine the actual calorie content of the reducing diet. Most reducing diets will range from 1000–1500 calories per day. Although most obese subjects are anxious to lose weight more quickly and often ask for a more restricted diet, it is generally unwise to agree to this. Diets below 1000 calories are often unappetizing and the patient may become hungry and tempted to stop his diet.

LESS WEIGHT LOST ON VERY RESTRICTED DIETS

The calculation just described is the one followed by most nutritionists and bariatricians. However, many patients claim that even though they have followed the reducing diet diligently, they have not lost weight. To evaluate this claim, the rate of calorie utilization during starvation has been used as

Table 11.1
Calories required for physical activity (percentage increase to be added to basal caloric requirement).

20%	BED REST AND EARLY CONVALESCENCE
30%	MODERATELY RESTRICTED ACTIVITY- LATE CONVALESCENCE
40%	SLIGHTLY RESTRICTED ACTIVITY
50%	LIGHT OCCUPATIONS (E.G. CLERICAL WORKERS)
60%	MANUAL LABORERS, TRUCKDRIVERS, ETC.
70-100%	HEAVY WORKERS-LUMBERJACKS, STEVEDORES

a measure of minimal needs to maintain weight. One group of researchers found that the minimal calorie use in their subjects was greater than 1000 calories[20] and thus a 1000-calorie diet should invariably result in weight loss. However, Wilkins and co-workers[21] report a bedridden 6-year-old who gained weight when he consumed more than 500 calories per day.

Furthermore, several recent studies have shown that during calorie deficit, there is both a decrease in basal metabolic rate and in the amount of exercise. Therefore, an obese patient may not lose 1 pound per week even if he strictly adheres to the diet prescribed. Bray[22] studied the energy expenditure of 18 obese subjects by analyzing expired air for oxygen and carbon dioxide and calculating oxygen consumption. When these subjects were not dieting, their caloric needs were 1100 calories per square meter of surface area. During a reducing diet, the calories required to maintain their current weight dropped to 900 calories per square meter. Thus, these obese patients would be expected to lose less weight than the loss calculated by the usual methods. For example, a patient who needs 2500 calories to maintain his obese state and adheres to a 1500-calorie reducing diet will probably lose less than 1 pound per week rather than the anticipated 2 pounds per week.

There are at least three possible explanations for this decrease in energy expenditure. The thermic effect of food which results in an increase in oxygen consumption following food ingestion might be smaller when less food is consumed. However, one study[20] showed that there was no change in oxygen consumption in the first few days, as would be expected if the decrease in thermic effect accounted for the decrease in calorie requirements. There may be a decrease in basal metabolism resulting from a decrease in the enzymes of the glycerophosphate cycle leading to a greater efficiency in the formation of adenosine triphosphate (ATP). Galton and Bray[23] found that the enzymes of the glycerophosphate cycle from adipose tissue of obese patients are half as active as those of normal weight individuals. With caloric restriction there was an even greater dimunition of activity of these enzymes. Thus, obese subjects on a reducing diet may be more efficient in forming ATP with a consequent fall in caloric needs.

Miller and Parsonage[24] studied 29 women who were unable to lose weight on a calorie-restricted diet. The patients were isolated and placed on a 1500-calorie diet; nine subjects did not lose weight and were found to have relatively low basal metabolic rates although none had clinical signs of hypothyroidism. The investigators did adipose tissue biopsies on 15 of their subjects. There was no correlation between fat cell size and basal metabolic rate, but there was a correlation between fat cell number and basal metabolic rate (although the authors do not give the exact figures). Patients with a greater number of fat cells had a higher basal metabolic rate. Thus, a patient with fewer fat cells might have a lower basal metabolic rate and have greater resistance to slimming. This study showed a correlation between lower basal metabolic weight and length of diet and lower body weight. Therefore, a patient who is on a diet for lengthy periods and who is close to his normal weight would be expected to have more difficulty losing weight than the very obese patient just starting a diet. These findings are consistent with the anecdotal reports of patients who reach weight plateaus and have difficulty continuing to lose; these patients may have adapted to reduced calorie intake with a decrease in basal metabolic rate.

It has also been noted that with a decrease in calorie intake there is a compensatory decrease in exercise. More than a decade ago, Mayer[25] demonstrated that at very low levels of exercise, food intake increases. However, at less marked decreases in caloric intake, energy expenditure from activity also decreases.[26] In some adolescent girls on a reducing diet, even when sitting there was a decrease in activity level and energy cost.[27]

Therefore, decreased calorie intake may result in a decrease in energy expenditure in at least three ways: a decrease in basal metabolic rate (perhaps via more efficient ATP production), a decrease in the thermic effect of food, and a decrease in activity level.

There is evidence that severe caloric restriction below 800 calories may result in an even greater adaptation to conserve energy. Conceivably such a mechanism might even halt weight loss in some patients. Therefore, not only is a more generous calorie intake more appetizing and nutritious, it may actually result in a greater weight loss than a very restricted diet.

GUIDELINES FOR REDUCING DIET

Several factors must be considered to determine the calorie content of a reducing diet in addition to those noted above. Women require fewer calories than men, but pregnant women require as much as 20% more calories. With age, basal metabolic rate decreases slightly and exercise often also decreases, so calorie needs decrease. These factors as well as the usual activity level of the patient are important.

Young,[28] a medical nutritionist, has studied diets and dieters for several decades and concludes that a successful low-calorie diet fulfills these criteria:

1. The diet should provide all the nutrition which the body needs, except calories.
2. The diet should come as close as possible to the individual's normal habits of eating.
3. The diet should protect the individual from between-meal hunger, give a sense of well-being, and not cause a tired feeling.
4. The diet should enable the individual to eat at home and away from home without feeling as if everyone is staring at him.
5. The diet should be one that can be lived with for the rest of the individual's new thin life.

Ensuring that the diet contains all the essential nutrients can be difficult. A simple rule is to include foods from all the major food groups. A diet which excludes major food groups or consists exclusively of only certain foods is likely to be dangerous. The recommended daily allowances (RDA) of the Food and Nutrition Board, National Academy of Sciences, National Research Council, are the standards used for planning reducing diets. These allowances specify the nutrient intakes needed to maintain good nutrition in practically all healthy persons. The allowances are generous so as to include people of different ages, sex, and activity levels. The allowances are revised approximately every 5 years to incorporate new research findings, e.g., zinc was added to the list as a required nutrient in the 1974 edition.[29] It is important to remember that probably not all the required nutrients have been identified and therefore a broad selection of foods is wise.

SELECTION OF APPROPRIATE REDUCING DIET

Despite numerous books and reports to the contrary, the most effective diet for weight loss is one that is calorie-restricted yet nutritionally balanced. The ideal ratio of carbohydrate, protein, and fat to total calories is 40–45% carbohydrate, 20% protein, and 35–40% fat. The low carbohydrate diet, also known as the "calories don't count diet" (Taller)[30] is touted as more effective than equicalorie carbohydrate-rich diets. Although in the first 10 days of a diet, more water may be lost on a low carbohydrate diet,[31] long-term studies have shown that rates of weight loss are the same on equicalorie diets regardless of composition.[32] Apparently the only advantage of a low carbohydrate diet is that restriction of carbohydrate results in voluntary restriction of fat.[33] Therefore, an appropriately balanced low calorie diet will be just as effective and markedly less dangerous than any diet which emphasizes particular nutrients.

EXCHANGE LISTS

The food exchange method[34] for following a reducing diet is usually more convenient for the patient and is more likely to result in a balanced intake of nutrients. This method has been promulgated by the American Diabetes Association and the American Dietetic Association. There are six food exchange lists and within each list various foods are specified that are approximately equal in calorie content to other foods in that list. The lists are: milk exchanges, vegetable exchanges, fruit exchanges, bread exchanges, meat exchanges, and fat exchanges. After determining the calorie content of the diet, the nutritionist or physician must assist the patient in planning his meals in food exchanges. A specific number of exchanges is allowed from each group daily (e.g., 2 milk, 2 vegetable, 2 fruit, 3 bread, 5 meat, and 1 fat exchange would constitute one variant of a 1000-calorie reducing diet). Table 11.2 lists three diets: 1000 calories, 1200 calories, and 1500 calories. The number of exchanges in each group provide adequate protein, fat, and carbohydrate for the usual reducing regimen but might be modified in some circumstances. The times at which various exchanges are consumed are not fixed and may be varied to suit the patient; e.g., many patients are less hungry and able to tolerate a diet better if snacks are allowed. In the 1000-calorie diet shown, an evening snack of 1 fruit exchange and ½ skim milk is allowed by omitting these from the evening meal.

The great advantage of the exchange lists is that it allows individual variation and can be easily learned by most patients. See Appendix 3 for details of the food exchange system. *Milk exchanges* contain approximately

Table 11.2
Three reducing diets using the food exchange system.

	1000 CAL/ DAY	1200 CAL/ DAY	1500 CAL/ DAY
BREAKFAST			
FRUIT	1	1	1
BREAD	1	1	2
MEAT	1	1	1
FAT	1	1	1
MILK	1/2 SKIM	1/2 SKIM	1/2 SKIM
LUNCH			
FRUIT	-	1	2
BREAD	1	1	2
MEAT	2	2	3
FAT	-	1	2
MILK	1/2 SKIM	1/2 SKIM	-
VEGETABLE	1	1	1
SUPPER			
MEAT	2	2	3
BREAD	1	2	2
VEGETABLE	1	1	1
FRUIT	1	1	2
FAT	-	2	2
MILK	1 SKIM	1 SKIM	1 SKIM

80 calories and include milk (non-fat, low fat, and whole), yogurt, and buttermilk. *Vegetable exchanges* are ½ cup each and contain approximately 25 calories. Some raw vegetables are allowed as desired and include chicory, lettuce, radishes, and watercress. *Fruit exchanges* contain approximately 40 calories, are served without sugar, and in varying amounts. *Bread exchanges* contain 70 calories and include bread, cereal and starchy vegetables. *Meat exchanges,* served in specified amounts, contain 55 calories and are divided into lean, medium fat, and high fat meats. If medium fat meat is eaten, ½ fat exchange is omitted and if high fat meats are consumed 1 fat exchange is omitted. *Fat exchanges* contain approximately 45 calories and include margarine, butter, oil, cream, bacon, nuts, and various dressings.

POPULAR DIETS

REASONS FOR INCREASED POPULARITY

In the past few decades the popular literature on diets has mushroomed. Despite repeated warnings by nutritionists, physicians, and various professional groups, huge numbers of obese patients follow fad diets, at least briefly. Even widely reported deaths from the notorious liquid protein diet did not deter large numbers of obese people from attempting this diet. Even though it has been repeatedly demonstrated that weight loss only occurs when calorie intake falls below calorie expenditure, fad diets have never been more popular. There are many causes of this apparent paradox. We are living in a culture that values slimness, yet there is an overabundance of food and a trend toward diminished activity. Small wonder that obesity is commonplace. Furthermore, the medical profession has been very ineffective in either the treatment or prevention of obesity. Such a situation enhances the appeal of diets that promise quick and easy weight loss.

In addition, there are several commonplace and scientific observations that suggest that there may be shortcuts to weight loss. For example, men can eat more than women yet remain slim. The fact that men have a greater lean body mass is not known to many dieting obese women who observe their husbands eating more than they do. There are numerous anecdotal reports of individuals who apparently eat large quantities yet gain no extra weight. The reasons for this are not always clear. The idea that certain foods may be more fattening than other equicalorie foods gains validity from several observations. After a binge of particularly salty foods, aldosterone is secreted and sodium is retained with water resulting in a very quick weight gain of up to several pounds. If there is increased sodium in the body and sodium is decreased, for example by fasting 1 or 2 days, diuresis occurs and there is a quick weight loss. These observations suggest that there may be some easy way to lose weight not yet discovered by the medical profession.

Many obese adolescents do not eat more than their slim peers but exercise less. The fact that an obese teenager may play tennis less vigorously than a slender teenager is not always convincing to the dieter. Dieters are very familiar with weight plateaus while dieting that are not consistent with any change in food or fluid intake. The reason for these weight plateaus is not known.

Furthermore, some researchers have been unable to account for weight gains or weight losses in their subjects. For example, in the experimental overfeeding study[35] the volunteers gained much less weight than anticipated from their calorie intake. Several theories have been proposed to account for this finding, including luxus konsumption, increased thermic effect of food, and calorie cost of growth of adipose tissue. None of these explanations has been proven and the finding itself gives credence to the idea that there is more to energy balance than is currently known.

BASIS OF EARLY WEIGHT LOSS ON FAD DIETS

In the first week on a new fad diet, most people lose approximately 8 pounds. The basis of this initial rapid weight loss is diuresis due to a loss of sodium and water.[36] Clarke[37] has determined the composition of the weight lost during a 28-day fast. Initially the major loss is water with significant amounts of protein. By day 14, water loss is minimal and protein loss also decreases while fat loss continues at nearly the same rate. By day 28, protein and water losses are minimal and fat losses continue relatively unchanged. In the first 2 days, approximately 5 pounds are lost and nearly 10 pounds are lost by the end of a week. Later, however, weight loss decreases. In addition, glycogen is lost early in the course of a reducing diet. For each gram of glycogen, 2.8 g of water are lost, which accounts for part of the initial weight loss in fad diets.

The quick weight loss diets are not only medically dangerous but may also be psychologically hazardous. The first few days are encouraging to the patient, but he may give up his diet when the weight loss decreases to 1 to 2 pounds per week. Or, he may try an even more radical diet in an attempt to continue the rapid weight loss. Most of the weight lost on fad diets is regained and initial weight may even be exceeded.

EXAMPLES OF POPULAR DIETS

Five hazardous popular diets and two safe diets will be described. There are a number of other diets available and for a more complete listing see Stern.[38] For a discussion of the Zen Macrobiotic Diet and Liquid Protein Diet see Chapter 9.

Dr. Atkins' Diet Revolution written by Dr. Robert C. Atkins[39] severely restricts carbohydrates while allowing unlimited amounts of protein and fat. He contends that obesity results from inability to properly metabolize carbohydrates. During the first week on this diet there is a quick weight loss of 8 to 10 pounds and ketosis occurs. Rapid weight loss soon ceases and the patient usually regains the weight. There are a number of medical risks associated with this diet, including fatigue, arrythmias, nausea, and fainting. Ketosis is hazardous in pregnant women and may influence later intellectual development of the infant.[40] The high protein content of this diet may be hazardous to individuals with kidney disease and may precipitate an attack of gout due to high uric acid levels. *The Drinking Man's Diet*[38] is a variant of a low-carbohydrate high-protein diet and has the same hazards.

Another dangerous diet was popularized by Taller, the *Calories Don't Count Diet.*[30] This is a tantalizing concept to many obese dieters but a fallacious one. In addition to a low-carbohydrate regimen, the dieter is advised to take polyunsaturated fat in the form of safflower capsules and margarine to stimulate the pituitary and burn off excess fat. This notion has no scientific basis and the low-carbohydrate aspect of this diet has the same hazards as similar regimens.

Another diet plan is *Simeons HCG* (human chorionic gonadotropin) diet plan.[41] In this plan, the obese patient follows a 500-calorie diet and receives a daily injection of HCG (a compound obtained from the urine of pregnant women). Despite claims of the effectiveness of this routine, HCG shots have not been demonstrated to be effective. One study[42] has shown that when an obese dieter is given any injection, whether it be sterile saline or HCG, he will tend to lose weight. Various factors probably contribute to the effectiveness of injections including placebo effect. Simeons also proscribed the use of cosmetics with oil, claiming that applied oils were absorbed and added to the fat stores; there is no evidence that this is true. The 500-calorie diet in this plan accounts for the weight loss achieved.

The grapefruit diet[38] is another low carbohydrate diet that is also known as the Magic Mayo diet. In this diet, a half a grapefruit or grapefruit juice is consumed at every meal. The grapefruit is allegedly a catalyst that activates the burning of fat. There is no evidence, however, that this is the case. The dieter is allowed all the meat, fish, and eggs desired and thus this diet is low in carbohydrate and high in cholesterol.

The *ice cream diet*[38] is a safe diet that includes two servings of ice cream per day on a 1000-calorie well-balanced nutritious diet.

The Weight Watchers diet has been used successfully by many group members and is a well-balanced and nutritious diet. It is part of a group approach that incorporates some of the principles of behavior modification. Other groups such as TOPS (Take Off Pounds Sensibly) and Diet Workshop also advocate sensible safe diets.

LOSS OF LEAN BODY MASS DURING WEIGHT LOSS

Even in very carefully designed weight loss programs there is usually some loss of lean body mass, especially early in the diet. Strang and colleagues[43] measured nitrogen excretion of obese subjects fed a reducing diet and during the early weeks the patients lost between 3 and 6 g of nitrogen daily, indicating the catabolism of 18 to 36 g of protein. After the first few weeks, however, an equilibrium was established and thereafter most of the loss was fat. Less than 4% of the nitrogen in the body was lost prior to the new equilibrium.

Children, adolescents, and pregnant women are in a state of anabolism, and weight reduction during these stages of life requires careful planning. As noted in Chapter 3, it was once popular to place obese pregnant women on a reducing diet in hopes of terminating pregnancy with a net loss of weight. However, recent work suggests that infant morbidity and mortality is increased when women gain less than the recomended 24 to 25 pounds.

Brook and colleagues[44] report on loss of lean body mass and deceleration of growth in height in children on a reducing diet in the hospital. Seven boys and 13 girls ages 1½ to 16½ years were hospitalized and placed on a 350-kcal diet to treat their obesity. Six obese children were treated as outpatients on 600- to 800-calorie diets. Both groups lost similar percentages of excess fat. The inpatients lost 41.9% in approximately 2 months and the outpatients lost 45.8% in nearly 6 months. However, the hospitalized patients on a very low-calorie diet lost a much larger percentage of lean body mass compared to the outpatients, 8.3% versus 2.5%, a threefold increase. These investigators also measured height before and after weight loss and this was converted to a yearly height velocity and compared to mean expected height velocity. Although individual variations are normally wide, only two of the 20 inpatients grew at even half the expected velocity. In the outpatient group, however, there was no difference between the observed and expected height velocities. Thus, very low-calorie diets associated with rapid weight loss, may significantly retard growth in some obese youngsters.

Rayner and Court[45] studied 26 obese children ranging from 3 to 12 years of age over the course of a year on a slimming regimen. Three therapeutic regimens were assessed: diet (1000 calorie), diet plus amphetamine derivatives, or diet plus fenfluramine. The group of children who lost weight on diet alone did not show a significant decrement in growth velocity, although the range was wide and some individual children may have had decreases in growth in height. There was a significant decrement in growth velocity in youngsters treated with diet plus fenfluramine. Although only a few children were studied, the implication is that diet alone (1000 calories) is less likely to retard growth than diet given in conjunction with anorexic drugs.

In adolescence, the effect of weight loss on growth will vary at different stages of growth. Heald[46] cites two examples. One is a 15-year-old girl, 5 years postmenarchial and biologically an adult woman. The second is a 15-year-old boy early in his growth spurt. Both are on 1000-calorie diets, and eat the same amount of protein; yet, the girl is in positive balance and the boy is in negative balance. There is some evidence that during catabolism in adolescence, growth is curtailed.[47] In a group of obese youngsters who lost weight at different speeds, it was shown that if loss of weight was less than 1% of the body mass over a unit of time, then adequate growth could still occur. If greater than 1% of body mass was lost, growth was curtailed. Thus, reducing regimens for obese teenagers must be carefully designed. Adolescence is basically a period of anabolism, but successful loss of body fat necessitates catabolism.

In summary, very restrictive low calorie diets are dangerous in children and may impede normal growth. Diets of at least 600 to 800 calories, depending on the age of the child, are necessary. In adolescents, the stage of puberty influences the caloric requirements to ensure growth in height. During the growth spurt, adolescents need more calories. Because of these problems, any child or teenager on a reducing regimen should be under medical surveillance.

FASTING

Fasting has a long religious and philosophical history but has only been subjected to scientific scrutiny as a treatment for obesity in the last 30 years. In 1959, Bloom[48] reported dramatic weight losses with no ill effects in a series of obese patients on short-term fasts. Since then there have been several studies which have documented the physiological changes that occur during fasting. Although patients lose weight rapidly and are not hungry during the fast, very few maintain the weight loss and they may regain even more weight than was initially lost. This disappointing result may relate to inappropriate selection of patients or inadequate post-fast medical surveillance. Several deaths have been reported during fasting or during the refeeding period, but these usually occurred during long-term fasts (more than 2 months). The more serious deleterious effects of fasting apparently do not occur during short fasts and therefore, if fasting has a place in the treatment of refractory obesity, it should be short-term.

SELECTION OF PATIENTS

The patient should have significant refractory obesity because the treatment has several possible dangerous complications. Because there is a sizeable loss of lean body mass during fasting, children and adolescents should probably not fast. Heyden and colleagues[49] have reported on the use of very carefully supervised intermittent fasts in adolescents but this should be considered still a research procedure. Pregnant and lactating women should not fast. Patients with a history of previous psychotic episodes should not undertake long-term fasts; Drenick[50] reports that of six patients with a history of psychosis, three became psychotic during the fast and one attempted suicide. Any patient contemplating a fasting regimen should have a psychiatric evaluation.

The other contraindications relate to physical health. Patients with gout, hyperuricemia, or a family history of gout should not fast because uric acid levels rise in all patients and may precipitate a clinical episode of gout even in an apparently normal patient. This may be a relative contraindication since the use of allopurinol may prevent attacks. Patients with a myocardial infarction or cerebral vascular accident of recent origin should not attempt to fast; hypotension and syncope occur in almost all patients and may decrease perfusion of the brain or heart and lead to ischemia or infarction. Fasting requires a number of renal adaptations and patients with chronic renal disease should not fast. Patients with anemia or nutritional deficiency diseases should not fast because even greater anemia or deficiency may result. The anemia that occurs in Pickwickian syndrome is an exception because it may improve with radical weight loss. Hepatic disease is a relative contraindication; there is bile stasis and worsening of bromsulphalein (BSP) retention with fasting that may worsen pre-existing hepatic disease, but the fatty infiltration of the liver that occurs in many very obese patients may improve with fasting.

WEIGHT LOSS WITH FASTING

Weight loss is precipitous during the first week of a fast; it is greatest in heavier patients, in men, in patients with edema and fluid retention, and those on a previous unrestricted salt intake. In Drenick's[50] study of 137 subjects, the average fast lasted 56 days and weight loss averaged 65 pounds with a range of 28–167 pounds. The amount of weight lost is proportional to the extent of the initial surplus weight. The weight lost in the average 300-pound subject averaged at least 1 pound per day over a 2-month fast.

The composition of the weight lost changes during the course of the fast[50] (Fig. 11.4). Glycogen, reflecting energy stored as carbohydrate, is lost during the first 3 days. Protein losses initially are high, about 75 g of protein per day, but this decreases to 18–24 g of protein per day in the first 30 days of the fast. The protein loss accounts for several of the clinical findings in fasted subjects. There is an arrest of hair growth and after 2 months the hair tends to fall out. The skin becomes dry and scaly and microscopic examination shows a narrowed epithelium; this effect reverses quickly with refeeding. Changes in the blood are also a consequence of protein catabolism. The

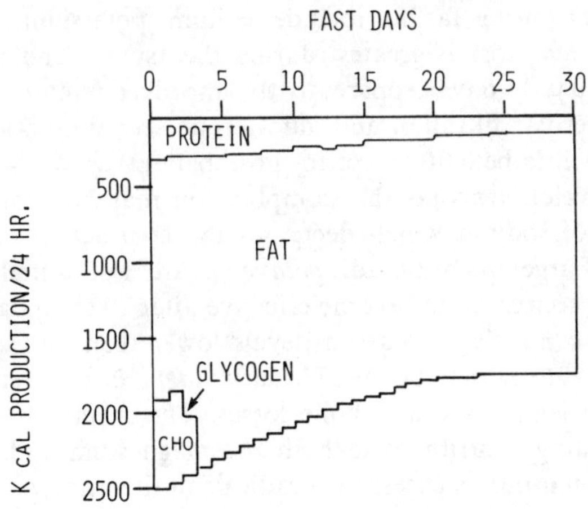

Figure 11.4. Composition of weight loss during fast. (Reprinted with permission from E. J. Drenick: Obesity in Perspective. Fogarty International Center Series on Preventive Medicine, Vol II, Pt II, edited by G. A. Bray. Washington, DC, Government Printing Office, 1976.)

mean hematocrit falls from 46.2 to 41.0 by the end of the 3rd month, although this is a falsely high reading because of concentration of the plasma compartment. There is also neutropenia which may be due to several factors, including folate deficiency and, in the later stages of fasting, an impairment of the bone marrow activity due to protein depletion. Fat losses during the fast account for the greatest loss of body fuels during the entire fast. After the first 3 days there is a rise in loss of fat which gradually declines to a steady level and accounts for 1000 to 2000 of the calories lost per day.

METABOLIC CHANGES

Net *body water* loss in a group of 10 obese subjects averaged 11.8 liters during the course of a 1-month fast.[50] It is estimated that two-thirds of the initial water loss originates from the extracellular fluid compartment including the vascular space and lumen of the gastrointestinal tract. Obese subjects who have retained fluid, with or without edema, tend to lose more fluid.

Calorie energy requirements decline during a fast for at least four reasons. Basal metabolic rate decreases and activity level declines. As weight is lost, the caloric cost of exercise decreases. Since food is not eaten, there is no calorie cost to process food intake (the thermic effect of food). The decline in basal metabolic rate with fasting may be responsible for part of the very rapid weight gain during refeeding and normal food intake may result in excessive weight gain.

Mineral losses during fasting include sodium, potassium, calcium, and magnesium. *Sodium* loss is greatest during the 1st day and ceases almost completely by 10 to 15 days. Apparently the improved retention results from decreased glomerular filtration and aldosterone secretion. Sodium supplementation is of little benefit except to those patients who lose weight very quickly and develop syncope; this complication may be avoided with the administration of sodium which decreases the contraction of the plasma compartment. Large quantities of *potassium* are lost initially but renal mechanisms for conservation become effective after 10 to 15 days of fasting. Most patients do not develop serum levels lower than 3mEq/L although actual potassium stores may be low. Urinary *magnesium* excretion increases and arises from lean tissue and bone losses. The metabolic acidosis that results from fasting contributes to both the magnesium and calcium loss which partially neutralizes excess acid radicals in the urine.

During fasting there is a *metabolic acidosis* which arises partially from phosphate and sulfate, that is, the acid residue of catabolized lean tissue. In addition, ketones (acetoacetic acid and beta-hydroxybutyric acid) are the major metabolic fuel during a fast and account for a large portion of acid radicals requiring neutralization in the urine. Increased fatty acid oxidation and decreased fatty acid synthesis during the fast result in the increased circulating levels of ketones. After adaptation to a fast, the circulating ketoacids[51] provide the major metabolic fuel (75%) for the brain. Some have thought that the ketosis is responsible for the surprising lack of hunger during a fast. Appearance of ketones in the urine can be used to assess the continuation of fasting; as little as 30 to 50 g of carbohydrate will eliminate the ketonuria.[52] The metabolic acidosis that occurs during a fast is partially offset by a compensatory respiratory alkalosis during the 1st month; hyperventilation occurs and results in a drop in pCO_2. Renal tissue acidosis also results in increased urinary ammonium excretion which balances some of the acid radicals and ketoacids.

Vitamin deficiencies may also occur. Drenick[50] reports a man who developed Wernicke's syndrome as a consequence of thiamine deficiency after 30 days of fasting. Folic acid levels also fall during the 1st month and may result in a macrocytic anemia after several months.

Hyperuricemia is another common finding and occurs because the ketoacids compete for excretion in the renal tubules. The rise in ketoacids during fasting thus reduces the excretion of uric acid and hyperuricemia develops; in some individuals this can result in gout or uric acid renal stones.

COMPLICATIONS

Several potential hazards may occur. Nausea is perhaps the most common complaint resulting in discontinuance of the fast. One-third of Drenick's 137 subjects had nausea by the end of 4 weeks and another 20% developed the symptom during the course of the 2nd month. Medication, rehydration, and supplementation were used to relieve the symptom, but were ineffective. Although it was intially feared that ulcer disease might follow a fast, this has not been observed.

Postural hypotension and syncope develop in most patients who adhere to the fast; this is most marked after waking in the morning. Hot showers or baths worsen the symptom as does the administration of diuretics.

Deaths have been reported and apparently have been the result of cardiac decompensation. In one case,[53] a 20-year-old woman, who had lost 128 pounds to attain her ideal weight of 132 pounds in 7½ months, died in the seventh refeeding day; electron microscopy revealed fragmentation of cardiac myofibrils. Cardiac complications appear to be much more common in longer fasts. Short-term fasts in patients without evidence of current or previous heart disease do not appear to be dangerous in terms of cardiac functioning.

Psychological complications appear to be more common during prolonged fasting. Depression and anxiety occurred in the patients studied by Kollar and Atkinson.[54] Rowland[55] also observed severe emotional changes during long fasts. During short fasts, inpatients who have been carefully selected appear to have few psychiatric problems. Drenick concludes that most patients on short-term fasts (less than 2 months) had improvement in psychosocial functioning, and 30 of 137 patients who were not employed prior to the fast were working 4 years after weight loss.[50] Thirty of the patients who were working at the time they started their fast had greater pay after their weight loss.

MANAGEMENT OF THE FASTING PATIENT

The fast should last no longer than 2 months and should be conducted in an inpatient setting, either a hospital or nursing home. Fasts on an outpatient basis have been unsuccessful. A team including an internist, psychiatrist, and nutritionist should be available during the fast and probably for 2 to 3 years after the weight is lost. Most weight is regained during the 2nd to 3rd year and follow-up treatment is needed during this period.

At the beginning of the fast, laxatives should be given because peristalsis may cease completely in the absence of food and result in fecal impaction. Ample fluid intake of at least 2 liters/day must be encouraged. Voluntary fluid intake drops precipitously during a fast and can result in severe metabolic complications. Allopurinol (600 mg/day) is routinely given to prevent gout and renal stones. Folic acid supplements of 5 mg/day prevents a deficiency of this vitamin. Vitamin and mineral capsules are routinely given. Potassium chloride solution is given daily.

Each day during the fast, the sitting and recumbent blood pressure should be taken to monitor orthostatic hypotension. Urine acetone is tested daily, in part to monitor adherence to the fast. Serum uric acid, serum creatinine, and a CBC are obtained weekly.

Even though most subjects will not lose down to their ideal weight during 2 months, longer fasts are inadvisable. Refeeding should start with tea and sugar and orange juice to prevent gastrointestinal upset. Then small amounts of regular foods, about 500 calories per day, are given; this amount seems to satisfy most patients because of the post-starvation anorexia. There is usually a marked weight gain with refeeding and there may be "refeeding edema." A spontaneous diuresis usually occurs in 10 days to 3 weeks.

POOR LONG-TERM RESULTS

Although predictably large amounts of weight are lost during the fast, long-term results have been disappointing. Campbell and colleagues[56] studied 70 patients who lost an average of 29.6 kg during a 14-week fast. The follow-up period averaged 28.2 months and the percentage of surplus weight rose from 28.2% at discharge to 62.7% at the end of the follow-up period. Drenick[50] followed 137 patients who lost a mean of 65 pounds during the fast; at the end of 1 year 105 subjects who could be evaluated had maintained their discharge weight but at the 6-year follow-up only nine of the 105 were at their reduced weight. Thus, very few patients maintain their lower weight. Drenick notes that there was an almost total absence of a continued treatment program after weight loss. It is possible that a short-term fast might be successful as part of a comprehensive treatment program that includes behavior modification to alter learned patterns of eating.

PROTEIN-SPARING MODIFIED FAST

Because many of the undesirable side effects of a fast are due to protein loss, several groups have investigated the use of protein and electrolytes to prevent loss of lean body tissue. Apfelbaum and associates[57] gave protein to fasting outpatients and reduced or eliminated nitrogen losses, yet weight loss continued. The protein supplement used has varied. One group[58] uses lean meat, fish, or fowl with a caloric content ranging from 400–700 calories and providing 1.3 to 1.5 g of protein per kilogram of ideal body weight. Another group[59] uses a dietary supplement of 45 g of casein, 30 g of glucose, and 0.25 mEq of potassium.

Reports of these regimens show encouraging results with 70% of 141 patients losing more than 40 pounds over the course of 40 to 52 weeks.[59] However, this plan has not yet received wide acceptance, in part because of the notorious liquid protein diet. As detailed in Chapter 9, the diet supplement in the so-called "Last-Chance Diet" is a poor quality protein and has often been used without medical supervision. Because deaths have resulted, even properly supervised protein-sparing modified fasts have become suspect. Also, although it has been thought that 1 g of protein per kilogram might prevent nitrogen loss, currently unpublished studies show that as much as 1.5 g of protein per kilogram will not produce nitrogen balance in some people for as long as 60 days.[60]

EXERCISE

In our sedentary society, the marked decrease in physical activity is partially responsible for the tremendous increase in the prevalence of obesity. Some obese individuals, often adolescents, eat less than their thin peers but exercise less. In 1968, Mayer et al.[61] compared body weight and calorie intake among workers in jobs with varying degrees of physical activity (See Fig. 11.5). The lowest voluntary intake is seen in workers who engage in

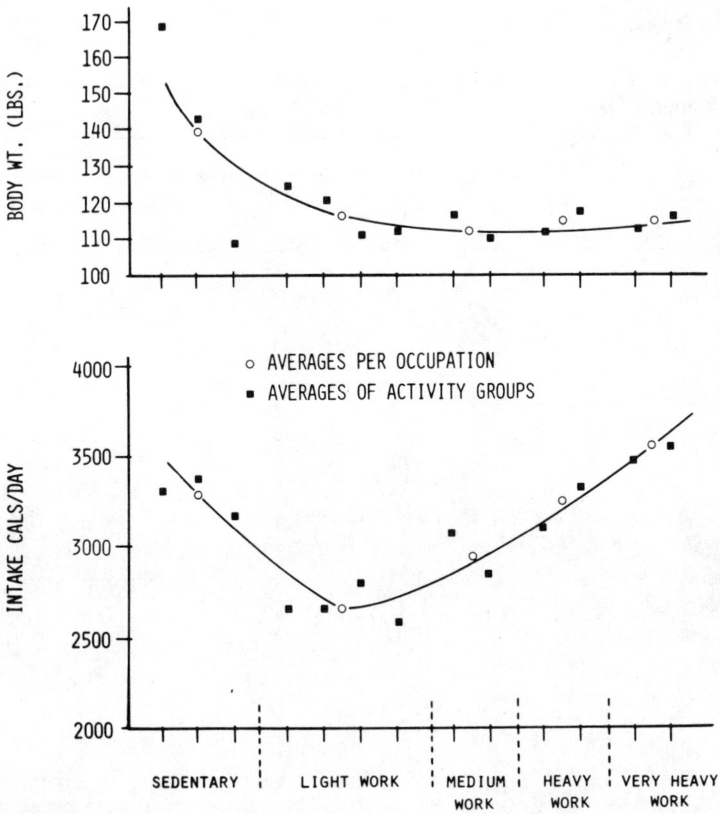

Figure 11.5. Body weight and caloric intake as a function of physical activity. (Reprinted with permission from J. Mayer, P. Roy, and K. P. Mitra: Am J Clin Nutr 4: 169–175, 1956.)

light work, such as clerks. Sedentary workers consume more than light workers and weigh more. Workers performing heavy work consume more than light workers but weigh less than sedentary workers. Thus, exercise influences food intake and body weight.

CALORIE COST OF EXERCISE

The role of exercise in the treatment of obesity has not been widely investigated. One reason for this is the dismal observation that to use up the calories from one moderate-sized hamburger would require 18 minutes of running, or 43 minutes of bicycle riding. To lose one pound of fat would require running for 3 hours or walking for 11 hours at 3.5 miles per hour. Table 11.3 lists the energy equivalents of selected food calories expressed in minutes of activities.[62] These figures are discouraging to all but the avid athlete. However, recent evidence suggests that these figures account only for the direct cost of exercise, and that exercise results in other effects that

Table 11.3
Energy equivalents of selected foods expressed in minutes of activity (adapted from Konishi[62]).

FOOD	CALORIES	ACTIVITY				
		WALKING	RIDING BICYCLE	SWIMMING	RUNNING	RECLINING
		MIN.	MIN.	MIN.	MIN.	MIN.
APPLE, LARGE	101	19	12	9	5	78
BEER, 1 GLASS	114	22	14	10	6	88
BREAD AND BUTTER	78	15	10	7	4	60
CAKE, 1/12, 2-LAYER	356	68	43	32	18	274
CEREAL, DRY, 1/2 C., WITH MILK AND SUGAR	200	38	24	18	10	154
CHICKEN, FRIED, 1/2 BREAST	232	45	28	21	12	178
COOKIE, CHOCOLATE CHIP	51	10	6	5	3	39
EGG, FRIED	110	21	13	10	6	85
ICE CREAM, 1/6 QT.	193	37	24	17	10	148
MALTED MILK SHAKE	502	97	61	45	26	386
MILK, 1 GLASS	166	32	20	15	9	128
ORANGE, MEDIUM	68	13	8	6	4	52
PANCAKE WITH SYRUP	124	24	15	11	6	95
PIE, APPLE, 1/6	377	73	46	34	19	290
PIZZA, CHEESE, 1/8	180	35	22	16	9	138
HAMBURGER	350	67	43	31	18	269
SPAGHETTI, 1 SERVING	396	76	48	35	20	305
STEAK, T-BONE	235	45	29	21	12	181
STRAWBERRY SHORTCAKE	400	77	49	36	21	308

dissipate energy, including a decrease in appetite and a prolonged elevation in metabolic rates after exercise.

The decrease in appetite with moderate exercise has been repeatedly documented, but the reasons for this have yet to be elucidated. There is a temporary elevation of temperature with exercise which may inhibit hunger. Hervey[63] postulates that food intake is inhibited by a lipostatic feedback mechanism when exercise mobilizes surplus fat. The finding that appetite decreases with exercise runs counter to the mistaken idea that appetite regularly increases after exercise, although there is some evidence that there may be a rebound increase in appetite 1 to 2 days after vigorous exercise.[64]

In addition to the direct caloric cost of activity and the attendant decrease in appetite, there is also a prolonged increase in basal metabolism after exercise. Allen and Quigley[65] report that the resting metabolic rate may be raised 25% above basal levels for 15 hours after strenuous activity such as football and raised 10% for as long as 48 hours after the activity. Thus, the caloric cost of strenuous exercise may be nearly double the usual calculated caloric cost.

Several studies have shown that exercise after a high-calorie meal markedly increases the thermic effect of food. In an early study,[66] it was found that the thermic response of food rose from 28% of the BMR with breakfast alone to 56% with breakfast and exercise. Bray and colleagues[67] studied six lean adult males who ingested 1000-calorie breakfasts with or without exercise. They found that the thermic effect of the food ranged from 10–30% above BMR, and with exercise the thermic effect was approximately doubled. The same subjects were also fed a 4000-calorie breakfast with and without exercise, but there was no additional increment in the thermic effect. Swindells[68] did not find an increase in thermic effect with exercise but Bray notes that the size of the meals in this study ranged from 600–900 calories. It may be that for this exercise-induced thermic effect to occur, very high-calorie meals are required.

CHANGES IN BODY COMPOSITION AND METABOLISM

Strenuous exercise has immediate effects and repeated exercise in physical training programs results in chronic adaptations.[69] Immediately after the start of exercise, the uptake of free fatty acids in the periphery is increased and decreases immediately after exercise stops. Free fatty acid mobilization starts to increase soon after exercise begins and remains elevated for a few minutes after exercise ceases. These are immediate effects of exercise on metabolism. After a number of exercise sessions, chronic adaptations occur. Plasma triglycerides and insulin both gradually decrease as fat stores decrease. These metabolic changes are illustrated in Figure 11.6.

Regular exercise without associated caloric intake change may not im-

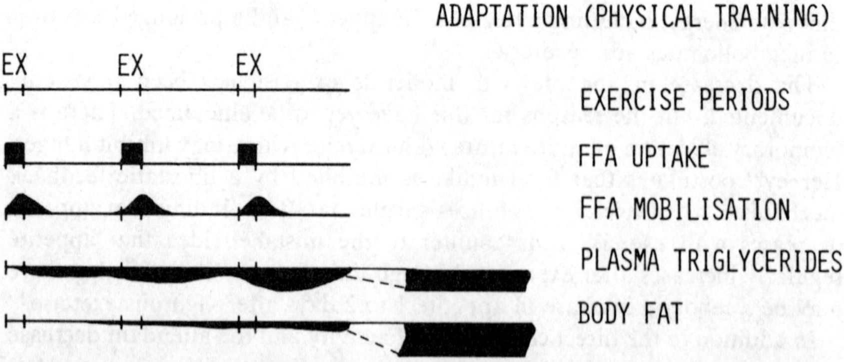

Figure 11.6. Metabolic changes induced by physical activity. (Reprinted with permission from P. Björntorp: Clin Endocrinol Metab 5: 431–453, 1976.)

mediately result in a loss of weight. Initially there may be an increase in lean body mass and a decrease in fat tissue without a change in body weight. The increase in lean body mass is primarily an increase in muscle mass. The capacity of muscle mass to increase with activity is limited and eventually there will be a net loss in weight. The initial delay in weight loss can be very frustrating to the obese patient, but advance warning may help. In men, an increase in waist measurement usually parallels increase in fat content. Therefore a decrease in waist measurement in men prior to weight loss can be encouraging. Triceps skinfold measures may also reveal a decrease in fat stores prior to very significant weight losses. The time required for body weight to fall with moderate exercise and no change in food intake varies but may require a month or more.

Exercise also results in a decrease in fat cell size but not in fat cell number. In one study of patients who received physical training after myocardial infarction, Sanne[70] found that fat cell size variation was limited after training. Some of the subjects had lost no weight but as a group, the body fat content decreased by 40%. In analyzing this data, Björntorp[69] concludes that some of the patients who did not lose weight may already have had the post-physical training fat cell size to begin with, and that fat loss in the other subjects was from enlarged fat cells. He notes that with dietary treatment on an outpatient basis, weight loss continues until a certain fat cell size is attained, and weight loss below this is very limited.

Exercise improves glucose tolerance in normal subjects and in obese post-myocardial infarction patients.[70] This effect has been known for decades and is probably due to a decrease in body fat and an increased insulin sensitivity. This improvement may not be due to a decrease in body fat alone. Patients with hyperplastic obesity who received vigorous physical training on an ad libitum diet had no change in body fat content, yet there was a marked increase in insulin sensitivity. The reasons for this have yet to be elucidated.

Exercise also lowers plasma triglycerides.[71] It is not known whether this is an immediate effect or a chronic adaptation to physical training.

Thus, several metabolic changes have been noted following physical training. There is an increase in lean body mass, primarily due to an increase in muscle mass, a decrease in fat cell size but not fat cell number, improvement in glucose tolerance with increased insulin sensitivity, and a decrease in plasma triglycerides.

Patients with hyperplastic obesity (i.e., with an increased number of fat cells) may be resistant to some of the metabolic effects of exercise. Björntorp and colleagues[72, 73] have studied several groups of hyperplastic obese subjects who have received physical training without a change in diet. These patients did not demonstrate a decrease in body weight or body fat content, although there was the expected increase in maximal working capacity and marked decreases in plasma insulin. The fat cell size in these patients also remained higher than that in other groups of obese patients. Björntorp[69] hypothesizes that there may be some defect in appetite regulation related to the steady-state fat cell size in these hyperplastic obese subjects. It may be that when hyperplastic obese subjects exercise there is an increase in appetite. In these patients exercise may not be a viable therapeutic approach, at least in terms of fat or weight reduction.

References

1. Agras WS, Ferguson JM, Greaves C, et al: A clinical and research questionnaire for obese patients. In: Obesity: Behavioral Approaches to Dietary Management. Williams BJ, Martin S, Foreyt JP (eds). New York, Brunner/Mazel Publ, 1976, pp 168–176.
2. Simonson M: Lecture at Conference: The Management of Obesity. Johns Hopkins Medical Institutions, Feb 13–16, 1978.
3. Bray GA, Jordon HA, Sims EAH: Evaluation of the obese patient. 1. An algorithm. JAMA 235: 1487–1491, 1976.
4. Stunkard AJ, Rush J: Dieting and depression re-examined: a critical review of reports of untoward responses during weight reduction. Ann Intern Med 81: 526–433, 1974.
5. Kelly MT: Nutrition History Developed at Johns Hopkins Medical Institutions. Presentation at Conference: The Management of Obesity. Johns Hopkins Medical Institutions, Feb 13–16, 1978.
6. Stunkard AJ, McLaren-Hume M: The results of treatment of obesity. A review of the literature and report of a series. Arch Intern Med 103: 79–85, 1959.
7. Stunkard AJ: Behavioral treatment of obesity: the current status. Int J Obesity 2: 237–248, 1978.
8. Stunkard AJ, Penick S: Behavior modification in the treatment of obesity: the problem of maintaining weight loss. Arch Gen Psychiatry 36: 801–806, 1979.
9. Romanczyk RG, Tracy DA, Wilson GT, Thorpe GL: Behavior techniques in the treament of obesity: a comparative analysis. Behav Res Ther 11: 629–640, 1973.
10. Stunkard AJ, personal communication.
11. Sobell MB, Sobell LC: The need for realism, relevance and operational assumptions in the study of substance dependence. Presentation at International Symposia on Alcohol and Drug Research, Addiction Research Foundation. Toronto, Canada, October 1973.

12. Bookbinder LJ: Simple conditioning vs the dynamic approach to symptoms and symptom substitution: a reply to Yates. Psychol Rep 10: 71–77, 1962.
13. Yates AJ: Symptoms and symptom substitution. Psychol Rev 65: 371–374, 1958.
14. Stunkard AJ: The management of obesity. NY J Med 58: 79–87, 1958.
15. Feinstein AR: The measurement of success in weight reduction: an analysis of methods and a new index. J Chron Dis 10: 439–456, 1959.
16. Jolliffe N, Alpert E: The "performance index" as a method for estimating effectiveness of reducing regimens. Postgrad Med 9: 106–115, 1951.
17. Boothby WM, Berkson J: Food nomogram. In: Rynearson EH, Gastineau CP: Obesity. Charles C Thomas, Springfield, Ill, 1949.
18. Manno B, Marston AR: Weight reduction as a function of negative covert reinforcement (sensitization) versus positive covert reinforcement. Behav Res Ther 10: 201–207, 1972.
19. Stunkard AJ: Behavioral treaments of obesity: failure to maintain weight loss. In: Behavioral Self-Management, Stuart RB (ed). Brunner/Mazel, New York, 1977, pp 317–350.
20. Bray GA: The Obese Patient. Philadelphia, WB Saunders, 1976, p 304.
21. Wilkins L, Blizzard RM, Migeon CJ: The Diagnosis and Treatment of Endocrine Disorders in Childhood and Adolescence. Ed 3. Springfield, Charles C Thomas, 1963, p 565.
22. Bray GA: The myth of diet in the management of obesity. Am J Clin Nutr 23: 1141–1148, 1970.
23. Galton DJ, Bray GA: Metabolism of α-glycerol phosphate in human adipose tissue in obesity. J Clin Endocrinol Metab 27: 1573–1580, 1967.
24. Miller DS, Parsonage S: Resistance to slimming: adaptation or illusion? Lancet 1: 773–775, 1975.
25. Mayer J, Thomas DW: Regulation of food intake and obesity. Science 156: 328–337, 1967.
26. Bray GA: Effect of caloric restriction on energy expenditure in obese patients. Lancet 2: 397–398, 1969.
27. Bullen BA, Reed RB, Mayer J: Physical activity of obese and nonobese adolescent girls appraised by motion picture sampling. Am J Clin Nutr 14: 211–223, 1964.
28. Young CM: Weight control in a college situation. Postgrad Med 51: 116–120, 1972.
29. National Academy of Sciences: Recommended Dietary Allowances. Ed 8. Washington, DC, Food and Nutrition Board of the National Academy of Sciences, National Research Council, 1974.
30. Taller H: Calories Don't Count. New York, Simon and Schuster, 1961.
31. Kekwick A, Pawan GLS: Calorie intake in relation to body-weight changes in the obese. Lancet 2: 155–161, 1956.
32. Pilkington TRE, Gainsborough H, Rosenoer VM, Carey M: Diet and weight reduction in the obese. Lancet 1: 856–858, 1960.
33. Stock AL, Yudkin J: Nutrient intake of subjects on low carbohydrate diet used in treatment of obesity. Am J Clin Nutr 23: 948–952, 1970.
34. Exchange Lists for Meal Planning. Prepared by Committees of American Diabetes Assoc, Inc and American Dietetic Assoc in cooperation with National Institute of Arthritis, Metabolism and Digestive Diseases and the National Heart and Lung Institute, National Institutes of Health, Public Health Service, US Dept of Health, Education and Welfare, 1976.
35. Sims EAH, Goldman RF, Gluck CM, et al: Experimental obesity in man. Trans Assoc Am Physicians 81: 153–170, 1968.
36. Hood CEA, Goodhart JM, Fletcher RF: Observations on obese patients eating isocaloric reducing diets with varying proportions of carbohydrate. Br J Nutr 24: 39–44, 1970.
37. Clarke S: Composition of weight loss during fasting. Presentation at Conference: The Management of Obesity. Johns Hopkins Medical Institutions, Feb 13–16, 1978.
38. Stern JS: Weight control programs. Curr Concepts Nutr 5: 137–155, 1977.
39. Atkins RC: Dr. Atkins' Diet Revolution. New York, McKay, 1972.
40. Churchill JA, Berendes DW: Intelligence of children whose mothers had acetonia during pregnancy. In: Perinatal Factors Affecting Human Development. Pan American Organization Committee on Medical Research, Pan American Sanitary Bureau, Washington, DC, Sci Pub No. 185: pp 30–35, 1969.

41. Simeons ATW: The action of chorionic gonadotrophin in the obese. Lancet 2: 946–947, 1954.
42. Carne S: The action of chorionic gonadotropin in the obese. Lancet 2: 1282–1284, 1961.
43. Strang JM, McClugage HB, Evans FA: The nitrogen balance during dietary correction of obesity. Am J Med Sci 181: 336–349, 1931.
44. Brook CGD, Lloyd JK, Wolff OH: Rapid weight loss in children. Br Med J 3: 44–45, 1974.
45. Rayner PHW, Court JM: Effect of dietary restriction and anorectic drugs on linear growth in childhood obesity. Arch Dis Child 49: 822–823, 1974.
46. Heald FP: Juvenile obesity. Curr Concepts Nutr 3: 81–88, 1975.
47. Wolff OH: Obesity in childhood. Q J Med New Series 24: 109–123, 1955.
48. Bloom WL: Fasting as an introduction to the treatment of obesity. Metabolism 8: 214–220, 1959.
49. Heyden S, DeMaria W, Barbee S, Morris M: Weight reduction in adolescents. Nutr Metab 15: 295–304, 1973.
50. Drenick EJ: Weight reduction by prolonged fasting. In: Obesity in Perspective. Fogarty International Center Series on Preventive Medicine, Vol II, Pt II. Bray GA (ed). Washington, DC, US Government Printing Office, 1976.
51. Owen OE, Morgan AP, Kemp HG, et al: Brain metabolism during fasting. J Clin Invest 46: 1589–1595, 1967.
52. Bray GA: The Obese Patient. Philadelphia, WB Saunders, 1976, p 331.
53. Garnett ES, Barnard DL, Ford J, et al: Gross fragmentation of cardiac myofibrils after therapeutic starvation for obesity. Lancet 1: 914–916, 1969.
54. Kollar EJ, Atkinson RM: Responses of extremely obese patients to starvation. Psychosom Med 28: 227–245, 1966.
55. Rowland CV Jr: Psychotherapy of six hyperobese adults during total starvation. Arch Gen Psychiatry 18: 541–548, 1968.
56. Campbell CJ, Campbell IW, Innes JA, et al: Further follow-up experience after prolonged therapeutic starvation. In: Obesity. Burland WL, Samuel P, Yudkin J (eds). London, Churchill Livingstone, 1974, pp 281–292.
57. Apfelbaum M, Boudon P, Lacatis D: Effets métaboliques de la diète protidique ches 41 sujets obeses. Presse Med 78: 1917–1920, 1970, cited in Bray GA: The Obese Patient, Philadelphia, WB Saunders, 1976, p 336.
58. Blackburn GL, Bistrian BR, Flatt JP, et al: Role of a protein-sparing modified fast in a comprehensive weight reduction program. In: Recent Advances in Obesity Research I, Howard A (ed). London, Newman Publ., pp 279–281, 1975.
59. Genuth SM, Castro JH, Vertes V: Weight reduction in obesity by outpatient semistarvation. JAMA 230: 987–992, 1974.
60. Stunkard AJ, personal communication.
61. Mayer J, Roy P, Mitra KP: Relation between caloric intake, body weight, and physical work: studies in an industrial population in West Bengal. Am J Clin Nutr 4: 169–175, 1956.
62. Konishi F: Food energy equivalents of various activities. J Am Diet Assoc 46: 186–188, 1965.
63. Hervey GR: A hypothetical mechanism for the regulation of food intake in relation to energy balance. Proc Nutr Soc 28: 54A–55A, 1969.
64. Edholm OG, Fletcher JG, Widdowson EM, McCance RA: The energy expenditure and food intake of individual men. Br J Nutr 9: 286–300, 1955.
65. Allen DW, Quigley BM: The role of physical activity in the control of obesity. Med J Aust 2: 434–438, 1977.
66. Miller DS, Mumford P, Stock MJ: Gluttony. 2. Thermogenesis in overeating man. Am J Clin Nutr 20: 1223–1229, 1967.
67. Bray GA, Whipp BJ, Koyal SN: The acute effects of food intake on energy expenditure during cycle ergometry. Am J Clin Nutr 27: 254–259, 1974.
68. Swindells YE: The influence of activity and size of meals on caloric response in women. Br J Nutr 27: 65–73, 1972.
69. Björntorp P: Exercise in the treatment of obesity. Clin Endocrinol Metab 5: 431–453, 1976.
70. Sanne H: Exercise tolerance and physical training of non-selected patients after myocardial

infarction. Acta Med Scand Suppl 551, cited in Björntorp P: Exercise in the treatment of obesity. Clin Endocrinol Metab 5: 431–453, 1976.

71. Lopez-SA, Vial R, Balart L, Arroyave G: Effect of exercise and physical fitness on serum lipids and lipoproteins. Artherosclerosis 20: 1–9, 1974.
72. Björntorp P, deJounge K, Krotkiewski M, et al: Physical training in human obesity. III. Effects of long-term physical training on body composition. Metabolism 22: 1467–1475, 1973.
73. Björntorp P, deJounge K, Sjöström L, Sullivan L: The effect of physical training on insulin production in obesity. Metabolism 19: 631–638, 1970.

APPENDIX 1

Stanford Eating Disorder Clinic Questionnaire

(Reprinted with permission from WS Agras, JM Ferguson, C Greaves, et al[1])

Name: ________________ Sex: M F Age: ___ Birthdate: __________
Address: ______________________________ Home phone: __________
______________________________ Office phone: __________

WEIGHT HISTORY:

1. Your present weight _____ height _____
2. How would you describe your present weight? (circle one)

   very overweight — slightly overweight — about average

3. At what weight have you *felt* your best or do you think you would feel your best?

   ______

4. How much weight would you like to lose? ______________
5. How dissatisfied are you with the way you look at this weight? (circle one)

   Completely Satisfied — Moderately Satisfied — Neutral — Moderately Dissatisfied — Very Dissatisfied

6. Do other people react to your weight problem? Yes ____ No ____ If yes, how do they react?

   ____
   ____

7. Why do you want to lose weight at this time? ______________________
   ____

8. What are the attitudes of the following people about your attempt(s) to lose weight?

	Negative (e.g., disapprove, resentful)	Indifferent (e.g., don't care, don't help)	Positive (e.g., encourage, understanding)
Husband			
Wife			
Children			
Parents			
Employer			
Friends			

9. Do the attitudes or behavior of your spouse or children affect your weight loss or gain? Yes__ No__ If yes, please describe: ________________

10. Indicate the periods in your life when you have been overweight on the following table. *Where appropriate*, list your maximum weight for each period and number of pounds you were overweight. Briefly describe any methods you used to lose weight, e.g., diet, shots, pills, in that five-year episode. Also list any significant life events you feel were related to either your weight gain or loss, e.g., college tests, marriage, pregnancies, illness.

Age	Maximum Weight	# Pounds Overweight	Methods Used to Lose Weight	Significant Events Related to Weight Change
Birth				
0–5				
5–10				
10–15				
15–20				
20–25				
25–30				
30–35				
35–40				
40–45				
45–50				
50–55				
55–60				
60–65				

11. How do you feel your weight affects your daily activities? (circle one)
    No effect Some effect Often interferes Extreme effect

12. How physically active are you? (circle one)
    Very active Active Average Inactive Very inactive

13. What do you do for physical exercise and how often do you do it?

FREQUENCY (daily, weekly, monthly)	ACTIVITY (swimming, jogging, dancing)

14. A number of different ways of losing weight are listed below. Please indicate which methods you have used by filling the appropriate blanks.

	Ages Used	Number of Times Used	Max. Wt. Lost	Comments: Length of time weight loss maintained; success; difficulties
TOPS				
Weight Watchers				
HCG shots				
Pills				
Supervised diet				
Unsupervised diet				
Starvation diet				
Behavior mod				
Psychotherapy				
Hypnosis				
Other				

15. Which method did you use for the longest period of time? ____________

16. In your attempts to lose weight, have you ever had a physical or emotional reaction of such severity that it impaired your family and/or work relationships or functioning?

Yes___ No___ If yes, please describe the symptoms and how long they lasted.

____

____

____

17. Have you had a major mood change after a significant weight loss?

Yes___ No___ If yes, indicate on the following checklist those changes:

	Not at All	A Little Bit	Moder-ately	Quite a Bit	Ex-tremely
a. Depressed, sad, feeling down or unhappy?	___	___	___	___	___
b. Feeling anxious, nervous or restless?	___	___	___	___	___
c. Feeling weak?	___	___	___	___	___
d. Feeling elated?	___	___	___	___	___
e. Feeling easily irritated, annoyed, or angry?	___	___	___	___	___
f. Feeling fatigued, worn out?	___	___	___	___	___
g. Being preoccupied with food and eating?	___	___	___	___	___

h. Feeling a lack of self-confidence? ____ ____ ____ ____ ____

18. What usually goes wrong with your weight loss programs? ____________

MEDICAL HISTORY:

19. What are your present medical problems? ____________

20. What medications or drugs are you taking? ____________

21. Are you allergic to medications, drugs, or foods? ____________

22. Please list any hospitalization or operations. Indicate your age for each hospital admission.

Age	Reason for hospitalization

23. Please list, by age, any serious illnesses you have had which have not required hospitalization or operations:

Age	Illness

24. Please describe any medical problems you have which are complicated by your weight.

25. When did you last have a complete physical examination? ____________

26. Who is your current doctor?____________________

27. How much alcohol do you usually drink per week?____________________

28. Please list any psychiatric contact, individual counseling, or marital counseling that you have had or are now having.

Age	Reason for contact and type of therapy

SOCIAL HISTORY:

29. Please describe your present occupation ____________________

30. How long have you worked for your present employer?____________________

31. Circle the last year of school attended:
    1 2 3 4 5 6 7 8 9 10 11 12 1 2 3 4 M.A. Ph.D. Other__________
    Grade School High School College

32. Present marital status: (circle one)
    Single Married Divorced Widowed Separated Engaged

33. Please answer the following questions for each marriage:

Date of marriage			
Date of termination			
Reason (death, divorce, etc.)			
Number of children			

34. Please describe your present spouse's occupation in detail ____________________

35. Spouse's age_____Weight_____ Height_____

36. How would you describe your spouse's weight? (circle one)

very overweight	slightly overweight	about average	slightly underweight	very underweight

37. Please list your children's age, sex, height, and weight and circle whether they are overweight, average, or underweight. Include any children from previous marriages, whether they are living with you or not.

Age	Sex	Weight	Height	Overweight		Average	Underweight	
____	___	____	____	very	slightly	average	slightly	very
____	___	____	____	very	slightly	average	slightly	very
____	___	____	____	very	slightly	average	slightly	very
____	___	____	____	very	slightly	average	slightly	very
____	___	____	____	very	slightly	average	slightly	very

38. Who lives in your house with you? ____________________

39. Is your father living? Yes__ No__ Father's age now or age and cause of death ____________________

40. Is your mother living? Yes__ No__ Mother's age now or age and cause of death ____________________

41. Describe your father's occupation ____________________

42. Describe your mother's occupation ____________________

43. Describe your father's weight while you were growing up: (circle one)

very overweight	slightly overweight	about average	slightly underweight	very underweight

44. Describe your mother's weight while you were growing up: (circle one)

very overweight	slightly overweight	about average	slightly underweight	very underweight

45. Please describe your family attitudes toward food and eating while you were growing up

____

____

____

46. Were your parents ever separated or divorced? Yes__ No__ If yes, how old were you?______

47. Who raised you as a child? ____________________

48. What was your relationship with your father like? (circle one)
Excellent Good Average Below average Poor

49. What was your relationship with your mother like? (circle one)
Excellent Good Average Below average Poor

50. Please list your brothers' and sisters' ages, sex, present weight, and height and circle whether they are overweight, average, or underweight.

Age	Sex	Weight	Height	Overweight		Average	Underweight	
____	___	____	____	very	slightly	average	slightly	very
____	___	____	____	very	slightly	average	slightly	very
____	___	____	____	very	slightly	average	slightly	very
____	___	____	____	very	slightly	average	slightly	very

51. Please write any other information you feel is relevant to your weight problem below. This would include interactions with your family and friends that might sabotage a weight loss program, or any part of your family history that is related and/or relevant to your weight problem.

____
____
____
____
____
____
____
____
____
____
____
____
____
____
____
____

APPENDIX 2

Nutrition History

(Reprinted with permission from Millicent Kelly, RD, Johns Hopkins Outpatient Nutritional Clinic, 1977)

Please be as Detailed as Possible in Answering the Following Questions. This Information is used as the Basis for your Diet.

(1) Date: ______________________ Age: ________
Name: ______________________ Sex: ________
Address: ______________________ Marital Status: ________
Number in Household
Adults: ________
Occupation: ______________________ Children: _____ Ages: ______

(2) Height:____ Weight:____ Any Weight Change in the Past Year? If so, Describe:

(3) Do You Take any Prescribed Medications? If so, Please Indicate:

(4) Have you ever been on a Diet? If so, What Type of Diet, when was it given and by whom, and what were the Results?

(5) Indicate Where You Eat Most of your Meals. (i.e., Home 70%, Restaurant 30%)
Morning:
Noon:
Night:
Between Meal Snacks:

(6) Food Preparation:
At Home Who Prepares Meals?
Are your Vegetables Prepared with Meat, Butter, Margarine, or any Fat?
If so, Estimate the Amount of Fat in your Serving:
Do You Eat Fried or Breaded Foods? What and How Often?

(7) Food and Health:
Do You Have Food Allergies? If so, Please Describe:
Do You Have Food Intolerances or Difficulty with Digestion? If so, Describe:
Do You Have Problems With Constipation and/or Diarrhea?
At What Time of Day Are You Most Hungry: Morning Noon Night Late Evening

Describe Your Physical Activities on a Daily and Weekly Basis. Include Work-Related Activities

Are There Any Foods Which You Dislike and Will Not Eat? Please Indicate:

(8) Describe a Typical Day's Food Intake. Include Times of Meals (or Approximate Times) and the Types of Foods Usually Eaten and Method of Preparation. Give Approximate Portions for All Times. *See Example Below.*

Morning Noon Evening Snacks

EXAMPLE:

BREAKFAST (7:00)	NOON MEAL (12:00–2:00)	EVENING MEAL (6:00–7:00)
½ cup unsweetened orange juice	2 or 3 ounces sliced chicken	4 ounces cooked-weight fried fish
1 cup cornflakes with ½ cup whole milk &	2 tsp. mayonnaise	vegetable salad (1 cup, with 1 Tbs. French dressing)
2 tsp. sugar	lettuce leaf	½ cup cooked green beans with 1 tsp. margarine
2 cups coffee with 1 tsp. milk in ea. (no sugar)	2 slices tomato	1 med. white baked potato with 1 Tbs. sour cream
	2 slices bread	½ cup Jello
	1 serving fresh fruit	1 cup tea with 2 tsp. sugar
	1 small bag potato chips	
	1 8 ounce diet soda	

(9) Describe your Fluid Intake Per Day Per Week

Water: ______________________________

Coffee: ______________________________

Tea: Iced and Hot: ______________________________

Juice (Types): ______________________________

Milk: (Whole/Skim or Others): ______________________________

Beer: ______________________________

Alcohol: ______________________________

Others: ______________________________

(10) Is there anything else about eating habits that you think we should know? Please write it in this space:

(11) Circle the items below which you eat. Estimate the amount you would have in a week or a day, if they are frequently used foods.

MILK AND MILK PRODUCTS:

Milk for: Drinking
Cereal
Cooking
Coffee or Tea

Cream
Sour Cream
Cheese (Type)
Cottage Cheese
Cream Cheese
Custard
Ice Cream
Ice Milk
Pudding
Sherbert
Yogurt (Type)

MEAT OR SUBSTITUTES:

Bacon
Beef
Chicken
Dried Beans or Peas
Egg
Fish
Hot Dogs
Lamb
Luncheon Meats
Peanut Butter
Pork
Sausage
Scrapple
Soybean Meat Products
Turkey

GRAIN PRODUCTS:

Bread: Commercial
Homemade
Biscuits
Cereal: Cooked
Dry (Type)
Crackers (Type)
French Toast
Macaroni
Muffins
Noodles
Pancakes
Rice
Rolls
Spaghetti
Waffles
Flour
Cracker Crumbs

FRUIT:

Fruit: Canned
Dried
Fresh
Juice

VEGETABLES:

Vegetables: Raw
Cooked (Type)
Salads

SOUPS-ENTREES-SALADS:

Casseroles (Type)
Salads (Meat or Pasta)
Chicken or Turkey
Egg
Ham
Tuna
Potato
Macaroni
Soup (Type)
Stews (Type)

FATS:

Butter
Margarine
Salad Dressing (Type)
Shortenings
Oil

SWEETS:

Cake
Candy
Chewing Gum
Cookies
Honey
Jam, Jelly, or Preservatives
Jello
Pies
Sugar (Used with What Foods)
Sweet Rolls

MISCELLANEOUS:

Artichokes
BBQ Sauce
Catsup
Diet Foods (Type)
Gravy
Nuts
Pickles (Type)
Sauces (Type)
Seeds (Type)

APPENDIX 3

The Food Exchange System

(Adapted from Exchange Lists for Meal Planning[34])

List 1: MILK EXCHANGES

Includes nonfat, lowfat, and whole milk

Each item contains approximately *80 calories,* 12 grams of carbohydrate, 8 grams of protein, and a trace of fat.

Starred items are higher in fat. When eating these you should eat less servings from the fat group.

1	C	Skim or Nonfat Milk
1/3	C	Nonfat Dry Powdered Milk
1/2	C	Canned Evaporated Skim Milk
1	C	Buttermilk made from Skim Milk
*1	C 1%	Fat Fortified Milk
*1	C 2%	Fat Fortified Milk
*1	C	Yogurt made from 2% Fortified Milk
*1	C	Whole Milk
*½	C	Canned Evaporated Whole Milk
*1	C	Buttermilk made from Whole Milk
*1	C	Yogurt made from Whole Milk

List 2: VEGETABLE EXCHANGES

Each item contains approximately *25 calories,* 5 grams of carbohydrate, and 2 grams of protein.

All items listed are for ½ C.

Starchy vegetables are listed in the Bread Exchange List.

½ C serving:

Asparagus
Bean Sprouts
Beets
Broccoli
Brussels Sprout
Cabbage
Carrots
Cauliflower

Greens:
Beets, Chards,
Collards, Dandelion,
Kale, Mustard,
Spinach, Turnip

Mushrooms
Okra

String Beans (Green or Yellow)
Summer Squash
Tomatoes
Tomato Juice
Turnips
Vegetable Juice cocktail
Zucchini

Celery	Onions
Cucumbers	Rhubarb
Eggplant	Rutabaga
Green Pepper	Sauerkraut

List 3: FRUIT EXCHANGES

Each item contains approximately *40 calories* and 10 grams of carbohydrate

Apple	1 small	Grape Juice	1/4 C
Apple Juice	1/3 C	Mango	1/2 small
Applesauce (unsweetened)	1/2 C	Melon	
		Cantaloupe	1/4 small
Apricots, fresh	2 medium	Honeydew	1/8 med.
Apricots, dried	4 halves	Watermelon	1 C
Banana	1/2 small	Nectarine	1 small
Berries		Orange	1 small
Blackberries	1/2 C	Orange Juice	1/2 C
Blueberries	1/2 C	Papaya	3/4 C
Raspberries	1/2 C	Peach	1 med.
Strawberries	3/4 C	Pear	1 small
Cherries	10 large	Persimmon, native	1 med.
Cider	1/3 C	Pineapple	1/2 C
Dates	2	Pineapple Juice	1/3 C
Figs, fresh	1	Plums	2 med.
Figs, dried	1	Prunes	2 med.
Grapefruit	1/2	Prune Juice	1/4 C
Grapefruit Juice	1/2 C	Raisins	2 Tbs.
Grapes	12	Tangerine	1 med.

Cranberries may be used as desired if no sugar is added.

List 4: BREAD EXCHANGES

Includes bread, cereal, and starchy vegetables

Each item contains approximately *70 calories*, 15 grams of carbohydrate, and 2 grams of protein

Bread		Cereal	
White (including French and Italian)	1 slice	Bran Flakes	1/2 C
Whole Wheat	1 slice	Other ready-to-eat Unsweetened Cereal	3/4 C
Rye or Pumpernickel	1 slice	Puffed Cereal (unfrosted)	1 C
Raisin	1 slice	Cereal (cooked)	1/2 C
Bagel, small	1/2	Grits (cooked)	1/2 C
English Muffin, small	1/2	Rice or Barley (cooked)	1/2 C
Plain Roll, bread	1	Pasta (cooked), Spaghetti, Noodles, Macaroni	1/2C
Frankfurter Roll	1/2		
Hamburger Bun	1/2		

Bread (cont.)	
Dried Bread Crumbs	3 Tbs.
Tortilla, 6"	1
Crackers	
Arrowroot	3
Graham, 2½″ sq.	2
Matzoh, 4″ × 6″	1/2
Oyster	20
Pretzels, 3-1/8″ long × 1/8″ dia.	25
Rye Wafers, 2″ × 3½″	3
Saltines	6
Soda, 2¼″ sq.	4
Starchy Vegetables	
Corn	1/3 C
Corn on Cob	1 small
Lima Beans	1/2 C
Parsnips	2/3 C
Peas, Green (Canned or Frozen)	1/2 C
Potato, White	1 small
Potato, Mashed	1/2 C
Pumpkin	3/4 C
Winter Squash, Acorn or Butternut	1/2 cup
Yam or Sweet Potato	1/4 C
For each of the following items omit 1 Fat Exchange	
Biscuit 2″ diameter	1
Corn Bread, 2″ × 2″ × 1″	1
Corn Muffin, 2″ diameter	1
Crackers, round butter type	5
Muffin, plain small	1
Potatoes, French Fried, length 2″ to 3½″	8
Pancake, 5″ × 1/2″	1
Waffle, 5″ × 1/2″	1
For the following, omit 2 Fat Exchanges	
Potato or Corn Chips	15
Cereal (cont.)	
Popcorn (popped, no fat added)	3 C
Cornmeal (dry)	2 Tbs.
Flour	2½ Tbs.
Wheat Germ	1/4 C
Dried Beans, Peas, and Lentils	
Beans, Peas, Lentils (dried and cooked)	1/2 C
Baked Beans, no pork (canned)	1/4 C

List 5: LOWFAT MEAT EXCHANGES

Includes lean meats, poultry, seafood, and lowfat cheeses
Each item contains approximately *55 calories*
Each 1-oz. meat serving contains 7 grams of protein and 3 grams of fat
1-oz. serving:

Beef: Baby Beef (very lean), Chipped Beef, Chuck, Flank Steak, Tenderloin, Plate Ribs, Plate Skirt Steak, Round (bottom, top), All cuts Rump, Spare Ribs, Tripe
Lamb: Leg, Rib, Sirloin, Loin (roast and chops), Shank, Shoulder
Pork: Leg (Whole Rump, Center Shank), Ham, Smoked (center slices)
Veal: Leg, Loin, Rib, Shank, Shoulder, Cutlets
Poultry: Meat without skin of Chicken, Turkey, Cornish Hen, Guinea Hen, Pheasant
Fish: Any fresh or frozen

Fish: Canned Salmon, Tuna, Mackerel, Crab, and Lobster	1/4 C
Clams, Oysters, Scallops, Shrimp	5 or 1 oz.
Sardines, drained	3
Cheeses containing less than 5 % butterfat	1 oz.
Cottage Cheese, dry and 2% butterfat	1/4 C
Dried beans and peas (omit 1 Bread Exchange)	1/2 C

List 5: MEDIUM FAT MEAT EXCHANGES

For each item omit ½ Fat Exchange

Beef: Ground (15% fat), Corned Beef (canned), Rib Eye, Round (ground)	1 oz.
Pork: Loin (all cuts Tenderloin), Shoulder Arm (picnic), Shoulder Blade, Boston Butt, Canadian Bacon, Boiled Ham	1 oz.
Liver, Heart, Kidney and Sweetbreads	1 oz.
Cottage Cheese, creamed	1/4 C
Cheese: Mozzarella, Ricotta, Farmer's cheese, Neufchatel,	1 oz.
Parmesan	3 Tbs.
Egg	1
Peanut Butter (omit 2 Fat Exchanges)	2 Tbs.

List 5: HIGH FAT MEAT EXCHANGES

For each item omit 1 Fat Exchange

Beef: Brisket, Corned Beef, Ground Beef (more than 20% fat), Hamburger (commercial), Chuck (ground, commercial), Roasts (Rib), Steaks (Club and Rib)	1 oz.
Lamb: Breast	1 oz.
Pork: Spare Ribs, Loin (Back Ribs), Pork (ground), Country-style Ham, Deviled Ham	1 oz.
Veal: Breast	1 oz.
Poultry: Capon, Duck, Goose	1 oz.
Cheese: Cheddar Types	1 oz.
Cold Cuts	4 ½″ × 1/8″ slice
Frankfurter	1 small

List 6: FAT EXCHANGES

Each item contains approximately *45 calories* and 5 grams of Fat

Margarine, soft, tub, or stick*	1 tsp.
Avocado (4″ dia.)†	1/8
Oil, Corn, Cottonseed, Safflower, Soy, Sunflower	1 tsp.
Oil, Olive†	1 tsp.
Oil, Peanut†	1 tsp.
Olives†	5 small
Almonds†	10 whole
Pecans†	2 large whole
Peanuts†	
Spanish	20 whole
Virginia	10 whole
Walnuts	6 small
Nuts, other†	6 small
Margarine, regular stick	1 tsp.
Butter	1 tsp.
Bacon Fat	1 tsp.
Bacon, crisp	1 strip
Cream, light	2 Tbs.
Cream, sour	2 Tbs.
Cream, heavy	1 Tbs.
Cream Cheese	1 Tbs.

* Made with corn, cottonseed, safflower, soy or sunflower oil only.
† Fat content is primarily monounsaturated.

French Dressing‡	1 Tbs.
Italian Dressing‡	1 Tbs.
Lard	1 tsp.
Mayonnaise‡	1 tsp.
Salad Dressing, mayonnaise-type	2 tsp.
Salt pork	3/4-inch cube

‡ If made with corn, cottonseed, safflower, soy, or sunflower oil, it can be used on fat-modified diet.

CHAPTER 12

Treatment of Obesity: Drugs and Surgery

DRUG THERAPY

The use of drugs in the treatment of obesity is controversial for several reasons. Although several agents have been shown to be effective during the first few weeks of treatment, notably amphetamine and related compounds, the long-term efficacy of any of the drugs has yet to be demonstrated. Patients treated with any of the anti-obesity agents almost always regain the weight that was lost. Furthermore, the amphetamines are notorious for their drug abuse potential and CNS-stimulant properties. The widespread abuse of amphetamines has virtually eliminated their use for obesity in the United States and most physicians now prescribe this drug only for hyperkinesis in children, narcolepsy, or for the rare patient with Kleine-Levin syndrome.

With most of the anti-obesity drugs, tolerance to the anorexic effect soon develops, and the drug becomes no more effective than placebo. Despite these generally negative findings, it is possible that the design of many of the trials obscures possible therapeutic effectiveness of some of the drugs. Most of the studies compare an anorexic drug with a placebo and sometimes the anorexic drug is combined with diet instruction and compared to a placebo. Drugs may be ineffective alone or with diet, but in combination with other treatment approaches, such as behavior modification, may be useful. One recent study[1] has shown that phentermine resin (Ionamin) prescribed at judiciously selected times during the course of psychotherapy can be highly effective. Craddock,[2] a general practitioner in England who has treated obese patients for years, uses certain drugs at highly selective times during the weight loss program.

Drugs could theoretically reduce body fat in several different ways. Food intake may be decreased by affecting several mechanisms which alter appetite; amphetamine is thought to decrease appetite via an effect on the neurotransmitters norepinephrine and dopamine. Intestinal absorption of nutrients may be decreased or delayed; e.g., agents that produce steatorrhea decrease intestinal absorption. Drugs that delay the transit of food out of the stomach; e.g., trans-epoxyaconitic acid,[3] theoretically would result in a decreased food intake. Another possible mode of action is to affect lipid metabolism either by decreasing lipid synthesis or increasing lipid utilization and mobilization. In animals, dihydroepiendosterone, an inhibitor of glucose-6-phosphate dehydrogenase, reduces lipogenesis.[3] Agents that make lipid or carbohydrate metabolism less effective might be useful. Finally, drugs which decrease insulin and increase growth hormone might be useful.

Although amphetamines are in disrepute as anti-obesity agents, they are very important in understanding current research with other anorexic agents. Also, they occupy a pivotal point in much of the current neutrotransmitter research as well as research into the mechanisms modulating hunger and satiety. The four drugs currently considered suitable for use in obesity are diethylpropion (Tenuate), mazindol (Sanorex), fenfluramine (Pondimin), and phentermine resin (Ionamin). The usefulness of each of these drugs in terms of effectiveness and side effects will be described. Finally the use of hormones in the treatment of obesity will be reviewed.

ANOREXIC AGENTS

AMPHETAMINES

Amphetamine was first synthesized by Edeleano in 1887 but it was not until the late 1930's that it was used in the treatment of obesity. Harris and colleagues[4] demonstrated that the weight loss was due to a decrease in food intake. In one part of their investigation, amphetamine was administered to subjects who ate the same amount of food whether or not they took the drug. Under these circumstances, the subjects did not lose weight, demonstrating that the effect of amphetamines is to decrease food intake. The structure of d-amphetamine is shown in Figure 12.1. Another reason that

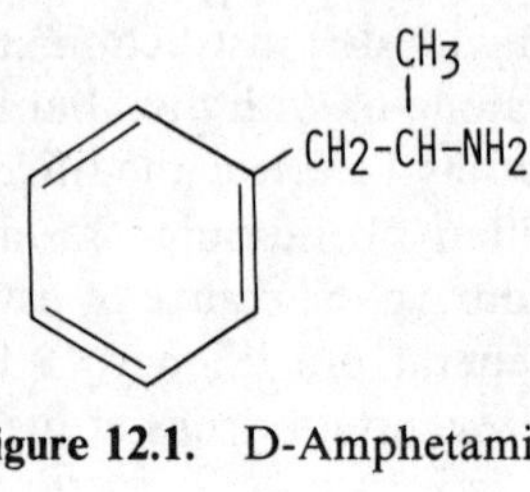

Figure 12.1. D-Amphetamine.

amphetamine is crucial to any discussion of anorexic drugs is that virtually all the agents that have been developed are modifications of the basic structure of a phenyl ring and side chain. However, drugs that are structurally similar do not necessarily have similar effects.

Amphetamines produce both short- and long-term effects.[5] As shown in Figure 12.2, amphetamine acts by enhancing the release of norepinephrine from the axon and by slightly reducing its re-accumulation. Evidence for this conclusion is as follows. The anorexia is inhibited by complete blockade of norepinephrine synthesis. Also the anorexia is enhanced by desmethylimipramine, a drug which blocks the re-uptake of norepinephrine by the nerve ending.

SIDE EFFECTS OF AMPHETAMINE

There are three major categories of side effects of amphetamines. The most important is central nervous system stimulation which results in nervousness, restlessness, high spirits, insomnia, decreased sense of fatigue, euphoria, and irritability. These side effects may result in *drug abuse* in susceptible patients. Jones[6] reported six cases of women who were dependent on amphetamines originally prescribed for obesity, and Craddock[2] reported three obese patients addicted to amphetamines. The potential for addiction with amphetamine and related compounds is the major reason these drugs are rarely recommended for obesity.

Penick[7] has noted that the incidence and importance of these CNS side effects may have been overemphasized. For example, it has been repeatedly noted that weight loss in dieters is frequently associated with depression, and some consider the high spirits and euphoria of the amphetamines to be a therapeutic effect rather than an undesirable side effect. Also, not all studies report a high incidence of stimulant side effects. It may be that patient expectation influences incidence of side effects. In one study,[8] 40 patients received phenmetrazine (Preludin) believed to have the same CNS effect as amphetamines. Another 40 control subjects received a placebo. Only two drug patients and one placebo patient complained of side effects. In a later study in the same clinic with different patients, the subjects were warned about possible side effects and 40% of the drug patients complained of side effects and only one placebo patient had side effects. It is possible that in the first study, the subjects had side effects but did not attribute them to the drug, or it may be that anticipation of an effect increases the likelihood of its occurrence.

Another group of side effects is due to *stimulation* of the *sympathetic nervous system* and includes dry mouth, blurred vision, lightheadedness and dizziness, tachycardia, palpitation, sweating, and elevation of blood pressure. One comprehensive comparative study[9] has shown that amphetamine, meth-

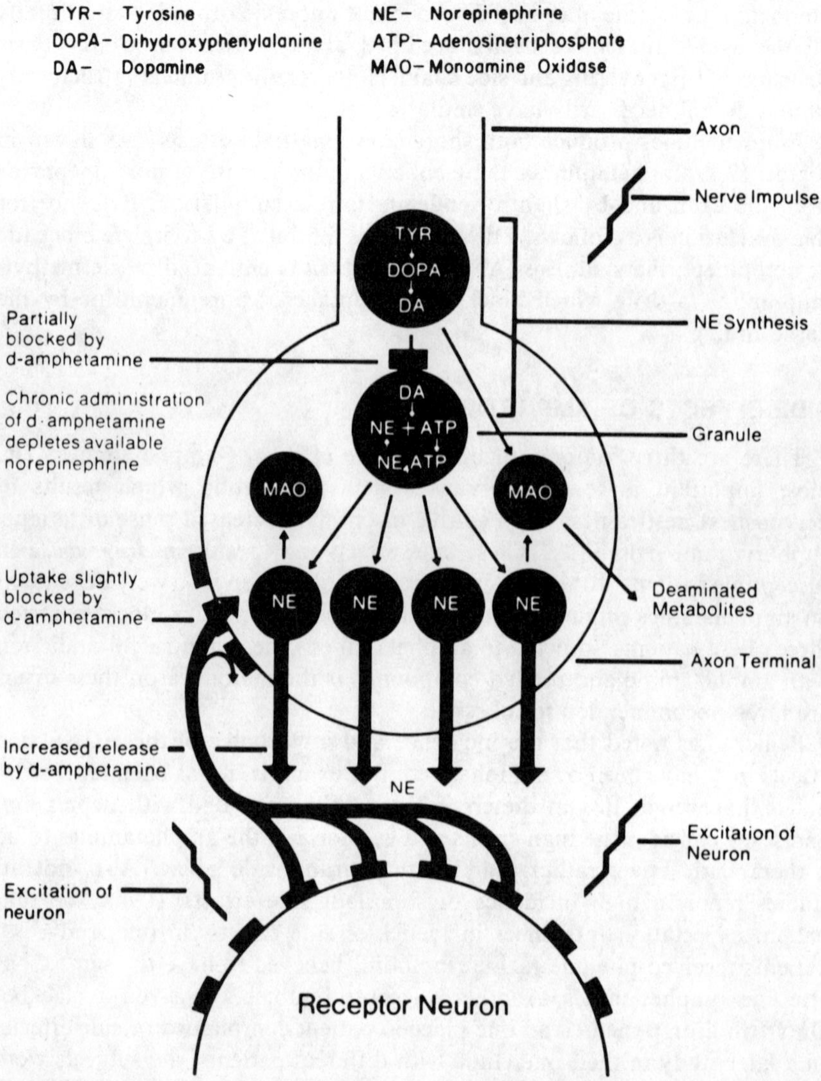

Figure 12.2. Site of action of amphetamine at the synaptic junction. Amphetamine acts by enhancing the release of norepinephrine from the axon and slightly reducing its reaccumulation. (Reprinted with permission from Sandoz Manual on Sanorex, 1974.)

amphetamine, ephedrine, phenmetrazine, and methylphenidate all produce a dose-related increase in blood pressure. Both systolic and diastolic blood pressure were increased as well as respiratory rate. All produced initial tachycardia, yet there was a relative bradycardia with amphetamine as blood pressure increased. This bradycardia may have been of reflex origin. Therefore, the use of amphetamine in hypertensive patients or those with cardiovascular disease must be cautious.

There are several psychiatric side effects. As noted earlier, there is a potential for drug addiction. However, a *toxic psychosis* can also occur on amphetamines, although the dose required to produce this effect is generally greater than that used for obesity. This psychosis closely mimics acute paranoid schizophrenia and has been used by Snyder[10] as a model of schizophrenia. The patient is frightened, suspicious, deluded, and may have auditory hallucinations. The following case illustrates the point:

> Carmen is a 16-year-old girl who took several tablets containing amphetamine and injected "speed" (IV amphetamine) at the behest of a group of friends. She was brought to the hospital a few hours later because she was found searching diligently through the leaves in the front lawn, was restless, and unable to sit quietly, and complained that there were bugs crawling on her arms. During the examination she was suspicious, believed the hospital attendants were in league to harm her, and said she could hear people saying she was a bad person for using drugs. She was severely agitated initially, but over the next 48 hours she recovered completely.

Another psychiatric complication of amphetamine use is seen most often in drug abusers. When amphetamine is stopped, a *serious depression* associated with suicidal ideation may follow. The cause of the depression is often not recognized by the physician since the patient may not admit to an overuse of amphetamine. The usual anti-depressant medication will often alleviate the depressive symptoms. In the following case, the cause of depression was not recognized during several hospitalizations and suicide attempts:

> Paula is a 23-year-old divorced woman who was initially started on amphetamines at age 18 to assist in losing weight. By that age she had seen several psychiatrists for depression and had been hospitalized three times, once following a suicide attempt. Initially she took the amphetamines as prescribed and lost weight and had a marked improvement in mood. Gradually she increased the dose and finally began buying street drugs and injecting IV amphetamines. For more than a year she was a prostitute and used some of the funds to buy drugs. When she was unable to use amphetamines, she became depressed and needed hospitalization. At the time she presented to our clinic, she admitted to drug use and complained of severe depression and constant visual misperceptions. Complete evaluation revealed a continuous temporal lobe spike. She was started on Dilantin and the misperceptions ceased and the EEG became normal, but she was still very depressed. Anti-depressants resulted in a marked improvement of mood and she has not used amphetamines for more than a year.

In this patient, a careful history of previous psychiatric problems might have prevented her subsequent amphetamine addiction. It may be that amphetamines have a place in the treatment of obesity, but at this time reports of deleterious side effects are so widespread that they cannot be recommended.

ANOREXIC DRUGS IN CURRENT USE

The four anorexic drugs that are used in weight reduction programs are: diethylpropion, mazindol, fenfluramine, and phentermine. Craddock[2] has suggested the following guidelines for the use of any anorexic drugs. In patients who have been initially well motivated to diet and have lost weight, drugs may be given to boost flagging motivation. In these patients the drug is used as a temporary expedient, usually for 3 to 6 months, as part of an individualized holistic treatment program. It may also be appropriate to use drugs in patients who have initial difficulty in adhering to a diet, assuming that there is a strong, positive doctor-patient relationship. A third indication is in patients who have successfully lost down to their normal weight but begin to relapse. A fourth indication has been cited by Roberts.[1] In patients in intensive insight psychotherapy, obesity itself was a hindrance to therapy and treatment with drugs resulted not only in weight loss but rapid progress in psychotherapy.

DIETHYLPROPION (TENUATE)

Diethylpropion has fewer CNS stimulant effects than amphetamine, yet is nearly as effective in reducing food intake. The basic chemical structure of amphetamine is modified by addition of a keto group onto the beta carbon and substitution on the N-terminal to result in diethylpropion (Fig. 12.3).

Several reports have established that it is an effective anorexic. Cunningham[11] studied 16 patients who lost 13 pounds in 12 weeks on the drug, and during a control period on placebo, 13 patients gained weight. McKay[12] and Craddock[2] contend that tolerance does not develop to the anorexic effect and it may continue to be useful for several months. Intermittent use of this drug may be the preferred method of use.

The addition of the keto group to the beta carbon decreases the incidence of CNS stimulant symptoms and 1% felt drowsy and 4% felt more relaxed.[13] Silverstone and Cleary[14] showed that this drug did not affect the quality of sleep. The addiction potential appears to be low although there are isolated reports of abuse in an occasional patient addicted to other drugs. Craddock[2] notes that although about 20 million patients have used this drug there has been only one death due to an accidental overdose in a child.

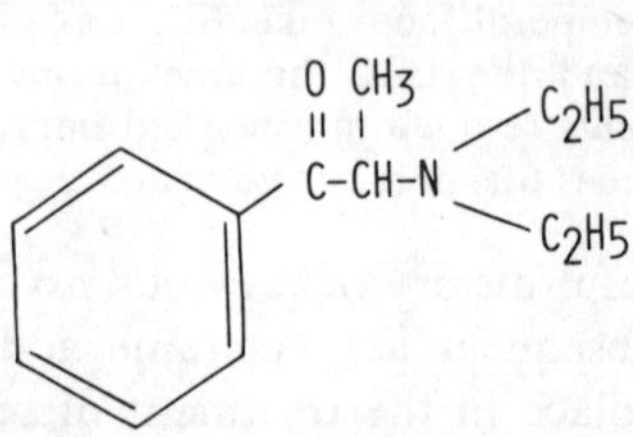

Figure 12.3. Diethylpropion (Tenuate).

The plasma half-life of diethylpropion is about 2 to 3 hours and the sustained action tablets are effective for 8 to 12 hours. The usual dose is 25 mg, three times a day not later than 6 p.m. or one sustained tablet (75 mg) before noon.

MAZINDOL (SANOREX)

Mazindol (Sanorex) is a tricyclic compound which probably inhibits the re-uptake of norepinephrine and thus prolongs its action. Its structure is shown in Figure 12.4.

Weight loss with this drug is greater than with placebo but similar to loss using the other anorexic drugs. There is a suggestion that the cardiovascular side effects are less with this drug than with diethylpropion but this has not been established with certainty. Although this drug does not belong to the same pharmacological group as amphetamine, it has CNS-stimulant properties including insomnia, euphoria, and restlessness. Dry mouth is a common side effect. Evans and Wallace[15] report that side effects caused 11.3% of the subjects to drop out in a large general practice trial and an additional 18.5% were lost to follow-up. Despite the CNS-stimulant side effects of this drug, cases of addiction have not yet been reported.

The plasma half-life of mazindol is 33 to 55 hours and the usual dose is one or two 2-mg tablets before noon. Intermittent dosage has been recommended for this drug.

FENFLURAMINE (PONDIMIN)

Fenfluramine has recently been evaluated in a number of trials. It is chemically related to amphetamine but has an ethyl group on the N-terminal

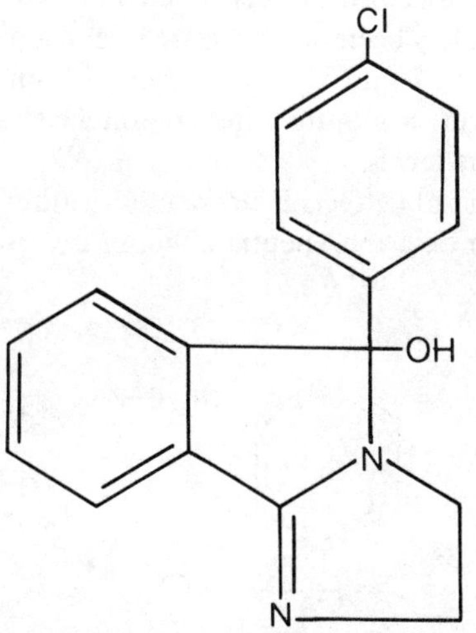

Figure 12.4. Mazindol (Sanorex).

and CF_3 has been introduced on the phenyl ring (See Fig. 12.5). Both these changes reduce the CNS-stimulant effects but do not interfere with the anorexic properties of the drug. Fenfluramine has been shown to reduce the brain concentration of serotonin and its metabolite, 5-hydroxy-indolacetic acid (5-HIAA) but has virtually no effect on norepinephrine or dopamine.[16] Since amphetamines affect primarily norepinephrine, with some influence on dopamine, the two anorexic drugs must differ strikingly in their central effect on appetite. Fenfluramine also appears to have a specific effect on carbohydrate metabolism. There is an increased muscle uptake of glucose with fenfluramine.[17]

There have been several trials of the effectiveness of fenfluramine. Hudson[18] used it in 176 patients for a year and noted an average weight loss of 23 pounds. However, 1 year later an average of 20 pounds had been regained. Stunkard and colleagues[19] compared the effectiveness and side effects of fenfluramine and amphetamine in 90 obese females. The drugs resulted in similar weight losses of approximately 1 pound per week over 7 weeks. The dropout rates were lower in the drug groups than with placebo. These investigators also found a higher frequency of side effects in the fenfluramine group than in either the amphetamine or placebo groups. Furthermore, half the fenfluramine dropouts left the group because of the side effects. It has been reported that tolerance to the anorexic effects of fenfluramine does not develop as rapidly as with amphetamine,[20] but this contention has not been confirmed. Court[21] has evaluated the effectiveness of fenfluramine in children ages 3 to 15 years and found that there was a significant weight loss or diminished weight gain in 14 of 19 children studied.

Although initially fenfluramine may be helpful to a tense hypertensive because of its pronounced side effect of sedation, no long-term improvement in the hypertension has been demonstrated. Hudson[18] found a sustained fall in blood pressure of 37 mm Hg systolic and 18 mm Hg diastolic over a 1-year period; however, 6 months after treatment stopped, the readings had returned to previous levels.

One of the major side effects is drowsiness, rather than CNS stimulation. Sometimes this can be a therapeutic effect in a very agitated obese patient.

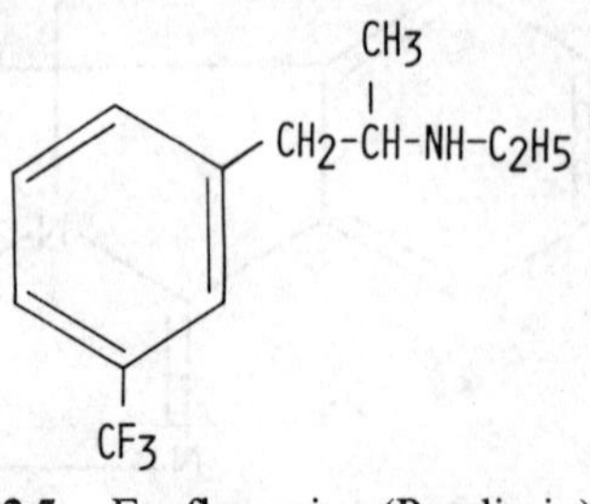

Figure 12.5. Fenfluramine (Pondimin).

Gastrointestinal symptoms, including diarrhea, vomiting, and abdominal pain appear to be more frequent with this drug than with amphetamine.[19]

One important difference between fenfluramine and the other anorexic drugs is that severe depression may follow approximately 4 days after the medication is stopped, even in people without a previous history of depression.[2] This is less likely to occur if the patient is taken off the drug gradually. Because of this post-drug use depression, intermittent therapy is unwise and it is therefore difficult to prevent the development of tolerance to the anorexic effect.

Insomnia has also been reported and five of 20 patients on normal dosage had frightening dreams.[22] Chronic administration results in a reduction in REM sleep with an abrupt rebound about 4 days after discontinuance of the drug. Depression may also occur while on this drug and depressed patients may become even more depressed. Thus, fenfluramine should never be given to depressed patients.

Although the addiction potential of fenfluramine is generally thought to be low, Levin[23] reported that 25% of 448 drug-dependent young men gave a history of fenfluramine abuse.

The plasma half-life is 13 to 30 hours and the effect of the drug is maximal after 6 to 10 hours. The usual dose is a 20-mg tablet twice daily. A sustained release 60-mg capsule is also available and can be taken once a day.

PHENTERMINE RESIN (IONAMIN)

Phentermine resin is the fourth common anorexic drug currently used in the treatment of obesity. Methyl groups have been substituted on the alpha carbon; its structure is shown in Figure 12.6.

The effectiveness of this drug is similar to that of amphetamine,[24] and it is as effective used intermittently as continuously.[25] Steel and colleagues[26] compared continuous administration of fenfluramine and phentermine resin and found them equally efficacious. However, when the drugs were given intermittently there was a much higher dropout rate in the fenfluramine group because cessation of this drug is associated with depression.

The stimulant side effects of phentermine are less because of the methyl substitution at the alpha carbon. However, 20% of patients in one clinical

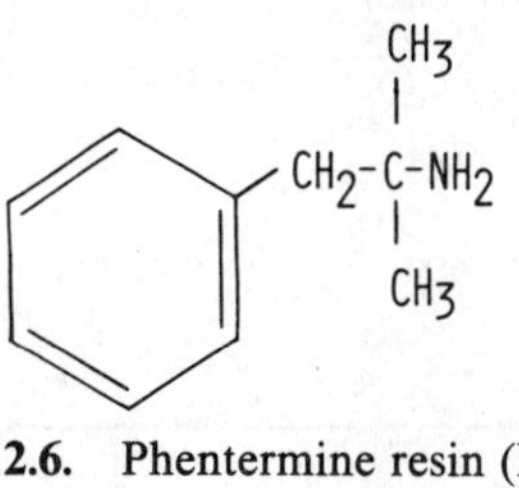

Figure 12.6. Phentermine resin (Ionamin).

trial had insomnia.[26] Dry mouth also occurs. Tachycardia and elevation of blood pressure are frequent.

The dosage is one 15- or 30-mg tablet before breakfast.

CHOICE OF ANOREXIC AGENT

In summary, the most efficacious anorexic drug with the fewest stimulant side effects is diethylpropion and it is probably a wise first choice in patients selected for drug treatment. Mazindol may have fewer hypertensive side effects but it has some stimulant side effects. It is as efficacious as the other drugs and may be the best choice for a hypertensive obese patient. Fenfluramine may be somewhat less effective in producing weight loss than diethylpropion. In a study[27] of 22 patients, there was an average weight loss of 8 pounds on diethylpropion, but only 5 pounds on fenfluramine. Craddock[2] also noted much greater weight loss on diethylpropion. The major disadvantage of fenfluramine is its tendency to worsen depression when the patient takes the drug and to cause depression when the drug is stopped abruptly. Phentermine resin is probably as effective as the other drugs but often causes insomnia. Table 12.1 lists these drugs and their indication.

These drugs are similar to the amphetamines in that weight loss decreases after a few weeks, although fenfluramine may be an exception. Intermittent dosage has been proposed as a means of prolonging effectiveness but is clearly contraindicated with fenfluramine because of the depression which follows cessation of the drug.

Table 12.1
Anorexic drugs currently used for treatment.

DRUG	INDICATIONS	CONTRAINDICATIONS	SIDE EFFECTS	INTERMITTENT USAGE
D - AMPHETAMINE (DEXEDRINE)	HYPERKINETIC REACTION OF CHILDHOOD KLEINE-LEVIN SYNDROME, NARCOLEPSY	OBESITY ESPECIALLY IF HISTORY OF PSYCHIATRIC PROBLEMS	• CNS STIMULATION • SYMPATHETIC NERVOUS SYSTEM STIMULATION	NO
DIETHYLPROPION (TENUATE)	ADJUNCT IN OBESITY TREATMENT		• OCCASIONAL CNS STIMULATION OR DROWSINESS	YES
MAZINDOL (SANOREX)	ADJUNCT IN TREATMENT OF OBESE PATIENTS WITH HYPERTENSION		• CNS STIMULATION • DRY MOUTH	YES
FENFLURAMINE (PONDIMIN)	ADJUNCT IN OBESITY TREATMENT	DEPRESSED PATIENTS	• DROWSINESS • GASTROINTESTINAL SYMPTOMS • INSOMNIA • ↓ REM SLEEP	NO
PHENTERMINE RESIN (IONAMIN)	ADJUNCT IN OBESITY TREATMENT	? HYPERTENSION	• INSOMNIA • DRY MOUTH • TACHYCARDIA • HYPERTENSION	YES

DRUGS THAT REDUCE INTESTINAL ABSORPTION

Cholestyramine and neomycin are two drugs that decrease fat absorption and produce steatorrhea. *Cholestyramine* is an ion-exchange resin which binds bile acids and results in increased excretion of fat. Bray[28] studied two grossly obese hospitalized patients on 1200-calorie diets with 80% of the calories from fat. These patients were given 36 g of cholestyramine daily for 9 days, but although there was a significant increase in fat excretion it was relatively low. Another study[29] of six patients demonstrated that this drug can produce a threefold increase in fat excretion on 30 g of cholestyramine daily. In an outpatient study,[30] use of this agent was not effective, probably because such large quantities of the unpleasant tasting resin must be taken even for mild effects.

Neomycin in doses of 6 to 12 g consistently produces steatorrhea.[31] However, the doses needed to produce this effect also cause morphological changes in the gastrointestinal tract which might be irreversible with long-term administration.

HORMONES IN THE TREATMENT OF OBESITY

Several hormones have been evaluated for the treatment of obesity; these include human chorionic gonadotropin, thyroid hormone, growth hormone, and progesterone. Although none is currently recommended for use in treatment, studies of both thyroid hormone and growth hormone may provide valuable data about the metabolism of adipose tissue.

HUMAN CHORIONIC GONADOTROPIN (HCG)

Simeons[32] first noticed that patients with Frohlich syndrome who were treated with human chorionic gonadotropin (HCG) had a loss of their ravenous appetite and also a change in body configuration. Extrapolating from this finding he treated obese patients with daily injections of HCG plus a 500-calorie diet and reported weight losses of 20 to 30 pounds in 40 days. He postulated that there was abnormal and normal fat and that chorionic gonadotropin was necessary to convert the abnormal fat to normal fat. His findings resulted in considerable interest, but thus far no well-controlled double-blind study has replicated his findings.[33] In one study,[34] control subjects received saline injections and 10 received human chorionic gonadotropin (HCG). In another part of this study, one group of patients received saline injections and one group received no injections. Patients receiving any injection lost more weight than those who received no injection, but HCG was no more effective than saline. The one positive part of this regimen is that there is apparently no deleterious side effect of the injections of HCG.

THYROID HORMONES

The literature on obesity is replete with reports on thyroid hormones. Not only has hypothyroidism been believed responsible for obesity, but thyroid hormones have been used to treat obesity even where no deficit has been demonstrated. However, there are several reasons why the use of thyroid hormones is usually inappropriate.[35]

First, thyroid function is usually normal in obese patients (See Chapter 4). Initial early reports of low basal metabolic rates in obese subjects were interpreted to indicate hypothyroidism, but since the normal values of BMR were determined in normal weight individuals, these findings do not necessarily indicate hypothyroidism. Later, more sophisticated evaluations of thyroid function in obese subjects have sometimes indicated an abnormality, but results have been inconsistent. The biological half-life of thyroid hormones may be abnormal in some obese patients[35] but the significance of this finding is not known. One study showed a decreased rate of thyroxine removal,[36] yet another study[37] showed a more rapid metabolic degregation of thyroxine. Bray[38] found that the activity of both soluble and mitochondrial alpha-glycerophosphate dehydrogenase decrease in adipose tissue with caloric restriction. Administration of T_3 prevented the decrease in this enzyme. Conceivably, this finding could have implications for the treatment of obesity.

A major limitation in the use of thyroid hormones in obesity is that although weight loss may occur with the drug, there is a rapid reaccumulation when thyroid hormone is stopped. Although Hollingsworth et al.[39] found an early increase in weight loss in hospitalized subjects on an 800-calorie diet and thyroid hormone, this effect decreased after the first few weeks and weight was quickly regained when patients were discharged from the hospital.

Another disadvantage of treatment with thyroid hormones is that weight lost is lean body mass rather than adipose tissue. This has been demonstrated in a number of studies. In a study of two obese patients treated with thyroid, Kyle and colleagues[40] measured body density and concluded that most of the weight lost represented lean body tissue. In another study[41], nearly 80% of the weight lost was lean body tissue and only 20% was due to a decrease in adipose tissue. Significant amounts of calcium are also lost with thyroid treatment. In a group of normal adults, urinary excretion of calcium was doubled soon after initiation of treatment with tri-iodothyronine.[42] If this finding is applicable to children, thyroid hormone would be contraindicated since calcium needs during growth are critical.

Another problem in the use of thyroid hormones is their side effects and consequent hazards. Gwinup and Poucher[43] put alternate obese patients on thyroid hormone without dietary restriction and noted a 25 to 30 pound mean weight loss. However, the patients developed elevations in blood pressure, tachycardia, restlessness, and sweating. They concluded that ... "the use of therapeutic doses of thyroid analogues ... merely substitutes one clinical entity for another (thyrotoxicosis for obesity)." In this study, weight returned to pre-treatment levels shortly after the drug was stopped. Several reports have shown a high incidence of cardiovascular side effects. In one report,[44] angina was noted in 20% of the patients. ST segment and T wave changes have also been shown, although there were very few subjects in this study and they were also on a starvation diet.[45]

In summary, there is currently little place in the treatment of obesity for thyroid hormones. They do not result in a weight loss that is maintained, and when weight is lost it is lean body tissue rather than fat and there are potentially very serious cardiovascular and other side effects.

GROWTH HORMONE

Growth hormone may prove to be effective in the treatment of obesity because it mobilizes fatty acids depleting adipose tissue stores, is calorigenic, and its lipolytic effects are produced without causing loss of nitrogen. Also it has been shown that growth hormone levels are low in obese subjects. This finding is probably secondary to obesity rather than etiological but nonetheless it merits consideration.

Novak and colleagues[46] studied four male hypopituitary dwarfs before and after growth hormone administration. There was a rapid cellular growth and increase in height and weight, but no increase in body fat during the first 12 months of treatment. Studies of growth hormone in experimental animals[47] have shown that growth hormone increases metabolic rate (i.e., has a calorigenic effect) even after thyroidectomy.

Bray and colleagues[48] have taken advantage of the fact that nitrogen loss occurs with thyroid and nitrogen retention occurs with growth hormone. They initially administered tri-iodothyronine and noted an increase in oxygen consumption and a rise in nitrogen excretion. When growth hormone was added to the regimen, oxygen consumption increased even more, but nitrogen excretion returned to normal. Thus, the calorigenic effect of both thyroid hormone and growth hormone can be exploited without nitrogen losses.

The relevance of these findings to the treatment of obesity in the general population is not known. One current problem with growth hormone is that even if it proves to be efficacious, supplies of growth hormone are extremely limited and growth hormone from other animals is ineffective.

SUMMARY OF DRUG USAGE

In summary, the use of drugs in a well-designed comprehensive treatment plan may have some value. Although amphetamines are currently in disfavor, they remain the standard against which other anorexic drugs are compared. Diethylpropion, mazindol, fenfluramine, and phentermine resin are drugs that might be considered. Other drug approaches have not yet been demonstrated to be effective but offer future promise. Hormone treatment is both ineffective and dangerous.

JEJUNOILEAL BYPASS SURGERY

In the last several years, several surgical bypass procedures have been devised. In 1954 Kremen and colleagues[49] performed a jejunoileostomy on an obese patient who subsequently lost a significant amount of weight. In 1963 Payne, DeWind, and Commons reported 11 patients with anastomosis of the jejunum to the transverse colon.[50] Massive electrolyte loss due to diarrhea prompted a new procedure in which the distal cut-end of the jejunum was attached to the side of the terminal ileum.[51] Later, Scott and colleagues[52] modified this technique with an end-to-end anastomosis of the terminal jejunum to the terminal cecum.

PROCEDURE

Both the Payne procedure and the Scott revision have been widely used for large groups of patients. The end-to-side procedure is technically easier because there is only one anastomosis, between the jejunum and ileum. The side-to-side procedure requires two anastomoses, one to re-establish the continuity of the gastrointestinal (GI) tract by connecting the jejunum with the terminal ileum and one to anastomose the severed ilial end to the colon. Figure 12.7 illustrates the two procedures. Although the end-to-side procedure is technically easier, weight loss may be less: there may be some retrograde reflux of intestinal contents into the bypassed segment, and absorption may occur, resulting in a diminished weight loss. With the end-to-end anastomosis, secretions from the non-functional bowel enter the colon and reflux is less likely. Therefore, a greater weight loss with less likelihood of regaining weight occurs with the end-to-end procedure.

The remaining length of the terminal ileum is the primary determinant of subsequent weight loss. The longer the remaining functional GI tract the less weight loss. With 35 inches left there is virtually no weight loss and at 25 inches weight loss is slow.[53] The optimal combination of weight loss with few nutritional or metabolic consequences occurs when 14 inches of jejunum are anastomosed to the terminal 4 inches of ileum.[54] With shorter lengths of remaining ileum there are more nutritional problems.

INDICATIONS

Appropriate selection of patients for bypass surgery is crucial and is generally well-agreed upon among various investigators.[55, 56] The patient

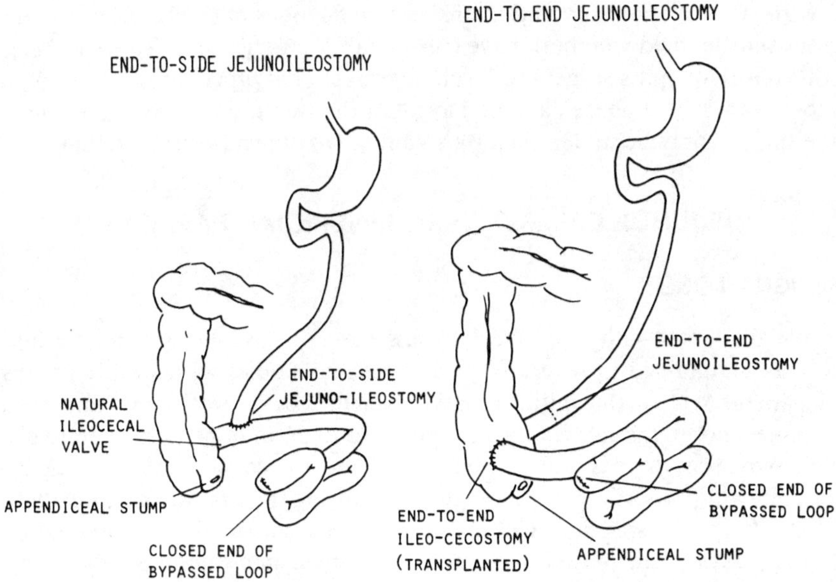

Figure 12.7. Jejunoilial bypass surgery: end-to-side and end-to-end procedures. (Reprinted with permission from R. T. Soper et al: J Pediatr Surg 10: 51–58, 1975.)

must be morbidly obese, by which is meant at least 100 pounds above ideal weight, according to usual height-weight tables, assuming a medium frame. In fact, most patients who come for bypass surgery are at least 100% greater than ideal weight. The patient must have been obese for at least 5 years. Most investigations have been with adults, but there are some recent reports of use of bypass surgery (either jejunoileal or gastric) on grossly obese adolescents. Generally patients over 50 years of age are not considered for the surgery, although gastric bypass has been performed on older patients. There must be evidence that other forms of treatment of obesity have failed. The patient must be relatively free of psychiatric disorders and have a stable life pattern. He should have evidence of one or more of the sequelae of obesity, including hypertension, Pickwickian syndrome, diabetes mellitus, or congestive heart failure. However, the patient should be free of renal failure, serious myocardial disease, inflammatory bowel disease, pulmonary emboli, cirrhosis of the liver, or active hepatitis. The patient must be highly motivated after having all the risks and all the complications of the procedure explained and must have the full support of his immediate family. Patients are encouraged to discuss the operation, its benefits and hazards, with patients who have had the procedure and may be given the address of the Intestinal Bypass Society (P.O. Box 6913, St. Louis, MO 63123). Also, the patient must agree to undergo revision if needed and must avoid pregnancy for 12 months.

In addition there must be an experienced team available, including a surgeon, internist, and psychiatrist, willing to follow the patient closely for

5 years. Good laboratory and intensive care facilities must also be available. Bray and Benfield who both have considerable experience as team members still consider bypass surgery to be an investigational procedure, even though more than 20,000 obese patients have had this surgery.[57] They recommend the surgery only be undertaken by a committed clinical research team.

JEJUNOILEAL BYPASS: BENEFICIAL EFFECTS

WEIGHT LOSS

Weight losses with jejunoileal bypass surgery have been dramatic and usually maintained in several well-documented studies with sizable groups of patients.[58, 59] In the initial months, weight loss is precipitous and then becomes more gradual, with a plateau at 12 to 36 months post-operatively. Following this, there is often a modest gain and an occasional patient regains a significant proportion of the weight lost. During the first weeks until about 3 months, malabsorption and malnutrition are maximal until adaptation begins. During this period, the functioning small intestine undergoes some elongation and marked hypertrophy of the villi. The jejunum elongates more than the ileum, but hypertrophy is similar in both. The weight plateau occurs when hypertrophy is complete. Figure 12.8 illustrates these major stages. Payne and colleagues[58] reported that the average rate of weight loss during the first 6 months was 11 pounds per month, and 6.1 pounds per month during the following 6 months.

An occasional patient (1%) will continue to lose below ideal weight and re-anastomosis may be required. Also, some patients do not have a satisfactory weight loss and the bypass has sometimes been reconstructed to further shorten the absorptive segment. Danowski and colleagues[60] report that 12 of their 125 patients required a second shortening procedure because of insufficient weight loss. One of their patients had gained weight from her operative weight of 204 pounds to 210 pounds at the time of the second procedure. Patients who do have a significant weight loss usually do not get down to their ideal weight. In a study of 200 patients, O'Leary and colleagues[61] found that on the average a patient can expect to lose one third of his weight. Thus, a 450-pound patient could anticipate stabilization at approximately 300 pounds. Danowski and colleagues[60] found that their patients stabilized about 34% above their ideal weight. However, these are average figures and individual patient weight loss varies greatly.

It is difficult to predict which patient will lose the greatest percentage of excess weight but, in general, the greater the pre-operative obesity, the greater the weight loss. Not only do these patients lose the greatest absolute amount of weight, but they actually lose a greater percentage of excess weight.[62] Also, a statistical correlation has been found between age and

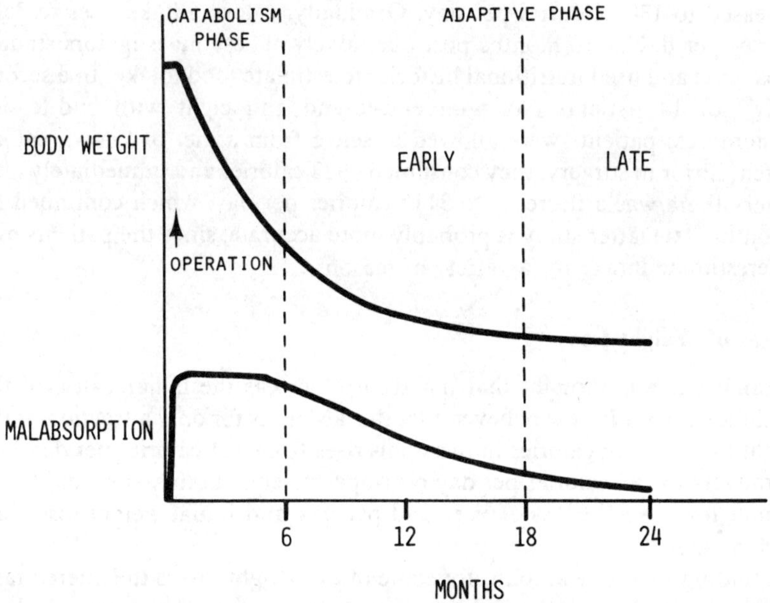

Figure 12.8. Stages of weight loss following jejunoilial bypass surgery. Malabsorption and malnutrition are maximal initially and gradually subside as the intestine adapts. When this happens weight loss slows and a new steady weight occurs. (Reprinted with permission from G. A. Bray: The Obese Patient. Philadelphia, W. B. Saunders Co., 1976, p 427.)

weight loss: younger patients lose more weight. The other factors correlated with weight loss are length of remaining functional gastrointestinal tract and time after surgery. In any given patient, however, it is impossible to predict weight loss accurately.

The cause of the weight loss is probably a combination of malabsorption, decreased food intake, and altered taste preferences. The patients have been reported to eat less food at each meal, snack less, eat fewer meals, have fewer binges, have a reduced craving for sweets, have less difficulty stopping eating, and have an increased frequency of breakfast consumption. Furthermore, patients become less susceptible to eating during times of emotional stress. In other words, the eating pattern of these patients became similar to those of non-obese subjects.[62] Bray and colleagues[63] found that after bypass surgery, patients ate significantly less liquid formula and ate it at a slower rate than before surgery. It has been suggested that these changes in eating patterns are all voluntary attempts on the part of the patient to avoid diarrhea, which is worse after dietary indiscretion. However, most patients said that these changes were achieved without much effort.

One study[64] estimated that caloric intake prior to surgery was approximately 6300 calories per day and during the first 6 months after surgery decreased to 1300 calories per day. Gradually, caloric intake rises to 3500 calories per day at 18 months post-operatively. These investigators studied 30 patients and used nutritional histories to estimate food intake. In a second study[64] of 14 patients (six with end-to-end and eight with end-to-side anastomoses) patients were allowed to select from a diet of known caloric content. Prior to surgery, they consumed 4922 calories and immediately after surgery there was a decrease to 3115 calories per day, which continued for 6 months. The latter study is probably more accurate, since the patients may underestimate intake for a variety of reasons.

Causes of Weight Loss

Initially, it was thought that malabsorption was the major cause of the weight loss, but it is now believed that this accounts for only a fraction of the weight loss. Loss of calories in the stools rises from 131 calories per day pre-operatively to 593 calories per day post-operatively, but this loss would only account for a weight loss of ⅛ pound per day and initial weight losses are much greater.[64]

A finding that may account for some of the weight loss is the altered taste preferences of these patients. In contrast to normal weight persons, at least some obese subjects prefer very sweet solutions, even after a meal. Prior to surgery, these very obese patients have similar abnormal preferences for sweet tastes, but post-operatively the subjective preference for a 40% sucrose solution declines significantly.[65] There is no change in the judged pleasantness of salty solutions, citric acid solutions, or quinine solutions after surgery.

DECREASE IN RISK FACTORS

Another benefit of bypass surgery is the decrease in risk factors that predispose very obese subjects to increased morbidity and mortality. In nearly all patients studied, there is a decrease in blood pressure, a decrease in blood glucose and insulin requirements, and a decrease in cholesterol and lipid levels; e.g., in a study by O'Leary and colleagues,[61] 46% of 200 patients had diastolic pressures greater than 90 mm Hg pre-operatively, and approximately one-third of these patients had lower pressures post-operatively. Pre-operatively, 70% of these patients were diabetic, using the oral glucose tolerance test and of those who had the IV glucose test, 90% were diabetic. One year after surgery, 13 of 119 patients tested were diabetic. Furthermore, all 12 patients who took insulin before the operation were no longer receiving hypoglycemic medication 1 year post-operatively. Other investigators[66, 67] have reported increased levels of circulating insulin in very obese subjects associated with an increase in insulin resistance. After surgery, serum insulin falls and insulin sensitivity increases. It is estimated that approximately 50% of patients have elevated lipid levels prior to surgery. Scott and associates[68] report a 50% decrease in cholesterol level after bypass and an 82% drop in triglyceride levels.

IMPROVED PSYCHOSOCIAL FUNCTIONING

A third group of benefits relates to improved psychosocial functioning. Several studies suggest that after weight loss there is generally an improvement in self-esteem, a decrease in psychiatric symptoms, an improved body image, and economic rehabilitation. Some patients do not have an improvement in mental state, but this is apparently much less common and can sometimes be predicted from a previous history of serious psychopathology.

Solow and colleagues[69] studied 29 patients and reported improved functioning in all areas of psychosocial functioning and contended that none of these patients developed substitute psychiatric symptoms following weight loss. Weiss,[70] on the other hand, reported the frequent occurrence of depression in 17 patients and Winkleman and colleagues[71] reported that six of 26 patients required psychiatric treatment following bypass surgery. In a study of 34 patients, Abram and colleagues[72] found that 76% were satisfied with the operation and were more self-confident after their bypass. However, 24% of these patients developed psychiatric problems, including an increase in neurotic symptoms and personal problems, or a psychosis. Statistically, male patients and those who lost the most weight were most vulnerable to psychiatric complications. Another group of investigators[73] found that 50% of the patients had significant post-operative psychological morbidity (judged by the need for post-operative psychiatric care or anti-depressants or patients' statements of being less happy now than prior to surgery). Of these patients, 20% had psychiatric therapy prior to surgery. These authors[73] note that most patients (72%) in their series of 21 patients had expected to lose more weight than they lost, and they were dismayed when they found they had to follow a reducing diet to reach their ideal weight. In summary, most studies show an improvement in self-confidence in a majority of patients, but the likelihood of deleterious psychiatric sequelae is significant. Patients with a prior history of psychiatric symptoms or treatment are at greatest risk.

There are alterations in body image after surgery. Most of the patients who come to bypass surgery have been obese during adolescence and probably half of the patients with adolescent obesity have body image disturbances. Either the attitudinal or perceptual aspect of body image may be disturbed (See Chapter 8). Kalucy and colleagues[74] reported that in 12 patients studied 2 years after bypass surgery, there was an improvement in the attitudinal aspect of body image in that they no longer felt ugly and disgusting, but the patients continued to behave as if they were still large.

However, in a careful recent study of 10 subjects, another group of researchers[75] found no improvement in the attitudinal aspect of body image.

The subjects were given the Draw-A-Person test and asked to draw a sketch of the "average" person and then a "self-sketch." The test was used to assess the perceptual aspect of body image and was administered prior to surgery, and 1 week, 3 months, and 1 year after surgery. A sentence completion test was used to evaluate the affective component of body image and included:

"Mirrors . . .

"When I am naked . . .

"When I am sad . . .

This study found no improvement in the attitudinal aspect of body image, but patients' estimates of their actual size and shape were reasonably accurate even before surgery, and gradually changed during the year following surgery, paralleling their actual loss of weight. This study is interesting, but the fact that none of their subjects demonstrated an abnormality in the perceptual aspect of body image prior to surgery is unusual.

SIDE EFFECTS AND COMPLICATIONS

The complications and side effects of jejunoileal bypass surgery are numerous and range from the trivial to life-threatening. The operative mortality rate has ranged from 0–6% and in more than 2500 reported cases has averaged just over 4%.[64] The very serious complications have included pulmonary embolization, serious wound infection, and renal failure. Other major complications include liver failure, urinary calculi, pseudo-obstructive megacolon, and polyarthritis. Other less serious complications include alopecia, diarrhea, and vitamin deficiencies.

Hepatic change is the most serious non-operative complication. From 60–98% of patients are reported to have fatty infiltration of the liver prior to surgery. After bypass, the hepatic triglyceride concentrations increase approximately 300%, although the architecture of the liver is maintained. As weight plateaus, there is a decrease in fatty infiltration. In 5% of the patients fatty liver progresses to fibrosis, and in 1%, fibrosis progresses to cirrhosis and death.[76] The etiology of the liver disease is not known, but may be secondary to malabsorption, or possibly due to release of a hepatotoxin from the bypassed segment of the small intestine. Patients who develop liver failure usually do so within the first 6 months after surgery. A sequence of liver changes has been described[77]: BSP dye retention occurs early, and then hypokalemia and hypoalbuminia occur. There is an associated rise in SGOT, SGPT, and alkaline phosphatase. Then hyperbilirubinemia may occur. This sequence has been observed in many patients who do not progress to liver failure. Later, there may be fluid retention with weight gain, peripheral edema, and ascites. It is important that jaundice does not occur until late in the course when intervention may be unsuccessful. Bray[78] recommends that patients be screened with monthly SGOT and SGPT determinations. If these enzymes remain elevated or rise, or albumin falls, or bilirubin rises, the patient should have hepatic scans and be considered for liver biopsy. Treatment of progressive liver failure is re-anastomosis. Two of the 125 patients studied by Danowski[60] who had restoration of their GI tract had cirrhosis of the liver. O'Leary and colleagues[61] report that four of their 200 patients required re-anastomosis to reverse progressive liver failure. The patients who are most susceptible to progressive liver failure are those who lose more than 10 to 15 pounds per month and who are the most obese pre-operatively. Statistically, male patients are at greatest risk.

A second major complication is *urinary calculi* which has been reported to occur in 1–30% of patients following bypass surgery. Payne's group[58] found that 12 of 156 patients developed renal calculi, and 30 of 125 patients studied by Danowski and colleagues[60] developed calculi. Several patients who developed calculi have had exhaustive metabolic studies. O'Leary's group[61] found that four of seven subjects had stones composed of calcium oxalate. Oxalate secretion was elevated, and urinary calcium, citrate, and magnesium secretion were lower than normal.

In 30 patients studied by Danowski's group[60] all had negative pre-operative pylography. There were 54 episodes of renal calculi in these 30 patients and 19 of the episodes were associated with renal colic. Twenty-seven calculi were passed spontaneously; 10 were removed by cystoscopy; seven required nephrostomy; and nine were left undisturbed. Thirteen of the stones were analyzed: 11 were exclusively calcium oxalate; one was apatite only, and one was a mixture. The interval between operation and detection of stones has varied between 24 days and 6 years with an average of 20 months. Neither the rate of weight loss nor frequency of diarrhea have been correlated with the development of renal stones. Dietary intake of oxalate may be important and reduction of fat and high oxalate food in the diet and increasing calcium may help prevent this complication. Intractable recurrent lithiasis may require re-anastomosis.

Pseudo-obstructive megacolon is another serious complication, and has been reported to occur in 25% of patients post-operatively.[79] Clinically, this condition is characterized by abdominal swelling and distention, sometimes associated with fever and air-fluid levels on x-ray. The symptoms are worsened after eating. The dilated segment is distal to the anastomosis between the jejunum and the ileum; either the distal ileum or colon may be dilated. The condition occurs in both the end-to-end and end-to-side varieties of the operation. Treatment is difficult, but involves suppression of anaerobic micro-organisms with metronidazole and antibiotics for the consequent overgrowth of aerobic microbes. This complication may be so troublesome as to require re-anastomosis.

Polyarthritis is an uncommon complication, ranging in various studies from 0–6%, and may be mild, or so serious as to prevent working, although it has not necessitated re-anastomosis. Usually the arthritis involves the extremities and is intermittent without deformities. No radiographic changes have been demonstrated and the standard laboratory tests are negative, including rheumatoid factor, antinuclear factor, and lupus erythematosis cells. Shagrin and associates[80] described seven patients all of whom had a tenosynovitis of the wrists; the fingers were also involved in five patients and the knees and ankles in three patients. Treatment with salicylates and rest are often effective, but some patients have required short courses of prednisone or triamcinolone.

Malnutrition occurs in various forms and degrees of severity in all patients post-operatively. Initially there is a hypoproteinemia in all patients and a decrease in serum level of all the essential amino acids except methionine.[81] This pattern develops in the early post-operative period but there is improvement 6 to 12 months after surgery. Alopecia is a common finding and is probably related to protein deficiency; regrowth of hair parallels improvement in protein levels. There is also a decrease in fat absorption associated with steatorrhea and a decreased absorption of the fat-soluble vitamins, especially vitamin B_{12}, but decreased levels of vitamins A and E have also been reported.[54] Liver compensation results in an increased production of bile salts from cholesterol with a consequent fall in cholesterol levels. There is also a loss of electrolytes in the stools with hypokalemia in nearly all patients. Serum calcium and magnesium levels may also fall. Treatment of the malabsorption during the first 6 months may include protein supplements, vitamin B_{12} by injection, multi-vitamins, potassium and calcium supplements, or anti-diarrheal medications.[82] The malabsorption is partly responsible for the dramatic weight loss in these patients, but includes loss of essential nutrients as well as fat. Malabsorption decreases as mucosal proliferation occurs in the remaining functional intestine and parallels the decline in weight loss.

Diarrhea is an almost universal occurrence after bypass surgery, and those who do not develop diarrhea usually have inadequate weight loss and may require a revision of the bypass with a shortening of the remaining ileum. In the first few weeks, the frequency of liquid stools ranges from 8–15 per day, and after 6 weeks this has decreased to 4–8 per day in most patients. Continuing diarrhea may result in more serious malnourishment and, if intractable, may require lengthening of the remaining bowel or re-anastomosis. A major problem with the diarrhea is the resulting painful hemorrhoids and occasional anal fissure or anal ulcer. Treatment with Lomotil (diphenoxylate) is often effective in decreasing the frequency of liquid stools, but is usually not needed beyond 6 to 8 weeks post-operatively. Separation of water intake from food intake reduces intestinal transit time and decreases the diarrhea.

Other complications have been reported but are less common or less serious. Epigastric distress, gastroenteritis, and gastroduodenitis have been reported in a significant number of patients but these problems are relatively easy to manage. There have been 9 reported cases of tuberculosis developing after intestinal bypass surgery, and 5 of these occurred in sites outside the lung.[83] Wound infection, incisional hematomas, and post-operative hernias are all direct consequences of the surgery itself.

In summary, jejunoileal bypass surgery is both the most effective and most dangerous treatment for massive obesity. Unlike the other available conservative treatment modalities there is a drastic weight loss that is maintained and many patients develop normal eating patterns and report satisfaction with the surgery. However, there is a significant operative mortality as well as several serious potential complications including liver failure, malnutrition, and pseudo-megacolon. Even those without serious complications are certain to suffer diarrhea and usually have several other side effects. Because of the many hazards, this surgery is only indicated in very refractory cases and should only be performed at institutions that can provide long-term follow-up by a team including a surgeon, internist, and psychiatrist.

GASTRIC BYPASS SURGERY

This surgical approach was initiated in Iowa City in 1967 by Mason,[84] and it has only recently been investigated by a number of groups. The procedure is technically somewhat more difficult and time-consuming than jejunoileal bypass, but two large comparative studies suggest that it is safer. Weight loss following surgery has been comparable in most studies using this method, but in some earlier studies patients lost less weight.[85] Selection of patients is the same: massive obesity, treatment failures, presence of the sequelae of obesity, and relatively good psychosocial adjustment.

OPERATIVE PROCEDURE

During the operation, the stomach is stapled together dividing the stomach into a proximal and a distal portion. The proximal portion is small with a 50- to 60-ml volume (10–15% of the stomach) and the distal compartment, which is in continuity with the duodenum, is non-functional (See Fig. 12.9). The small proximal pouch is anastomosed to the jejunum to re-establish continuity of the gastrointestinal tract. Alden has reported[86] that the operating time for jejunoileal bypass was 60 minutes and for gastric bypass 68 minutes. However, in Buckwalter's study,[87] operating time for jejunoileal bypass ranged from 2½–4 hours and for gastric bypass from 3½–6 hours.

RESULTS

After surgery, the patient learns to eat small amounts of solid foods and to avoid sweet beverages. Overdistention of the remaining functional gastric pouch results in nausea; vomiting follows if intake is not curtailed. Repeated

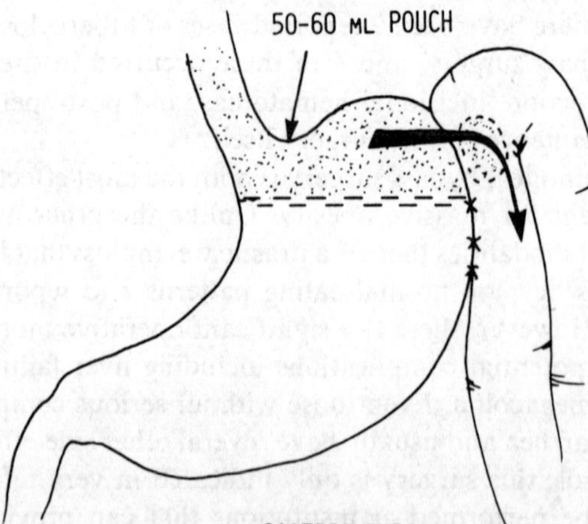

Figure 12.9. Gastric bypass surgery.

overdistention for a lengthy period of time increases the capacity of the gastric pouch and obviates the beneficial effects of the surgery. Hypertonic sweet solutions result in the dumping syndrome and diarrhea because the pyloric mechanism has been bypassed.

Average weight loss after surgery in many series is reported to be approximately 40 to 47 kg,[87, 88] although an early report of 17 patients with gastric bypass showed a weight loss at 1 year of only 24 kg.[85] Weight loss is usually gradual and steady at about 2 to 2½ kg/month. Body weight usually plateaus between 20 and 26 months after surgery. Buckwalter[87] reports that these patients also have a change in eating habits and prefer vegetables, fruits, and salads compared to their pre-operative preference for snack foods.

COMPLICATIONS

Operative mortality is similar to that of jejunoileal bypass and is approximately 3%.[89] However, there are markedly fewer complications with this procedure and the major reported complications are marginal ulcerations and reflux gastritis. Also, most patients have nausea and vomiting immediately after surgery until they learn to decrease their food intake. The incidence of psychiatric problems is not known with certainty, but it is possible that some patients may develop symptom substitution to compensate for the lack of oral gratification. It was initially feared that this procedure might result in ulceration, but this is a relatively rare occurrence (1.4%). Liver disease, diarrhea, polyarthritis, renal stones, and severe electrolyte disturbances have not been observed with gastric bypass surgery. The number of complications is decidedly fewer with this procedure.

BYPASS SURGERY IN ADOLESCENTS

Both jejunoileal and gastric bypass surgery have been used for very obese adolescents. The major hesitation in the use of these procedures stems from uncertainty about the effect on growth potential. It is known that even a modest reduction in weight with dieting can alter growth and therefore the large weight loss following surgery could be detrimental.

White and colleagues[90] report on three adolescents with jejunoileal bypass. All three children were massively obese with weight 3 to 4 times above ideal. All three developed diarrhea post-operatively and one had serious liver changes and urinary calculi. However, all three are reported improved in terms of functional capacity and social interactions. The authors conclude that each teenager continued to grow along his expected height curve but they give no details.

Gastric bypass has also been used for morbid adolescent obesity.[91] Twenty-two patients had gastric bypass surgery, including seven children with Prader-Willi syndrome. Their weight loss averaged 25% 36 months post-operatively among the genetically normal adolescents, but the Prader-Willi patients lost less weight. Complications were few and there were no deaths. The authors state that growth in height was not interrupted.

Bypass operations may be applicable to obese adolescents but even greater caution is warranted in these cases than in adults. The long-term effects of both procedures are not known and may be important, especially to teenagers with most of their lives to live. At this time, bypass operations for obese adolescents should only be performed in very carefully controlled situations; these operations are still a research procedure.

COMPARATIVE STUDIES OF BYPASS SURGERY

Two recent reports have compared the results of gastric bypass surgery to jejunoileal bypass. Both groups conclude that gastric bypass produces at least comparable weight loss and has fewer side effects than jejunoileal bypass. The same selection criteria were used for the two group studies.

Alden[86] studied 100 patients in each group; they had all been operated on by the same surgeon. Jejunoileal bypass patients had an average weight loss of 40.6 kg with a range from 17.7–77.0 kg. The jejunoileal bypass patients had many complications, including serious liver disease, which resulted in the death of one patient, polyarthritis in four patients, one of whom required re-anastomosis, and urinary calculi in 10 patients. Almost all patients had diarrhea and rectal discomfort, and electrolyte problems were common. Nine bypasses were re-anastomosed and there was a re-hospitalization rate of 32%. Gastric bypass patients had a comparable weight loss of 40.2 kg with a range of 20–67 kg. Complications included nausea and vomiting in the first weeks; one patient had a superficial erosion at the stapled gastroenterostomy stoma, and one patient had a large gastric hemorrhage from an ulcer in the functional gastric pouch. Three patients developed the dumping syndrome and one had reflux esophagitis. No deaths occurred and no gastric bypasses had to be taken down, and the hospitalization rate was only 12%.

Buckwalter[87] conducted a prospective randomized clinical trial comparing 19 gastric bypass patients and 19 jejunoileal bypass patients. He concluded that gastric bypass was superior and discontinued entry of new patients into the trial for jejunoileal bypass. Operating time was longer for gastric bypass. Weight loss was slightly better with the gastric bypass patients. Complications were very similar to those previously described in both groups. There was one death in the entire group in a woman with a gastric bypass who developed a pulmonary embolus post-operatively.

In summary, there is evidence that gastric bypass is comparable in terms of weight loss and has markedly less morbidity than jejunoileal bypass. Mortality may be less. For either surgical procedure, careful selection of patients is of paramount importance. Either operation produces dramatic anatomic, physiological, and probably psychological change and therefore must be performed only in suitably refractory patients.

References

1. Roberts CR: Psychological treatment of obesity with phentermine resin as an adjunct. Am J Psychiatry 135: 936–939, 1978.
2. Craddock D: Obesity and Its Management. Ed 3. Edinburgh and London, Churchill Livingston, 1978, pp 92–109.
3. Anonymous: Fighting obesity: developments you may have overlooked. Curr Prescribing, 103–106, 1978.
4. Harris SC, Ivy AC, Searle LM: The mechanism of amphetamine-induced loss of weight. JAMA 134: 1468–1475, 1947.
5. Bray GA: The Obese Patient. Philadelphia, WB Saunders, 1976, pp 359–361.
6. Jones HS: Fenfluramine used as a substitute for methylamphetamines and dexamphetamines in the treatment of dependence on these drugs. S Afr Med J (Suppl) 45: 31, 1971.
7. Penick SB: Amphetamines in obesity. Semin Psychiatry 1: 144–162, 1969.
8. Unpublished data, cited by Penick SB: Amphetamines in obesity. Semin Psychiatry 1: 157, 1969.
9. Goodman EL, Housel EL: The effect of d-amphetamine sulfate in the treatment of the obese hypertensive patient. Am J Med Sci 227: 250–254, 1954.
10. Snyder SH: Amphetamine psychosis: a "model" schizophrenia mediated by catecholamines. Am J Psychiatry 130: 61–67, 1973.
11. Cunningham GLW: Diethylpropion in the treatment of obesity. J R Coll Gen Pract 39: 347–349, 1963.
12. McKay RHG: Long-term use of diethylpropion in obesity. Curr Med Res Opin 1: 489–493, 1973.
13. Walsh AL: Side Effects of Anti-Obesity Drugs. Springfield, Ill, Charles C Thomas, 1962.
14. Silverstone T, Cleary T: Clin Trials 4: 837, 1967, cited by Craddock D: Obesity and Its Management. Ed 3. Edinburgh and London, Churchill Livingston, 1978, p 97.
15. Evans ER, Wallace MG: A multi-centre trial of mazindol in general practice in Ireland. Curr Med Res Opin 3: 132–137, 1975.

16. Garratini S: In: Recent Advances in Obesity Research. Howard A (ed). London, Cambridge Univ Press, 1975, p 354.
17. Butterfield WJH, Whichelow MF: Fenfluramine and muscle glucose uptake in man. Lancet 2: 109, 1968.
18. Hudson KD: The anorectic and hypotensive effect of fenfluramine in obesity. J R Coll Gen Pract 27: 497–501, 1977.
19. Stunkard A, Rickels K, Hesbacher P: Fenfluramine in the treatment of obesity. Lancet 1: 503–505, 1973.
20. Kneebone GM: Fenfluramine in the treatment of obesity. Med J Aust 2: 833–835, 1968.
21. Court JM: A trial of fenfluramine in children with obesity associated with reduced muscle activity. S Afr Med J 46: 132–133, 1972.
22. Mullen A, Wilson CWM: Fenfluramine and dreaming. Lancet 2: 594, 1974.
23. Levin A: Abuse of fenfluramine. Br Med J 2: 49, 1973.
24. LeRiche H: A study of appetite suppressants in a general practice. Can Med Assoc J 82: 467–470, 1960.
25. Munro JF, MacCuish AC, Wilson EM, Duncan LJP: Comparison of continuous and intermittent anorectic therapy in obesity. Br Med J 1: 352–354, 1968.
26. Steel JM, Munro, JF, Duncan LJP: A comparative trial of different regimens of fenfluramine and phentermine in obesity. Practitioner 211: 232–236, 1973.
27. Silverston JT, Cooper RM, Begg RR: A comparative trial of fenfluramine and diethylpropion in obesity. Br J Clin Pract 24: 423–425, 1970.
28. Bray G: The Obese Patient. Philadelphia, WB Saunders, 1976, pp 399–400.
29. Campbell UD, Juhl E, Quaade F: Treatment of obesity with cholestyramine. Nord Med 84: 1628–1629, 1970.
30. Unpublished study, cited in Bray G: The Obese Patient. Philadelphia, WB Saunders, 1976, p 399.
31. Faloon WW, Paes IC, Woolfolk D, et al: Effects of neomycin upon intestinal absorption. Ann NY Acad Sci 132: 879–887, 1966.
32. Simeons ATW: The action of chorionic gonadotrophin in the obese. Lancet 267: 946–947, 1954.
33. Albrink M: Chorionic gonadotropin and obesity? Am J Clin Nutr 22: 681–685, 1969.
34. Carne S: The action of chorionic gonadotropin in the obese. Lancet 2: 1282–1284, 1961.
35. Rivlin RS: The use of hormones in the treatment of obesity. Curr Concepts Nutr 3: 151–162, 1975.
36. Nicoloff JT, Drenick EJ: Altered peripheral thyroxine metabolism in severe obesity. Clin Res 14: 148, 1966.
37. Hung W, Gancayco GP, Heald FP: Thyroxine metabolism in obese adolescent males. Pediatrics 36: 877–881, 1965.
38. Bray G: Effect of diet and triiodothyronine on the activity of sn-glycerol-3-phosphate dehydrogenase and on the metabolism of glucose and pyruvate by adipose tissue of obese patients. J Clin Invest 48: 1413–1422, 1969.
39. Hollingsworth DR, Amatruda TT, Scheig R: Quantitative and qualitative effects of l-triodothyronine in massive obesity. Metabolism 19: 934–945, 1970.
40. Kyle LH, Ball MF, Doolan PD: Effect of thyroid hormone on body composition in myxedema and obesity. N Engl J Med 275: 12–17, 1966.
41. Bray GA, Melvin KEW, Chopra IJ: Effect of triiodothyronine on some metabolic responses of obese patients. Am J Clin Nutr 26: 715–721, 1973.
42. Lukensmeyer WW, Hege JG, Theil GB, Wilson WR: Calcium and phosphorus metabolic studies in triiodothyronine induced hypermetabolism. Am J Med Sci 259: 282–291, 1970.
43. Gwinup G, Poucher R: A controlled study of thyroid analogs in therapy of obesity. Am J Med Sci 254: 416–420, 1967.
44. Drenick EJ, Fisler JL: Prevention of recurrent weight gain with large doses of synthetic thyroid hormones. Curr Ther Res 12: 570–576, 1970.
45. Sabeh G, Bonessi JV, Sarver ME, et al: Hydrocortisone and/or desiccated thyroid in physiologic dosage. XVI. Therapy of obesity with starvation and desiccated thyroid. Metabolism 14: 603–611, 1965.

46. Novak LP, Hayles AB, Cloutier MD: Effect of HGH on body composition of hypopituitary dwarfs. Mayo Clin Proc 47: 241–246, 1972.
47. Evans ES, Simpson ME, Evans HM: The role of growth hormone in calorigenesis and thyroid function. Endocrinology 63: 836–852, 1958.
48. Bray GA, Raben MS, Londono J, Gallagher TF: Effects of triiodothyronine growth hormone and anabolic steroids on nitrogen excretion and oxygen consumption of obese patients. J Clin Endocrinol Metab 33: 293–300, 1971.
49. Kremen AJ, Linner JH, Nelson CH: Experimental evaluation of nutritional importance of proximal and distal small intestine. Ann Surg 140: 439–448, 1954.
50. Payne JH, DeWind LT, Commons RR: Metabolic observations on patients with jejunocolic shunts. Am J Surg 106: 273–289, 1963.
51. Payne JH, DeWind LT: Surgical treatment of obesity. Am J Surg 118: 141–147, 1969.
52. Scott HW Jr, Law DH IV, Sandstead HH, et al: Jejunoileal shunt in surgical treatment of morbid obesity. Ann Surg 171: 770–782, 1970.
53. Weismann RE: Surgical palliation of massive and severe obesity. Am J Surg 125: 437–446, 1973.
54. Scott HW Jr, Dean R, Shull HJ, et al: New considerations in use of jejunoileal bypass in patients with morbid obesity. Ann Surg 177: 723–735, 1973.
55. Phillips RB: Small intestinal bypass for the treatment of morbid obesity. Surg Gynecol Obstet 146: 455–468, 1978.
56. DeWind LT: Jejunoileal bypass surgery for obesity. In: Treatment and Management of Obesity. Bray GA, Bethune JE (eds). Hagerstown, Harper & Row, 1974, pp 132–140.
57. Benfield JR, Bray GA: Is obesity a surgical disease? West J Med 123: 396–398, 1975.
58. Payne JH, DeWind LT, Schwab CE, Kern WH: Surgical treatment of morbid obesity: sixteen years of experience. Arch Surg 106: 432–437, 1973.
59. Salmon PA: The results of small intestine bypass operations for the treatment of obesity. Surg Gynecol Obstet 132: 965–979, 1971.
60. Danowski TS, Bahl VK, Fisher ER, et al: Prospective study of jejunoileal bypass in obesity. VII. Clinical manifestations at 17–35 and 36–47 months. Obesity Bariatric Med 7: 99–106, 1978.
61. O'Leary JP, Weeks JB, Woodward ER: An overview of surgical intervention for obesity. J Fla Med Assoc 65: 95–97, 1978.
62. Mills MJ, Stunkard AJ: Behavioral changes following surgery for obesity. Am J Psychiatry 133: 527–531, 1976.
63. Bray GA, Zachary B, Dahms WT, et al.: Eating patterns of massively obese individuals. J Am Diet Assoc 72: 24–27, 1978.
64. Bray GA, Benfield JR: Intestinal bypass for obesity: a summary and perspective. Am J Clin Nutr 30: 121–127, 1977.
65. Bray GA, Barry RE, Benfield J, et al: Food intake and taste preferences for glucose and sucrose decrease after intestinal bypass surgery. In: Hunger: Basic Mechanisms and Clinical Implications. Wyrwyckee ND, Bray GA (eds). New York, Raven Press, 1976.
66. Bray GA, Davidson MB, Drenick EJ: Obesity: a serious symptom. Ann Intern Med 77: 779–795, 1972.
67. Crockford PM, Salmon PA: Hormones and obesity: changes in insulin and growth hormone secretion following surgically induced weight loss. Can Med Assoc J 103: 147–150, 1970.
68. Scott HW Jr, Dean RH, Younger RK, Butts WH: Changes in hyperlipidemia and hyperproteinemia in morbidly obese patients treated by jejunoileal bypass. Surg Gynecol Obstet 138: 353–358, 1974.
69. Solow C, Silberfarb PM, Swift K: Psychosocial effects of intestinal bypass surgery for severe obesity. N Engl J Med 290: 300–305, 1974.
70. Weiss L: Predicting post-operative psychopathological reactions in intestinal bypass candidates. Obesity Bariatric Med 3: 168–172, 1974.
71. Winkleman EI, Schumacher OP, Hermann RE, et al: Study raises question about ileal bypass. JAMA 231: 126–132, (Abs.), 1975.
72. Abram HS, Meixel SA, Webb WW, Scott HW: Psychological adaptation to jejunoileal bypass for morbid obesity. J Nerv Ment Dis 162: 151–157, 1976.
73. Rigden SR, Hagen DQ: Psychiatric aspects of intestinal bypass surgery for obesity. Am Fam Physician 13: 68–71, 1976.

74. Kalucy RS, Solow C, Hartman M, et al: Self reports of estimated body widths in female obese subjects with major fat loss following ileojejunal bypass surgery. In: Advances in Obesity Research. I. Proceedings of 1st International Congress on Obesity. Oct 9–11, 1974, London, Newman Publ Ltd, 1975, pp 331–332.
75. Schiebel D, Castelnuovo-Tedesco P: Studies of superobesity. III. Body image changes after bypass surgery. Int J Psychiatry Med 8: 117–123, 1978.
76. Phillips RB: Small intestinal bypass for the treatment of morbid obesity. Surg Gynecol Obstet 146: 458, 1978.
77. Brown RG, O'Leary JP, Woodward ER: Hepatic effects of jejunoileal bypass for morbid obesity. Am J Surg 127: 53–58, 1974.
78. Bray GA: The Obese Patient. Philadelphia, WB Saunders, 1976, p 431.
79. Barry RE, Benfield JR, Nicell P, Bray GA: Colonic pseudo-obstruction: a new complication of jejunoileal bypass. Gut 16: 903–908, 1975.
80. Shagrin JW, Frame B, Duncan H: Polyarthritis in obese patients with intestinal bypass. Ann Intern Med 75: 377–380, 1971.
81. Moxley RT III, Pozefsky T, Lockwood DH: Protein nutrition and liver disease after jejunoileal bypass for morbid obesity. N Engl J Med 290: 921–926, 1974.
82. Bray GA: The Obese Patient. Philadelphia, WB Saunders, 1976, pp 424–428.
83. Bray GA: Intestinal bypass surgery for obese patients: behavioral and metabolic considerations. Psychiatr Clin North Am 1: 673–689, 1978.
84. Mason EE, Ito C: Gastric bypass in obesity. Surg Clin North Am 47: 1345–1351, 1967.
85. Printen KJ, Mason EE: Gastric surgery for the relief of morbid obesity. Arch Surg 106: 428–431, 1973.
86. Alden JF: Gastric and jejunoileal bypass. Arch Surg 112: 799–806, 1977.
87. Buckwalter JA: A prospective comparison of the jejunoileal and gastric bypass operations for morbid obesity. World J Surg 1: 757–768, 1977.
88. Mason EE, Ito C: Gastric bypass. Ann Surg 170: 329–339, 1969.
89. Printen KJ: personal communication, cited in Bray G: The Obese Patient. Philadelphia, WB Saunders, 1976, p 435.
90. White JJ, Cheek D, Haller JA: Small bowel bypass is applicable for adolescents with morbid obesity. Am Surg 40: 704–708, 1974.
91. Soper RT, Mason EE, Printen KJ, Zellweger H: Gastric bypass for morbid obesity in children and adolescents. J Pediatr Surg 10: 51–58, 1975.

CHAPTER

13

Psychological Treatment Modalities

The medical and psychological treatment of obesity has been notoriously unsuccessful. Most patients do not lose large percentages of their surplus weight, and if they do, most patients regain most of the weight originally lost. Traditional insight psychotherapy has been thought to be useless in achieving significant weight loss although the patient may have a clearer understanding of the psychodynamic factors resulting in overeating. Recently Rand and Stunkard[1] have challenged this pessimistic view of psychoanalysis, reporting significant weight losses and improvement in body image in 84 obese patients in long-term analysis. Although most other studies report dismal results with traditional psychotherapy alone, it is noteworthy that Hilde Bruch[2] has repeatedly noted the effectiveness of intensive psychotherapy, particularly with developmentally obese adolescents. However, these two reports are the most notable exceptions in a field which generally reports failure in treating obesity.

This bleak outlook for the treatment of obesity was the impetus for investigating the new behavioral approaches to weight reduction. Although initial outcome reports were very encouraging, long-term follow-up studies have thus far shown only a modest overall advantage to these behavioral approaches. The same methodological problems abound in the voluminous literature on behavior therapy for obesity; obese subjects have been selected by widely different criteria, dropouts are frequent, and reporting of results has been inconsistent. Perhaps the most promising aspect of the behavior therapies is that there are a few patients that do very well both at losing weight and maintaining the loss. However, the parameters that determine which obese subjects will be responsive have not yet been elucidated.

EXTERNAL CUE THEORY

Aside from therapeutic potential, the behavior therapies have contributed enormously to our understanding of obesity by focusing on actual eating patterns and the events surrounding eating. Schachter[3] has described a series of studies which demonstrate the susceptibility of human eating behavior to environmental cues and he suggests that the obese are more sensitive to environmental cues associated with eating than are the non-obese. An important corollary of this theory is that elimination or alteration of various environmental cues would be expected to result in a decrease in inappropriate eating behavior and consequent loss of weight.

The external cue hypothesis was derived from three major sources: observation of obese ventromedial hypothalamic rats,[4] Stunkard's work on gastric motility,[5] and finally Schachter's[3] own work in which various environmental changes resulted in a change in eating behavior.

Rats who become obese after destruction of the ventromedial hypothalamus have been described as "finicky" and "lazy"; that is, they are more selective about which food they will eat than are lean rats and they are less likely to work to get food if some impediment is put in the way. They eat more if the food is good tasting and easily available and may be said to be more sensitive to environmental food cues. The food intake of these obese animals is apparently not controlled by internal factors (such as hunger or satiety) as much as the food intake of lean rats.

The gastric motility study, reported by Stunkard and Koch,[5] showed a correlation between gastric contractions and hunger in lean, but not in obese, human subjects. In this study, the subjects swallowed a gastric balloon and the investigators monitored the gastric contractions. Every 15 minutes the subjects were asked whether they were hungry. There was a close correlation between reports of hunger and gastric contractions in the non-obese but not in the obese.

Schachter and colleagues manipulated a number of variables to determine the effect on eating patterns. In one study of the effects of gastric preloading,[3] half the subjects were fed a sandwich and half were not. All the subjects were then given crackers and asked to rate their taste (to disguise the purpose of the study) while the investigators kept track of the number of crackers they consumed. The non-obese subjects consumed fewer crackers following a gastric pre-load than when they did not eat a sandwich first. In striking contrast, the obese subjects ate at least as many crackers following a gastric pre-load as they did on an empty stomach. In an experiment by Nisbett,[6] obese subjects tended to eat one or three sandwiches depending on how many were presented to them, even though they were told that there were many more sandwiches in a nearby refrigerator. In an experiment by Schachter,[7] a clock was designed to run either twice as fast or twice as slow as actual clock time. Obese subjects tended to eat more when they thought it was later than it was and less when they thought that it was earlier than it was.

Johnson[8] performed another study along the same lines with obese and normal subjects to determine the effect of food cue prominence on effort. Subjects were required to lift a 7-pound weight with their index finger in a harness in order to receive a quarter of a sandwich. Then subjects were tested in various conditions on the basis of prominence of food cues; e.g., in the "food visible" condition a desirable sandwich covered with a plastic wrap was placed beside the subject prior to the work trial to obtain a quarter of a sandwich to eat. In the "food invisible" trials, sandwiches were placed next to the subject wrapped in a non-transparent white paper. In another condition, half the subjects ate one quarter of a very good tasting sandwich and half the subjects ate white bread. In all the food cue prominent conditions, the obese subjects worked harder for the food, suggesting a susceptibility to external stimuli.

In short, obese subjects were found to eat more and work harder to obtain food when it was better tasting and more appealing visually. Schachter[9] concludes that in the obese, eating is controlled by the saliency of the environmental food-relevant cues rather than by psychogenic hunger triggered by unhappiness, boredom, or other unpleasant internal states. Schachter theorizes that the obese overeat because they are stimulus-bound, rather than because they are neurotic.

The externality theory has also been studied in the natural environment as well as in the laboratory. Nisbett and Kanouse[10] studied food-buying behavior in the obese and non-obese, with and without calorie deprivation. When hungry, the normal weight individuals bought more food than when they had eaten, but the obese bought the same amount of food whether calorie deprived or not. The study concluded that the obese were relatively insensitive to the internal cue of hunger. Schachter[9] studied obese and non-obese Occidentals in an Oriental restaurant; the obese were less likely to use chopsticks ostensibly because they were less likely to tolerate delay in eating.

Although this is a very interesting theory, more recent work has failed to confirm some of the predictions of this "externality" theory. One study[11] has shown that the lean as well as the obese are responsive to external food cues; hence the obese individuals' tendency to overeat may not be accounted for by an increased sensitivity to environmental stimuli. Another problem with these studies is that the subjects were generally mildly or moderately obese female college students, who may be a different subset than the patients seen in medical clinics. College students are likely to be from the middle or upper classes, whereas very obese patients are likely to come from the lower socioeconomic classes. Despite these problems in the selection of obese subjects, the externality theory has been a potent stimulus for research and many behavioral techniques rely on reducing the potency or prominence of food-relevant cues.

BEHAVIORAL CONTROL OF OBESITY

There are four major aspects of behavioral programs for obesity.[12] *First*, the behavior to be controlled is carefully described and documented, often via a daily food intake and exercise diary. *Second*, the stimuli that precede eating are identified; certain situational cues come to be associated with certain behavior and a certain reinforcing consequence with the result that the cue influences behavior more each time. E.g., if a child sees and smells an appetizing hamburger (the stimuli) and eats it (the behavior) and is then praised by his parents for eating well (reinforcement), the next time he sees or smells a hamburger he will be more likely to eat it. Another example would be that turning on the television may be a cue to begin eating snack foods. There may be a chain of behaviors that result in eating. The first link may be buying the food, the second preparing it, the next serving it, and finally eating it. Technically, the process that serves as a cue to eat something is called the stimulus control of eating; certain cues in certain situations result in eating. The *third* step in behavioral programs is development of techniques to control the act of eating. The techniques used are designed to shape behavior; that is, the changes stress one small achieveable step at a time. E.g., patients are taught to eat more slowly and to associate eating with highly specific stimuli. The *fourth* step is to modify the consequences of eating. A system of formal records for weight loss or changes in eating patterns is established.

MONITORING THE BEHAVIOR TO BE CHANGED

The first step is to determine the eating and exercise patterns that need to be changed and the stimuli associated with them. Figure 13.1 illustrates a typical *eating record.* The patient records the time at which he ate, what he ate, and the stimuli associated with the eating. These stimuli include the environment where he ate (e.g., home, work, restaurant), who was present (family, friends, or alone), his feelings, and whether or not he was hungry. The patient should be given a booklet with sufficient forms for at least 1 month. Some investigators[8] have found that failure to provide the patient with materials for record keeping may result in an early dropout from the program. Initially, the patient is told not to try to change his usual eating behavior, but simply to become aware of what he eats and the environmental or emotional cues that trigger eating. Many obese patients are surprised at the frequency and quantity of food that they consume. Some behavioral studies have focused solely on this aspect of behavior programs and found

EATING RECORD DATE ____________

TIME	FOOD	AMOUNT	STIMULI			
			PLACE	PEOPLE	FEELINGS	HUNGRY?

Figure 13.1. Eating record. (Adapted and reprinted with permission from D. R. Brightwell and Pennwalt Prescription Products).

that self-monitoring (record-keeping) alone has a small but detectable influence on eating patterns and may result in weight loss (although the effect is weak and of short duration).[13] Stunkard[12] has reported that although the effect may be weak in producing weight loss, some patients who have lost weight and start to regain have been able to achieve control over their eating patterns simply by reinstituting self-monitoring. Recording food intake and calories consumed also increases the patient's nutritional knowledge.

A *physical activity diary* is shown in Figure 13.2. The patient records the physical activity performed, minutes performed and the stimuli associated with physical activity (environmental and emotional cues); e.g., some people will participate in physical activities if they are with a group, but not alone, and some people exercise when they are tense. Some obese patients are overweight because they exercise less than their slim peers and the physical activity record may identify such individuals.

Food management behaviors include buying food, storing food, preparing food, serving food, eating, cleaning up, and snacking. Jeffrey and Katz[14] have developed a questionnaire which identifies some of the more common food management behaviors that are likely to contribute to obesity (See Appendix 4). Shopping behaviors that are likely to be part of a chain of

ACTIVITY DIARY DATE ____________

TIME	PHYSICAL ACTIVITY	MINUTES PERFORMED	STIMULI		
			PLACE	PEOPLE	FEELINGS

Figure 13.2. Activity diary. (Adapted and reprinted with permission from D. R. Brightwell and Pennwalt Prescription Products).

behaviors resulting in overeating include the following: shopping while hungry without a list or plan, impulse buying, and purchase of unnecessary quantities of food, especially high calorie foods. Food-storing behaviors likely to result in overeating include: storing food in transparent, easily accessible containers, and leaving food on the countertop or in the living room. A cook who prepares large quantities of high calorie foods is also likely to overeat. Food-serving practices can also contribute to overeating. Patients who serve themselves, have second helpings, and leave food containers on the table are more likely to overeat. Eating large mouthfuls quickly and "cleaning one's plate" may also result in increased food intake. Frequent snacks of high calorie foods also contribute to obesity. After the individuals's food management behaviors are determined, specific countermeasures can be designed.

CUES THAT ELICIT EATING

The food and activity records and food management questionnaire are then analyzed with the patient to determine the environmental or emotional stimuli that result in faulty eating patterns. The discriminative stimulus results in overeating which may lead to improved mood, a consequence that reinforces the likelihood of the behavior (overeating) recurring. Brightwell[15] has identified several sequences that may result in overeating using the formula S⟶B⟶E (a stimulus is followed by behavior which is followed by an event which reinforces the likelihood of the stimulus eliciting the behavior):

S ⟶	B ⟶	E
Hunger ⟶	Eating ⟶	Satisfaction
Nervous ⟶	Eating ⟶	Calmer
Angry ⟶	Eating ⟶	Calmer
Excited ⟶	Eating ⟶	Even better
Watching TV ⟶	Eating ⟶	Enjoyment
Food on counter ⟶	Eating ⟶	Satisfaction

Using the food intake record the patient and therapist can usually identify several cues that trigger eating. Often the patient has been unaware of his eating behavior and may be genuinely surprised at the number of stimuli that elicit eating.

TECHNIQUES TO ALTER EATING BEHAVIOR

Food Management Behavior

Once the stimuli that elicit eating are identified, a plan is devised to eliminate inappropriate stimuli and develop potent new discriminative stimuli. Changes in food management—the buying, storing, and preparation of food—can eliminate some of the environmental cues that trigger eating. The patient is advised to shop when he is not hungry using a carefully prepared low calorie list. Food is stored in opaque, inaccessable containers in the cupboards or refrigerator so that the patient is not tempted to eat every time he walks by the kitchen. Food is all kept in the kitchen away from the television, where snacking is common. If low calorie meals of moderate quantity can be prepared by someone other than the obese patient, this often eliminates nibbling while cooking which can result in the intake of a considerable number of calories. However, if the patient must do his own cooking, meals should be relatively simple to prepare, requiring only a short amount of time in the kitchen. Only enough should be prepared for a moderate sized serving for each person. Meals should not be prepared "family-style" with the containers on the table, as this provides another cue that may result in an unneeded "second-helping." After finishing the meal, food should be stored or thrown away immediately. Available food should require preparation and not be high calorie snack foods. One of our patients who loved cookies and described herself as the "cookie monster" was able to lose weight by never buying more than one cookie at a time: eliminating cookies altogether was apparently unthinkable, but she no longer had a box of cookies in the cupboard. All of these techniques are designed to eliminate or decrease the potency of environmental stimuli that elicit eating.

Techniques to Control the Act of Eating

Several techniques are used to decrease actual food intake, including eating slower and chewing each bite more times and swallowing each bite before eating another bite. Early researchers described an "obese eating style" characterized by rapid eating, relatively few but large bites, and a hypersensitivity to food-relevant cues.[16] However, several investigators[17] have been unable to confirm that the obese have a specific eating style. The obese may not be more rapid eaters than normal weight individuals and they do not seem to take fewer bites.

However, eating slower does tend to decrease actual food intake even if the obese patient did not eat quickly before. Several techniques have been devised.[18] One technique is to lay utensils down between each bite. Some people use smaller utensils, such as cocktail forks. Serving portions are arranged to appear as large as possible. Snacking is often a very difficult behavior to control. An obese person who snacks and plans to eliminate dessert to compensate, rarely is able to follow through on his plan. A better idea is to save a tidbit from a meal for a later snack.

Obese individuals are notorious for skipping meals, particularly breakfast. Often the result is overeating at the next meal. A major change is to plan and eat three meals a day and one snack, which often decreases the likelihood of a binge at the end of a food-deprived day. Many obese individuals have morning anorexia and may even be nauseous, especially if they have eaten several thousand calories the night before. Elimination of breakfast and often lunch as well, may perpetuate this pattern of night binging. There is also a psychological advantage to eating three meals a day. Some obese individuals who skip a meal during work come home and reward themselves with food for not eating all day.

An aspect of eating behavior that has been largely ignored is the process of stopping eating. Most theories have focused on the triggers that begin eating. However, it has been noted[19] that obese humans and rats eat no more often than their lean counterparts, but eat more when they do eat, suggesting a deficiency in the mechanism that terminates eating. Once obese individuals start eating they may not stop as soon as normal weight people do. One of our obese patients would continue eating until everything was finished, even if she wasn't hungry. She was a subject in a research project in which we observed the actual process of eating, and she had never recognized this eating pattern; she remembered that she had been taught as a child to belong to the "clean plate club" and had been admonished not to waste food. We asked her to try learning to leave some food on her plate at the end of each meal and she found she was very anxious when she did this. We have designed a systematic desensitization program for her: she will be taught relaxation therapy and intially will imagine increasing amounts of food on her plate until she is relaxed thinking of a full plate left uneaten. She will then practice leaving larger amounts of food on her plate in an "in vivo" laboratory situation. We hope that this technique in combination with the more conventional changes in eating behavior will result in a permanent weight loss for this patient.

In parallel with these techniques designed to decrease the power of certain environmental cues that trigger eating, new discriminative stimuli are devised to assist in the development of new eating patterns. The patient is asked to obtain a place setting which is distinctive and uniquely his and henceforth he is advised to eat only from this place setting. He is asked to select a plate and glass that are smaller than those he has usually used. The patient is asked to eat only in one place in his home and to isolate eating from all other activities such as reading, watching television, or listening to the radio. He is instructed to remove from the table all visual cues for eating such as crackers, cookies, serving dishes, etc. All food is to be consumed at his place setting, whether it is a full-course meal or a snack. The purpose of these changes is to develop a new set of discriminative stimuli that elicit eating. Some obese patients find that they eat more when they are alone and arranging to eat meals with someone else may be a way of decreasing food intake.

MODIFY CONSEQUENCES OF EATING

The final step in behavior modification programs is to modify the consequences of eating. Early studies rewarded loss of weight *per se* but recent investigations[20] have found that rewarding change in eating behavior, rather than weight loss, is more effective. It is important that reinforcement for changes in behavior be immediate and individualized. Often family members will promise extravagant rewards if the patient will lose significant amounts of weight; however, the constant and immediate temptations to overeat usually render any long-term reward unattainable. Also, what is a positive reinforcement for one person may be meaningless to someone else. The obese individual must be assisted in selecting a series of significant rewards for himself.

Most programs[12, 15] use positive reinforcement for change in eating behavior or weight loss. The person may be awarded a certain number of points for chewing slowly or saving parts of a meal for a later snack. Points can then be converted to concrete rewards such as money, clothes, etc. Each small improvement in eating behavior is immediately noted and rewarded. In addition, social feedback for all successes is important and can be achieved through friends, family, co-workers, or other dieters. If a patient lays down his utensils between bites, a family member might remark that this was a good idea, thereby providing positive social reinforcement that would increase the likelihood of the behavior recurring. Selection of appropriate rewards (positive reinforcement) is not always easy, however. Some people are embarrassed if someone comments on their eating behavior, and a remark from a family member might actually be punishment (i.e., decrease the likelihood of a new eating behavior recurring).

Relapse into customary eating patterns is usually ignored, and Brightwell[21] recommends that the patient never be criticized if he fails to follow the new plan. Instead, the eating diary is reviewed and the individual is assisted in designing new techniques that may be more effective and in selecting more potent positive reinforcements.

Consequences that decrease the likelihood of a behavior recurring (technically called "punishment") have also been used to eliminate inappropriate eating habits. If a patient prepares a batch of cookies for her husband and consumes several in the process, the husband might respond that he doesn't want her to bake him any more cookies. If the result of this remark is to decrease the likelihood of the wife consuming cookies, it is "punishment" in behavioral terminology. Other techniques have been used by some investigators. The patient may write a check to a certain very disliked organization (for instance, the Ku Klux Klan) which is kept by the therapist.[22] If the subject does not lose weight, or eating behavior remains unchanged, the therapist mails the check. If this consequence decreases the occurrence of inappropriate eating behavior, it is "punishment."

ALTERNATIVE WAYS TO COPE WITH EMOTIONS

Although both normal weight and obese subjects use food to cope with feelings, probably there is a tendency for obese people to do this more often. Learning to use alternative (non-eating) ways of handling feelings can be useful. Anxiety often elicits eating and can be dealt with in several different ways. Physical activity often counteracts tension and has the added advantage of calorie expenditure. It is often difficult for an obese individual to be in an active exercise program, but sometimes just going for a walk around the block when tense will obviate some overeating. A second method of combating tension is relaxation therapy and some investigators have suggested that relaxation therapy should be an integral part of any program for obesity. Many obese subjects report that they eat when they are tired; napping or increasing the hours sleeping at night can be helpful. Many people overeat when they are angry or irritated, rather than express their anger effectively and appropriately. Assertive training is a behavior-shaping program that has been successfully incorporated into many weight control clinics. The essence of all these techniques is to teach the patient to cope effectively with his emotions rather than to disguise them by overeating. Before using any of these methods, however, it is essential that a psychiatric evaluation be completed. Inappropriate selection of patients for an assertive training program can be hazardous.

RELAXATION THERAPY

This technique was initially described by Jacobson in 1938[23] and is used in a modified form by many therapists. The technique based on the principle of contrasting effects is as follows. The patient is asked to clench his right fist and to pay careful attention to all those areas in his hand and forearm that are tense. Then he is asked to gradually "let go" and allow all the tension created to ebb away. Then he is asked to compare the right hand and forearm to the left side and usually the patient will report that the right hand is relaxed, warm, and slightly heavier than the left side. Then the patient is asked to clench his other fist, note its tenseness, then gradually relax. As the patient breathes out, the therapist reiterates "let go" and tells the patient that he will gradually become more relaxed. The various muscles of the body are contracted and relaxed in a systematic fashion, including the muscles of the face and neck. During the entire procedure, the therapist reiterates that the patient will gradually become more and more relaxed. Progressive relaxation has been used in a variety of clinical situations, notably systematic desensitization, and has been useful to some obese patients who eat when they are tense.

Most subjects can learn this technique in one or two sessions with the therapist. Some investigators[24] suggest that the therapist demonstrate each step of the relaxation by actually doing it himself so that the patient can model his behavior according to the therapist. We have tape-recorded one session with the therapist teaching the individual patient relaxation therapy and we ask the patient to practice relaxation therapy at home listening to the tape-recording. If there is a strong positive doctor-patient relationship, this technique can be very useful. Once the technique has been mastered, the patient can use relaxation therapy at home or at work when tempted to eat to alleviate tension. Another advantage of an individual tape recording is that it can be tailored to the patient; most individuals have certain muscle groups that tend to reflect tension, and the physician can emphasize these areas during the tape recording.

ASSERTIVE TRAINING

Assertive training has also been used as part of a comprehensive treatment program for obesity. Many obese individuals are not effectively self-assertive in their daily lives. Often these patients feel guilty if they refuse to do something they don't want to do and may even be unable to refuse offered food when dieting for fear of hurting someone else's feelings. Patients with defects in assertiveness can be identified by certain questions. Wolpe[25] asks:

> "Suppose you are waiting in a line for theatre tickets and someone cuts in front of you. What would you do?"
>
> A patient in need of assertive training might respond:
>
> "Well, inside I'd be knotted up, burning. It would probably spoil my whole evening, and the knot in my stomach would still be there when I went to bed that night, but I wouldn't say anything—because I wouldn't want to make a scene."

One very obese woman who came to our clinic waited 3 hours before asking the receptionist why she had not been seen! Part of her treatment program was urgently needed assertive training. Some patients who benefit from assertive training describe themselves as "emotional time bombs"—they hold in all their feelings and explode in a useless self-defeating rage in response to a minor irritation.

In reference to food, some patients are unable to refuse food, or insist that food be served or prepared so that overeating can be avoided. An example of a question which would elicit this attitude is as follows:

> "If your hostess offers you a piece of cake that you do not particularly like, what would be your response?"
>
> A non-assertive obese patient might answer:
>
> "I would accept because my hostess's feelings would be hurt if I refused, even if I was on a diet.

The underlying principle of assertive training is behavior shaping. By a series of successive approximations, the patient is gradually taught to be more appropriately assertive. Some patients are afraid to express their own opinions and wishes because they believe they will become overly aggressive and insensitive to the needs of others. Behavior therapists stress that an appropriately assertive person considers the needs of others as well as himself and states his requests, not demands, in a forthright manner, accepting responsibility for his own emotions and requests. An appropriate response to someone cutting in front of you in line would be: "Excuse me, but I was here first." An inappropriately aggressive response would be to grab the person's shoulder and shove him out of line.

The techniques used include role playing and modeling behavior, usually in the context of group therapy.[26] Situations that actually occur in the everyday life of the patient are used as examples, and the therapist may model an assertive response. The appropriate response to the offer of an unwanted piece of cake would be "No thank you." The patient is repeatedly asked to practice responses to troublesome situations, each time more closely approximating the appropriate assertive response. After each response, the therapist offers gentle criticism pointing out soft or apologetic gestures. After the patient is able to role play assertive responses, he may be asked to use his new behavior in an "in vivo" situation, e.g., at a party where he is offered food he doesn't want on his diet. The idea that others' feelings will be damaged is usually incorrect and may reflect egocentricity or magical thinking on the part of the patient. The patient may erroneously believe that his own anger or irritation is very powerful and capable of hurting others. These beliefs are very common and often are not amenable to simple assertive training, but may require psychotherapy as well.

SUMMARY

Both relaxation therapy and assertive training are useful adjuncts in a behavioral program for obesity, but should not be used alone or without a thorough psychiatric evaluation. Passivity can be a reaction formation, a defense mechanism in which the patient behaves opposite to his real feelings. In this situation, elimination of the passivity with assertive training may result in inappropriate rage or aggression. Or, an angry paranoid patient may need help in suppressing his rage, rather than learning to express what may be a bottomless pit of fury. In any case, judicious selection of patients is critical.

COGNITIVE RESTRUCTURING

Mahoney and Mahoney[27] have pioneered a technique called cognitive restructuring for the treatment of obesity. Perfectionistic standards, negative beliefs, and private monologues can be obstacles to success in weight loss. These investigators have taught subjects to record, evaluate, and alter these negative monologues. The following are examples of negative thought patterns:

1. "This will never work—I have always regained whatever I lose."
2. "After tonight, no more desserts until I've lost 20 pounds."
3. "After Christmas and New Years Day, I'll diet."
4. "I blew it today; I'll be fat forever."
5. "I just have no will power."
6. "My whole family is fat—it must be in the genes."

The characteristic thought patterns of each subject are identified and the person is asked to revise his private monologue so it is more reasonable. If the person eats a forbidden cookie and then says to himself "I blew it today, I'll be fat forever," this sets up a self-defeating repetitive pattern where one mistake spells complete failure. An alternative thought that does not rest on an all-or-nothing philosophy might be: "That was one mistake on my diet, but if I follow my diet the rest of the day, I will continue to lose weight."

Mahoney and Mahoney describe this therapeutic technique as "cleaning up one's cognitive ecology." This technique is similar to a method used by Beck[28] in treating depressed patients by encouraging them to substitute positive thoughts for their usual gloomy, self-denigrating ruminations. Cognitive restructuring is essentially a method of improving self-esteem applied specifically to self-destructive thoughts about one's eating behavior.

RESULTS OF BEHAVIOR THERAPY

RESULTS AT END OF TREATMENT

Initially, behavior modification programs appeared to result in markedly greater weight loss than the usual dietary regimens. In 1959, Stunkard and McLaren-Hume[29] found that of the 1368 patients studied in the previous 30 years, only 16% lost 10–20 pounds, 12% lost 20–40 pounds, and 5% lost more than 40 pounds. In a pioneering study utilizing behavior techniques in 1967, Stuart[30] reported that 8 obese women had a mean weight loss of 37.75 pounds over a 1-year period. Two patients of the original group of 10 dropped out of treatment. Three of the patients (30% of the original group) lost more than 40 pounds and six lost more than 30 pounds. Although this represents a dramatic improvement in weight loss, Stuart's original study lacked a control group. Harris[31] soon replicated this study with mildly obese college students using a no-treatment control group. Although there was only a 10.5-pound weight loss in the experimental group, there was an average weight gain of 3.6 pounds in the control group.

Penick and colleagues[32] compared behavior therapy to the currently available traditional treatment. The behavior therapy program included documentation of behavior to be controlled, modification of stimuli governing eating, development of techniques to control the act of eating, and prompt reinforcement of behaviors that delayed or controlled eating. The traditional treatment included supportive group psychotherapy, diet and nutrition instruction, and drugs (appetite suppressants) if requested. Thirty-two subjects were studied, 15 in the behavior modification groups, and 17 in traditional therapy. There were 12 group therapy sessions over a 3-month period, once weekly, lasting about 2 hours for both the control and experimental groups. All patients were at least 20% overweight. The median overweight of patients treated with behavior therapy was 78%, and the median overweight of the control patients was 80%. The results with the control groups were similar to those reported in the 1959 review, with 25% losing more than 20 pounds, although none in the control group lost more than 30 pounds. However, 53% of the patients receiving behavior therapy lost 20 pounds, 33% lost more than 30 pounds, and 13% lost more than 40 pounds. This was a significant improvement over the usual findings in the treatment of obesity, but not as dramatic as Stuart's initial findings.

Currey and associates[33] studied a group of 144 patients who had been obese for an average of 20 years and who had medical problems associated with their obesity (e.g. hypertension or diabetes) or were at risk for major medical problems. Most patients were referred by physicians to this medically based eating disorders clinic. The immediate results were as follows: 43% lost less than 5 kg (11 pounds), 28% lost 5 to 9 kg (11 to 19.8 pounds), 23% lost more than 9 kg (19.8 pounds), and 6% lost more than 18 kg (39.6 pounds); these results are roughly the same as the results reported in 1959 for traditional medical treatment. Currey and colleagues conclude that older medically referred obese patients with associated health problems do no better with behavior modification than with the more traditional dietary regimens. Furthermore, of the initial 144 patients, only 64 patients completed treatment.

Another study of medically referred obese patients was reported by Musante.[34] Of a group of 229 obese patients, many of whom had been obese since childhood, 50% lost 20 pounds or more. No follow-up data are presented. Although this is an encouraging finding, the treatment approach described involves institutionalization at a day-treatment facility called "Structure House." There are four major goals at the day-treatment center: correction of misconceptions about food and eating behavior, changing maladaptive eating behavior, learning to manage time and activity, and coping with stress that leads to overeating. Perhaps the most important aspect of this program is the fact that learning new eating habits is conducted in a real life situation. Initially, patients eat 21 meals with no changes, and concern with diet is minimized. Then the patient plans his own menus around a certain number of calories. Patients learn to judge portion sizes correctly, and practice their new eating behaviors in potentially difficult situations such as buffets, cookouts, etc.

MAINTENANCE OF WEIGHT LOSS POOR

Recent follow-up reports of behavior modification techniques have been disappointing in terms of maintenance of weight loss. For example, Stunkard and Penick[35] have recently reported results of a 5-year follow-up of their initial behavior therapy report in 1971. At the end of treatment, weight losses were better with behavior therapy than with the traditional regimen (the control group). At a 1-year follow-up, the majority of patients in both groups weighed less than they had at the end of treatment, but during the next 4 years patients in both groups began to regain. Only 3 of the 12 behavior group and 4 of the 13 traditional treatment patients weighed less than they had at the end of treatment. As a group, at the end of the 5-year follow-up, the behavioral group had maintained a weight loss of 5.3 kg (11.6 pounds) and the traditional group had maintained a weight loss of 5.5 kg (12.1 pounds). Importantly, one of the behavior patients who had lost 8 kg (17.6 pounds) at the end of treatment continued to lose weight and had lost 33 kg (72.6 pounds) at the 5-year follow-up. The reasons for this success are not known.

In the follow-up of patients studied by Currey and associates,[33] 8 of the 64 who completed treatment were lost to later follow-up, and 12 additional patients refused to answer telephone inquiries. These 12 were assumed to have regained their pretreatment weight or more. Of the 56 patients contacted for follow-up at 12 months, 70% had regained their pretreatment weight or more, 10% had maintained the weight lost during treatment, and 20% had continued to lose an average of 4 kg (8.8 pounds).

Evaluation of follow-up studies is difficult for some of the same reasons noted in the 1959 review.[29] There is still no generally accepted standard for reporting weight reduction data, and various studies select subjects by widely differing criteria. Furthermore, follow-up has sometimes been less than 6 months, a time insufficient to judge maintenance of weight loss.

Brightwell and Sloan[36] reviewed more than 100 reports of behavior modification and found only 15 group studies that provided sufficient information to evaluate the effectiveness of the treatment. To qualify for inclusion in the review, these authors required the following information: data derived from at least six cases, sufficient data provided to compare results (at least pretreatment and post-treatment weights, and ideal weight), duration of 26 weeks actual treatment, and a follow-up period of at least 26 weeks after all contact with the therapist had ceased. Of the 15 group studies which met these criteria, there was a maintenance of weight lost in only seven studies. Of the subjects in these seven studies, not all maintained the weight loss and most of the subjects were not grossly overweight to begin with.

Another difficulty in evaluating follow-up reports is that clinically significant weight losses in group studies are rare. Of the nine follow-up studies reviewed by Stunkard and Penick,[35] only four had median weight losses at the end of treatment greater than 14 pounds, and weight losses were not well maintained at follow-up.

MAINTENANCE STRATEGIES

Although maintenance of weight loss with behavior programs has been disappointingly low, it has focused research attention on a fact long recognized by obese patients: weight loss is relatively easy to achieve, but maintenance of that weight loss is often extremely difficult and probably depends on a number of complex interacting factors. Behavior modification probably represents a significant advance in producing an initial weight loss, but the problem of maintaining this loss has yet to be solved.

Some behaviorists have investigated various maintenance strategies. Booster sessions in which behavior techniques are continued after treatment, although at less frequent intervals, have been tried as a technique to improve the maintenance of weight lost at the end of treatment. Ashby and Wilson[37] assigned post-treatment subjects to several different groups. Two groups met with a behavioral therapist every 2 weeks and one group met with a therapist every 4 weeks in what was essentially a continuation of the treatment program. (These groups were the booster groups.) Two groups met either every 2 weeks or every 4 weeks in a non-specific support group and subjects in the control group had no contact with the therapist except at weigh-ins at 3, 6, 9, and 12 months. Unfortunately, the booster groups maintained weight losses no better than the other groups. Although Kingsley and Wilson[38] found that booster sessions facilitated the maintenance of treatment produced weight reduction in groups in a 12 month follow-up, this was independent of the specific group treatment modality used. Although there was a better initial weight loss in the behavior group compared to a social pressure group, the weight losses achieved were maintained equally well with booster sessions.

SUMMARY

In summary, at present there is very little evidence that behavior modification is more efficacious in maintaining significant weight loss than other methods. However, some studies show that behavior modification results in greater weight loss during treatment than other methods, although this loss is not maintained. Also several behavior methods lend themselves to keeping patients in treatment longer than with dietary regimens. Maintenance strategies have thus far been ineffective, but offer future promise. There may be a subset of obese patients who are particularly sensitive to behavior modification techniques, but means of identifying such patients have not yet been devised.

BEHAVIOR MODIFICATION IN CHILDREN

There is ample evidence that in our society obesity is becoming more prevalent among children because food intake is increasing and physical activity is decreasing. Since some studies have suggested that adipose cell number remains constant after adolescence, treatment measures that reduce the prevalence of obesity in children are urgently needed. It is only in the last few years that behavior modification methods have been tried with children and thus far success has been modest. A major characteristic of most programs has been involvement of one or both parents. Theoretically, such parental participation would seem essential since children model the eating behavior of important people in their life. A child is unlikely to eat a balanced, healthful, slenderizing diet if his parents regularly consume cookies, desserts, McDonald's hamburgers, and french fries.

A behavior therapy program for seven girls and three boys aged 7 to 13, conducted by Rivinus and colleagues,[39] resulted in an average weight loss of 6.2 pounds; in the 10 weeks prior to treatment these same children had gained an average of 3.5 pounds. During treatment, the children and mothers met in individual sessions for 10 weeks. Children kept a log of food eaten and their mothers were instructed in rewards, contracts, and modeling of appropriate behavior. An interesting sidelight was that the children with normal weight mothers lost more weight than the children of obese mothers.

A study by Kingsley and Shapiro[40] investigated the importance of parental participation. There were four groups: child-only group, mother-only group, mother and child together group, and no treatment control group. In the three treatment groups, the members were taught the principles of behavior modification during 8 weekly sessions, during which a deposit of $30.00 was refunded, contingent on attendance at the group. The children in the treatment group all lost more weight (1.6 kg) than those in the control group but there was no significant difference among the three experimental groups. However, in the mothers-only group, mothers lost an average of 2.8 kg during the treatment period, which was significantly more than the mothers in the other groups. Although the children lost similar amounts of weight in all the experimental groups, the mothers' satisfaction with treatment was greatest in the mother-child together group. Although this study does not support the idea that parental participation is essential, the experimental groups were small (only 10 subjects in each) and follow-up was short (20 weeks).

An important point to remember in evaluating future reports of behavior therapy of obese children, is that weight loss *per se* may not be necessary for treatment to be effective. Since children are growing, a decline in the rate of weight gain may be all that is required of treatment. In fact, as noted earlier, even relatively small weight losses may result in a decrease in expected height velocity. Thus, reports with only minor changes in weight in children may be significant.

CLASSICAL CONDITIONING TECHNIQUES

Classical conditioning paradigms have not been as widely used as operant conditioning programs, but have recently been re-investigated and offer promise for future research and treatment. Early investigators attempted to produce an aversion to food by introducing an electric shock or unpleasant odor every time food is eaten.[41] Others tried to produce a generalized state of tension or anxiety whenever food was consumed.[42] In this study rapid weight loss was produced initially but not maintained and, as might be expected, the dropout rate was high.

TRANSSWITCHING

A recent study[43] has investigated a variant of classical conditioning termed "transswitching" which does not rely on aversive measures. In classical conditioning, an unconditioned stimulus results in an unconditioned response (e.g., food in the mouth is an unconditioned stimulus which results in salivation, an unconditioned response). If a buzzer is sounded (the conditioned stimulus) at the same time that the unconditioned stimulus is presented (food in the mouth), after several trials the buzzer alone will elicit the response (now termed the conditioned response). In transswitching,[44] the same conditioned stimulus (CS) can be conditioned to different (or even opposite) conditioned responses (CR's) at the same time in different contexts. Dogs can be conditioned to salivate to a buzzer CS and to respond with leg flexion to a tactile CS. Next, in a different chamber the conditions can be reversed making the buzzer a signal for a leg flexion CR and the tactile stimulus a signal for salivation. The dogs are able to master the discrimination and respond to the buzzer with salivation in one chamber and leg flexion in the other. In this case, the chamber served as a switching agent to modify the meaning of the conditioned stimulus.

In an experiment with obese subjects, the sight and smell of food were the conditioned stimuli (CS's) and salivation the conditional response (CR). The switching agent was sunglasses. It was predicted that the sunglasses would modify the meaning of the food cues (sight and smell of food) and determine whether or not the conditioned response (salivation) would occur. Food cues were expected to elicit salivation when sunglasses were on, but not when sunglasses were off.

Two obese subjects were studied in a single case design. Initially the subjects were tested in the baseline condition. Food was placed in front of them and they were told to think about food, look at it, and smell it. If it was a "sunglasses-on" trial, they were told they would be allowed to eat, but if it was a "sunglasses-off" trial they were told they would not be allowed to eat. Before the experiment, these two subjects' salivation bore no relationship to whether it was a situation in which they would be allowed to eat or not. Then, during the experimental phase, in a series of more than 100 trials, food was presented and eating was allowed only in the "sunglasses-on" condition but not in the "sunglasses-off" condition. After the experiment, the salivation tests were repeated, and there was a striking correlation between salivation level and presence or absence of sunglasses. When sunglasses were on, salivation was greater than when sunglasses were off (See Fig. 13.3).

Each subject was then "deconditioned." In this portion of the experiment, eating was permitted on a random basis unrelated to the presence or absence of sunglasses. In some instances the investigators said that the subjects would be allowed to eat after a trial and they were not allowed to eat, or they were told they would not be allowed to eat and then they were allowed to take a bite. Salivation was then re-tested, and there was no relationship between level of salivation and presence or absence of sunglasses. In a final phase of the experiment, each subject was "reconditioned" and salivation levels were again positively correlated with the presence of sunglasses.

An interesting sidelight of this experiment was the subjects' reactions during the "deconditioning" phase of the experiment. They were irritated, as expected, but also couldn't remember the instructions for 60 seconds and ate when they were told they couldn't eat, or vice versa, and couldn't remember if they had already taken a bite.

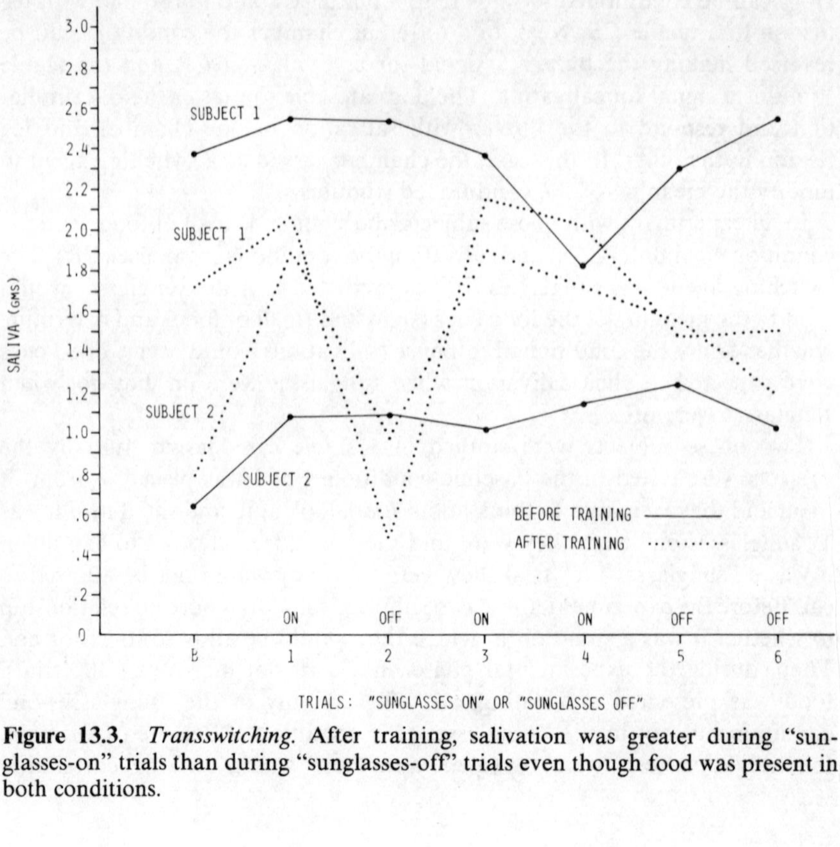

Figure 13.3. *Transswitching.* After training, salivation was greater during "sunglasses-on" trials than during "sunglasses-off" trials even though food was present in both conditions.

The goal of this pilot study was to demonstrate that the transswitching paradigm could be used to alter certain alimentary responses to food cues. Salivation was the conditioned response chosen since it is relatively easy and inexpensive to measure. However, other autonomic and endocrine responses of digestion may be even more important and will be the focus of further study. Insulin secretion, which lowers blood sugar and enhances appetite, may be stimulated by the sight or smell of food. If insulin secretion were lowered only when appropriate, not merely to the sight and smell of food, this might simplify dieting. A dieter passing a candy shop wafting out a delicious smell may respond with insulin secretion and a lowered blood sugar which enhances appetite; if a person could be conditioned to respond with insulin secretion only when he plans to eat, this might facilitate dieting. There is evidence that salivation levels parallel insulin levels so it is possible that the transswitching paradigm may be useful in conditioning insulin responses.

Subjects in this project were selected by a screening process designed to identify obese subjects whose salivation response had no relationship to whether or not it was appropriate to eat. It was predicted that the salivation patterns of normal weight subjects would be greatest when eating was permitted and lowest when eating was not permitted; however, this was not the case. The lean subjects, like the obese subjects, had salivation patterns that bore no relationship to whether eating was permitted or not. Despite this finding, it is likely that modifying salivation patterns to suit the dieting situation would be helpful to the obese patient attempting to reduce.

In summary, although classical conditioning techniques have not been widely used in the treatment of obesity, they offer promise. Techniques that rely on aversive stimuli are likely to be of little clinical value because of the very high dropout rate. However, new approaches which are less unpleasant to the patient, such as the transswitching procedure, may prove valuable.

HYPNOSIS

Hypnosis has often been suggested as a treatment for obesity, but there are few objective studies of its effectiveness. Winkelstein[45] reported a study of 42 obese women who were between 10 to 60 pounds over their ideal weight with an average of 32 pounds excess weight. The subjects were in good physical health and were not psychotic, although no other statement is given about their psychological health. During the first two sessions, the principles of weight reduction were discussed with the patients and a hypnotic trance was induced. Those subjects who could not achieve a deep trance during the first two sessions were eliminated from the study. Once the trance state was established, many different post-hypnotic suggestions were made. All were aimed toward changing maladaptive eating behavior and included elimination of snacks, refusal of high calorie foods, and decrease of hunger. After the first few sessions, the post-hypnotic suggestions lasted only a few hours or days, but after several sessions lasted for days or weeks.

All subjects lost weight and all completed the experiment. This alone is a significant finding. The maximal weight loss during treatment was 58.5 pounds and the minimum 9.25 pounds and the 6-month average for the entire group was 27 pounds. The active treatment period was 14 weeks and at follow-up at 6 months not one of the subjects had returned to pre-treatment weight. Rate of weight loss was not consistent week to week, and sometimes different post-hypnotic suggestions were needed. Time required on the part of the therapist was less than 2 hours for the first two sessions and approximately 15 minutes per session during the following weeks.

The results of this study were outstanding compared to the usual results in obesity studies, including behavior modification. However, the author does not give exact weight loss at the end of treatment and it may be that 6 months is too brief a follow-up.

A more recent study[46] of 40 obese subjects found that mean weight loss at the 3-month follow-up was 12.6 pounds (range +13 to −50 pounds). This weight loss was not maintained at 6 months and there was a decrease to a 9.5 pound loss (range +10 to −50 pounds) from the initiation of treatment. This study reports only group statistics and does not give results at the end of treatment. The ideal weight for individual subjects is not given nor is the size of the original sample.

Hypnosis has a relationship to relaxation therapy. The repetitive monotonic instructions used during relaxation therapy are soporific and in susceptible patients may induce a trance. Relaxation therapy has been used successfully in the treatment of obesity, and it may be that subjects who respond would also find hypnotherapy useful. This is an area that has yet to be investigated.

GROUP APPROACHES

Group interaction is an integral part of several types of treatment of obesity, including the patient self-help groups and some behavior modification programs. Relatively few controlled studies have investigated the role of group therapy. Some researchers have found that there is a lower attrition rate in group programs for obesity, but not necessarily more successful weight reduction.

London and Schreiber[47] compared the effectiveness of group discussions and an appetite suppressant over a 6-month period with 240 obese patients who were at least 20% above their ideal weight. There were six regimens. One group took drugs (d-amphetamine sulfate-prochlorperazine), one group took a placebo, and one group took no drugs. Three other groups combined these conditions with group discussion. The treatment period was 6 months. The attrition rate in the groups that met for discussion biweekly was markedly less than for those who did not meet in groups. Each group started with 40 patients and the highest dropout rate was in the condition with no drugs and no group discussion (only nine of the original 40 patients completed the experiment). The condition with the active drug combined with group discussion had the lowest attrition rate (32 subjects completed the experiment). Patients in groups lost the most weight during treatment. Patients who received group discussion and drugs lost an average of 18.8 pounds compared to an average loss of 10 pounds with drugs alone. Even the patients who received no medicine and group discussion were more successful in weight loss than the patients in any of the drug conditions without group discussion.

Although most studies of group methods have had lower attrition, not all have been more successful in promoting weight loss. Munves[48] compared individual nutrition education interviews with group interaction using the discussion-decision methods described by Lewin. Of 48 initial subjects, 43 completed the experiment, a surprisingly low attrition rate. During the 4-month treatment period, weight loss was similar in the two conditions, but at the end of the subsequent 4-month follow-up, the subjects who had received individual nutritional instruction performed better in terms of continued weight loss. However, weight loss was often small, less than 5 pounds, and only one subject attained his ideal weight. Thus, in this study, a group method was less effective than individual treatment. However, Munves' subjects were college students and most were not impressively obese. Furthermore, subjects were not screened for psychiatric problems and the group technique used was the discussion-decision method rather than group psychotherapy.

In another study that compared group therapy and individual nutrition counseling, no differences were found in effectiveness[49] at the 2-year follow-up. At the end of 1 year, 40% of the patients who had received individual instruction, 27% of the group patients, and 19% of the control patients had lost 10% or more of their initial overweight. At the end of the 2-year follow-up, some patients had regained the weight they had lost and the figures decreased to 26%, 20%, and 10%, respectively, of the patients who maintained a loss of 10% or more of their initial overweight.

Psychoanalytic group psychotherapy has not been proven more efficacious in weight reduction than the traditional nutritional counseling. Holt and Winick[50] studied six obese middle-aged women in analytic therapy. There were 22 sessions over the course of 6 months and the average weight loss at follow-up at 30 months was 4.3 pounds. Although weight loss was not impressive, the authors note that there was an improvement in general adaptation and emotional well-being of these six patients.

Although there is less attrition in the group studies, there has been no demonstration of improved effectiveness. However, in the studies cited, little attempt has been made to choose group members who are particularly suited for group therapy, nor has any systematic study of the psychodynamics of the individual members or group process been undertaken. A more careful attention to factors known to be important in group therapy might result in a selection of group members responsive to this form of treatment.

SELF-HELP GROUPS

In view of the dismal results of the medical management of obesity, it is not surprising that there are several self-help groups for obesity. These include Weight Watchers, TOPS (Take Off Pounds Sensibly), Overeaters Anonymous, and Diet Workshop.

Weight Watchers, Inc. is a commercial organization founded by Jean Nidetch. It is a privately owned company with regional offices around the nation. The effectiveness of this group in producing weight loss is not known as no figures have been released. Bray[51] reports that of 267 women in their obesity clinic, 118 had been to Weight Watchers. They attended an average of 25 weeks and lost an average of 21 pounds, but almost all regained weight. It is possible, of course, that these figures represent only a small unsuccessful subset of the Weight Watchers group.

TAKE OFF POUNDS SENSIBLY (TOPS)

TOPS is a non-profit, self-help organization that maintains cordial relationships with the medical profession and has been studied by several investigators. The group was founded more than 30 years ago in 1947 by a Milwaukee housewife, who has had a lifelong battle with obesity. TOPS has grown in size to more than 330,000 members distributed in 12,000 chapters in all 50 states and in several foreign countries. Primarily, the group has middle-class members with a few lower-class members. Most group members are women although groups in Chicago called "Sir Tops" include businessmen and executives. Stunkard and colleagues[52] have characterized the average member as a 42-year-old woman with an ideal weight of 119 pounds who enters TOPS weighing 188 pounds, leaves after 16 months, and loses 15 pounds during this time. There is of course wide variability in the length of time that members belong, but there is apparently a core group of members who belong for long periods and a group of members who belong for brief periods. There is a correlation between length of membership and initial weight loss; the greater the initial weight loss the longer the membership.

In an early study, Stunkard[53] reported that different chapters were widely divergent in effectiveness. For example, in one chapter, 62% of the members lost 20 pounds and in the least successful chapter only 10% of the members lost at least 20 pounds. However, a later survey[54] showed that these differences were not due to enduring characteristics of the chapters; different chapters showed different weight losses at different times. In both studies the same 22 chapters were evaluated, and there were widely different weight loss averages in the same chapter at different times. Also, although there was an overall increase in TOPS members in the geographical area studied, this was due to the formation of new chapters; membership of the original groups actually declined.

Many members drop out of the TOPS program. Approximately 30% of the membership is stable over a 2-year period, indicating a very high attrition rate.[54] Those who remain are apparently those who are able to lose weight successfully with the TOPS program—less than one-third of those who initially join. Also, those who are most overweight are most likely to remain. The closer an individual is to normal weight, the less likely he is to remain in the group.

The program[55] itself centers around a weekly group meeting lasting 1½ to 2 hours. The meetings usually start with a song or a pledge attesting to the common goal of "controlling emotions" to prevent overeating. The remainder of the time is devoted to a program that may be educational. Each individual is weighed and the pounds lost or gained are reported to the group. Members who have lost weight are praised and there is applause and much approval. When a member has gained weight there may be mild censure or booing and derision. In some groups, the member who has gained the most weight is called "Pig of the Week" and may be required to sit in the "Pig Pen." The chapters we have seen do not use such strong punishment but do criticize the person who gains weight. Thus, both positive reinforcement (approval, praise) and punishment (public humiliation) are elements of the program. The weigh-in is the key ritual and some members leave after this part of the meeting. There is also a group called KOPS (Keep Off Pounds Sensibly) which is composed of successful TOPS members who encourage others in the group.

The TOPS program focuses on food intake rather than energy expenditure. Most sessions are devoted to strategies that decrease food intake but there is little said to encourage physical activity. The group will not allow intestinal or gastric bypass patients to join nor do they permit members to take anorexic drugs or belong to any of the health spas.

TOPS has an interesting relationship with the medical profession. The founder was encouraged by her physician during the formation of the group. The group has allowed physicians and researchers to study their program and even intervene. The majority of TOPS members have had contact with their physicians prior to joining a chapter and continued to consult their physicians during their membership, but less than 3% were referred by their physicians.[12] Even fewer of the members (less than 1%) have consulted mental health workers, psychiatrists, psychologists, or social workers. The reason for this is not clear, since the group considers overeating an emotional problem indicative of a lack of emotional control. Sometimes physicians or dieticians are invited to speak during the program and they are usually warmly welcomed. However, anger at the attitude of the medical profession toward obesity often surfaces during meetings. Members comment on the apathy of their physicians toward obesity or the derogatory remarks that their physicians have made. Many think their physicians did not adequately evaluate for the presence of either physical or emotional factors which might contribute to their obesity. Thus, the relationship TOPS has with the medical profession is an ambivalent one that probably reflects many of the feelings physicians have toward obesity.

Levitz and Stunkard[56] have reported on a novel attempt to combine behavior modification and patient self-help. Sixteen chapters of TOPS in the Philadelphia area participated in the study, in which 234 subjects received one of four treatments: behavior modification conducted by a professional therapist, behavior modification conducted by a TOPS leader, nutrition education conducted by the TOPS leader, or continuation of the usual TOPS program (control group). During treatment, fewer patients dropped out of the two behavior modification groups. At the 12-month follow-up 38% and 41% had dropped out of the behavior modification groups; 55% had dropped out of the nutrition education group; and 67% had dropped out of the control (usual TOPS program) group. During treatment more weight was lost by subjects in the behavior group conducted by the therapist (average of 4.2 pounds) than in the behavior group conducted by the TOPS leader (average of 1.9 pounds). The nutrition education group lost an average of only 0.2 pounds and in the TOPS control groups, subjects actually gained weight (average of 0.7 pounds). Furthermore, at follow-up at 12 months, subjects in groups led by a professional not only maintained their weight loss, but lost slightly more weight. In the behavior group led by a TOPS leader the subjects regained the weight they lost and the nutrition education group members had gained 4 pounds at the end of 12 months. The TOPS control group gained an average of 2.8 pounds by follow-up. In summary, the behavior modification groups led by professional therapists had the lowest attrition rate, the best success during treatment, and maintained and even increased the weight lost at the 1-year follow-up. However, even the best results in the behavior modification groups were poorer than other studies have reported. The authors suggest several reasons for this including the fact that the subjects were older and had usually already lost some weight prior to the study. Also, TOPS members may be more resistant to treatment as they have usually made several previous unsuccessful attempts at weight loss. Although weight losses were modest, if these results were extended to the 330,000 persons who belong to TOPS and the dropout rate were halved, this would be a significant contribution to the management of obesity.

In summary, TOPS has not yet been proven to be much more effective than other methods in producing weight loss, but there may be ways of improving its effectiveness. The willingness of TOPS to work with the medical profession may provide an opportunity to investigate combinations of various treatment approaches.

OVEREATERS ANONYMOUS

Overeaters Anonymous is another patient self-help group that is modeled on Alcoholics Anonymous. It has not been as widely successful as TOPS or Weight Watchers, but there may be some patients who are particularly suitable referrals. Like TOPS, this group recommends consultation with a physician before starting their diet plan. Each new member is assigned a sponsor and every day the new member contacts his sponsor and they agree on the following day's menu. The daily contact continues for at least the first few weeks of the program and some people continue calling their sponsor daily for more than a year. The diet suggested is a sensible one ranging from 800–1800 calories.

The major premise of this group is that its members are compulsive overeaters who feel powerless over food.[57] Like Alcoholics Anonymous, this group has 12 steps which are suggested as a program of recovery (Table 13.1). These include admission that the individual is powerless over food,

Table 13.1
Overeaters Anonymous: The 12 steps suggested as a program of recovery. (Reprinted with permission of AA World Services, Inc., P.O. Box 459, Grand Central Station, New York, NY 10017.)

1. We admitted we were powerless over food—that our lives had become unmanageable.
2. Came to believe that a Power greater than ourselves could restore us to sanity.
3. Made a decision to turn our will and our lives over to the care of God as we understood Him.
4. Made a searching and fearless moral inventory of ourselves.
5. Admitted to God, to ourselves and to another human being the exact nature of our wrongs.
6. Were entirely ready to have God remove all these defects of character.
7. Humbly asked Him to remove our shortcomings.
8. Made a list of all persons we had harmed, and became willing to make amends to them all.
9. Made direct amends to such people wherever possible, except when to do so would injure them or others.
10. Continued to take personal inventory and when we were wrong, promptly admitted it.
11. Sought through prayer and meditation to improve our conscious contact with God as we understood Him, praying only for knowledge of His will for us and the power to carry that out.
12. Having had a spiritual awakening as the result of these steps, we tried to carry this message to compulsive overeaters and to practice these principles in all our affairs.

belief in the power of God to restore sanity, and admission of various shortcomings. Abstinence is the guiding principle of the Overeaters Anonymous programs. This means that the person eats *only* what he and his sponsor have agreed upon for that day. During the meetings members are known only by each other's first names and the sessions are pervaded with confessions of overeating. Group members who successfully lose weight describe themselves as "saved" and "really happy for the first time" in their lives.

This group attempts to incorporate the obese person's family into the treatment plan and there are a few O-anon groups (analogous to the Alanon groups for families of alcoholics). The family is cautioned that their dieting relative will change not only his eating behavior but will also be attempting to establish his own self-worth. Thus far, these family groups have not been well attended, but the idea is interesting.

GROUP PROGRAMS AND EXERCISE

DIFFICULT TO STUDY

Exercise programs in the treatment of obesity have been given little attention. In the behavior modification programs, attention is focused almost exclusively on food intake rather than energy expenditure. Part of the reason for this is that physical activity is a behavior that does not occur as frequently in many obese persons and it is therefore more difficult to study the consequences which reinforce or punish exercise. In contrast, food intake is a behavior that is easily observed and the consequences can be analyzed. To determine why physical activity occurs less in some obese people usually requires a careful history or observation of the person when he does exercise. Many obese people tire easily when they exercise (a negative consequence which decreases the likelihood of the person exercising again, i.e., punishment) or exercise may remove a positive consequence and thus decrease the likelihood of exercise recurring. Many very obese individuals have a disturbance of body image and exercise increases their awareness of their body and often their disgust at their appearance (i.e., the consequence is punishment) and exercise becomes less likely. This sequence of events is particularly common among obese adolescent girls who refuse to take part in gym classes. Several consequences serve as punishment in this situation. Not only does the girl become more aware of her own feelings about her body, but she is frequently ridiculed by her peers, a potent punisher. Thus, she refuses to take part in sports, and she decreases her caloric expenditure even further. Since eating may remove feelings of loneliness or unhappiness (negative reinforcement) eating may occur more often and further increase the girl's obesity.

As noted earlier, exercise increases energy expenditure in several ways and thus a program which incorporates an increase in activity level may be helpful in weight reduction. Several methods for achieving this goal have been attempted, but none has been dramatically successful. These include commercial enterprises such as figure salons, exercise clubs, and health spas, as well as medically-sanctioned programs such as exercise groups for patients with particular health problems.

COMMERCIAL ENTERPRISES

The commercial enterprises designed to result in weight loss through exercise have suffered from poor management and sometimes outright charlatanism. However, the idea of some exercise programs is sound. One exercise salon in Tampa requires a physician's permission to join, then gives each new member a diet tailored to his ideal weight and a series of exercises. Although the exercises are primarily designed to improve the figure rather than increase energy expenditure, for many obese subjects this very mild activity has several beneficial effects. First, it begins an increase in physical activity at a level that can be tolerated. Second, it results in a decrease in hunger immediately after exercise. Third, and perhaps most importantly, it alters the routine of many obese subjects who overeat at night; instead of sitting home watching television and snacking, the obese person who attends the spa in the evening may avoid the most tempting eating situation. Several of the best exercise programs have incorporated the principles of behavior modification. If weight or inches are lost, the attendants congratulate the person and they may be awarded tickets for a drawing for every pound or inch lost (positive reinforcement). Also, the names of successful individuals and inches or pounds lost are posted. Encouragement is given to members who have not lost weight and they are not criticized. Diet suggestions are offered by the leaders and group attendance is encouraged.

Not all the treatment offered at exercise salons is helpful. Nearly all utilize various devices to produce spot reduction in hips, waist, or thighs. These include massage, rollers, belts, etc. Early studies in the 1930's[58] suggested that massage might have a metabolic effect. However, Kalb[59] studied 40 patients on an 800-calorie diet during which 20 patients received massage twice a week. There was a loss of weight in both groups and reduction in the size of the arms and thighs, but the group that received massage did not have greater reduction.

EXERCISE PROGRAMS FOR OBESE CORONARY PATIENTS

Groups of obese patients with specific ailments, particularly post-coronary subjects, have sometimes formed exercise groups. At the University of South Florida a group of moderately obese coronary patients belong to a medically supervised jogging group. The level of exercise is monitored and increased in accordance with the individual's pulse rate. This exercise plan is designed primarily to increase the functional capacity of the heart, but is also predicted to result in a decrease in fat stores. This is a pilot project and results are not yet available. In any such project it is, of course, vital that patients be carefully selected and monitored since overenthusiastic exercise can be lethal. Also, obese coronary patients are more prone to sudden death, and exercise could be a stress that triggers the terminal event.

AEROBIC DANCING

Another group approach that may hold promise for obese patients is aerobic dancing.[60] Developed by a former dancer, this is a technique that allows the person to increase his tolerance to exercise in an enjoyable group. Members of the group must have their physicians' permission to join the group. The founder choreographs new dance steps to certain tapes and records, and leaders in individual chapters teach group members the new dance routines. Each member determines the working pulse range of his heart and periodically takes his pulse to ensure that he is not exceeding a safe range; if so, the group member either rests temporarily or is less energetic in the dance routine. Although this program was designed for the normal weight individual, with medical supervision certain selected obese patients might benefit from a modified program of aerobic dancing.

Unfortunately most of these group approaches have not been scientifically investigated. The plethora of groups—aerobic dancing, coronary jogging, clubs, and dance therapy—suggests that exercise groups may become part of a holistic treatment program for obesity.

IMPORTANCE OF FAMILY COOPERATION

The family is of crucial importance in the treatment of obesity. A dieter often finds it very difficult to remain on his diet if he is surrounded by people who eat as they wish. Sometimes families actively discourage relatives from dieting and may say they look frail or sick if they do lose weight and encourage them to overeat. This may reflect a cultural or ethnic attitude toward body appearance, and encouragement to eat may represent genuine caring for the dieter. However, at times the motivation for encouraging the person to eat may arise from the family member's own unconscious needs. One obese teenage girl came to our clinic for evaluation with her slender, attractive mother who said she had given up trying to encourage her daughter to diet. She would purchase cookies and sweets and bring them home to her daughter who watched hours of television. After several psychotherapy sessions with the mother, it was learned that mother and daughter were in competition for the father's affection, and that the mother was fearful that if her daughter lost weight she would successfully eliminate her mother from the competition for the father. In this situation, a diet and exercise program were initially inappropriate. The first step was to engage the father and mother in therapy to solidify their relationship so that the mother could genuinely encourage her daughter's weight loss.

Marital interactions can have a tremendous impact on eating practices. One obese 32-year-old woman weighed 250 pounds and began losing weight on a behavior modification program. When she was under 200 pounds and began to wear attractive clothes and make-up, her husband began to accuse her of having sexual affairs and subtly sabotaged her diet by taking her out to French restaurants and bringing her gifts of high calorie foods. It became increasingly clear that her husband feared that if she were attractive and self-confident that she would leave him for someone else. Marital therapy was started and the patient's husband eventually accepted his wife's genuine affection for him and was able to encourage her in her new eating behavior.

Another couple had a more complex difficulty. The patient was a 20-year-old woman who was 20 pounds overweight with the binge-eating syndrome and an obsessive-compulsive personality. She lived with a 54-year-old man who looked like her father and had the same interpersonal style as her father. She related to him in a child-like way, begging him to help her lose weight and control her binges one day, and the next day pleading with him to go to the store to buy her various high calorie snacks. He found himself in an intolerable position because when he refused to shop for her she became tearful and angry and accused him of not loving her. If he did shop for her she felt guilty about eating and castigated herself unmercifully. She was in individual psychotherapy and he came to sessions intermittently. When he finally realized the no-win doublebind situation he was in vis-à-vis shopping for her, he was able to refuse to shop for her and she called her psychiatrist to talk about her consequent feelings of rejection. This young woman faithfully reproduced her hostile dependent relationship with her father in her relationship with her boyfriend.

In patients who have developmental obesity as described by Bruch,[2] the family interaction may actually be the cause of the child's obesity and should be the focus for therapy. The obese adolescent teenager is often the identified patient. Bruch believes these obese youngsters are used to meet the parents' own needs, and these youngsters grow up unaware of their own thoughts and feelings and are also unaware of their own internal bodily states. Consequently, overeating may be used to assuage loneliness or depression, to alleviate boredom, or to hide anger. This theory has not been proven, but Bruch reports very successful results in developmentally obese youngsters treated with family and individual psychotherapy. Although she gives very lucid descriptions of the families she has seen, she offers no overall statistical results of treatment, either in terms of weight loss or psychosocial functioning.

Family therapy can be useful in the treatment of obesity. The principles of this form of treatment are beyond the scope of this book, but two approaches that have been helpful will be reviewed.[61] Some families with an obese youngster are overly involved with the problem. One technique that has been useful to us is to focus on the problems of other family members during the family therapy sessions. If an obese girl has come as the identified patient, the sessions may be spent discussing the asthmatic attacks of the younger brother and the emotional factors that intensify the asthmatic episodes. When the obese girl is no longer the focus of the family attention, she may be able to become more independent or feel less guilty. Another approach that has proven even more useful is to help the family establish intergenerational boundaries. The mother and obese daughter may be overinvolved, with the mother choosing the daughter's clothes, friends, etc. A reestablishment of the husband-wife dyad as separate from the children may facilitate the growth and development of the daughter.

In some situations, the family factors that encourage overeating seem to be less psychiatrically ominous and may only represent lack of knowledge or habit patterns. Several techniques have been used to increase the nutritional knowledge and emotional support of relatives. Some programs require the most important family member to visit the dietician with the obese patient. Jordan and Levitz[62] treated one group of obese adolescent girls by teaching their mothers the principles of behavior modification. An interesting finding in this study was that the children of normal weight mothers lost more weight than the children of obese mothers. It may be that successful treatment of obese youngsters may be impossible without involvement of significant family members.

Brownell[63] has studied spouse involvement in the management of obesity, and has recently reported a pilot study comparing the results of three behavior modification groups. The spouses of all subjects were asked if they would attend the group sessions and participate in additional training. In one group there were couples training, with spouses attending the group sessions and receiving additional training, including learning to model appropriate behavior, assisting in stimulus control, and employment of behavior incompatible with overeating. The second group consisted of obese subjects only, but their spouses had agreed to attend the group sessions. These two groups were called the cooperative spouse groups. The third group consisted of the obese subjects alone, whose spouses had not agreed to attend the group or receive additional training (the non-cooperative spouse group). At the end of treatment, there was an average 20-pound weight loss in the cooperative attending spouse group, a 15-pound average weight loss in the cooperative non-attending spouse group, and only a 10-pound weight loss in the non-cooperative spouse group. At the 3-month follow-up, these trends continued, with additional losses in each group, but least in the non-cooperative spouse group. These findings signal the need for family participation in any program designed to treat obesity.

TREATMENT OF BODY IMAGE DISTURBANCES

The pediatrician and family physician can sometimes help prevent the development of a body image disturbance. Disturbances in the attitudinal aspect of body image may be fixed during adolescence and subsequent treatment is very difficult. Most relatives do not realize that teasing about weight or belittling the obese youngster's appearance can have lasting deleterious effects. If the physician enlists the support of the family and encourages them to accept the person as he is, a body image disturbance may be averted, even if no weight is lost.

PSYCHOANALYSIS

Achievement of ideal weight does not necessarily result in an improvement of body image disturbance. The individual may behave as though he is still large or may still consider his or her body unattractive or grotesque. Successful bypass patients may still consider their bodies loathesome or abnormally large. Initially it was suspected that weight loss may have been too rapid for the body image to adjust. However, no marked improvement has been noted in body image disturbance in some patients even after weight has been stable for many months (See Chapter 12). Since an emotional disturbance seems to be a necessary but insufficient condition for the development of a body image distortion, it seems likely that this emotional disturbance must be corrected to treat the body image problem. These ideas are supported by the findings of Rand and Stunkard[1] who studied obese patients in psychoanalysis for several years. Not only did they lose weight, but their self-concept and body image improved. Bypass patients generally do not participate in intensive psychotherapy, and hence, underlying emotional conflicts are not resolved and this may be a prerequisite to an improved body image.

DANCE THERAPY

In addition to psychoanalysis, several other methods may prove useful as part of the treatment for body image disturbances. Dance therapy[64] or movement therapy is a relatively new treatment modality that has yet to be fully integrated into the mainstream of psychiatry. Dance therapists contend that verbal therapy is effective only for problems that have a verbal representation, and they feel that many symptoms arise from non-verbal conflicts. Movement is believed to both reflect and influence emotions. For instance, a patient who is depressed may stare at the ground, move slowly, and have a circumscribed kinesphere. A kinesphere is the area around a person that can be reached by any part of his body. Some people never put their arms over their heads or reach behind themselves or toward other people, and are thus said to have a circumscribed kinesphere. Obese patients who are less active may be particularly likely to have such circumscribed movements. Dance therapy designed to increase their range of movements would increase their level of activity as well as awareness of their own body. Conceivably, this might result in an improved perception of their body, although verbal psychotherapy would doubtless be needed as part of a comprehensive treatment program.

The major problem with dance therapy has been its close association with certain extreme elements in psychiatry that sometimes border on charlatanism. Wilhelm Reich[65] posited that people have character armour which may be expressed in the presence or absence of certain body movements. He believed that what the person meant could be best understood by how he said it and his actions. This very valid point has been enthusiastically endorsed and elaborated by movement therapists. Unfortunately, other less valid ideas of Reich's have also been incorporated into dance therapy philosophy. The infamous orgone box was designed by Reich and consisted of a box covered with alternating layers of rock and steel wool that supposedly trap orgone energy from the atmosphere. Reich believed that people with various diseases, including cancer, could be cured by being placed in the orgone box and he distributed these boxes around the country. Although this was demonstrated to be nonsense long ago, it is a current topic of lively interest in dance therapy circles. Such uncritical acceptance of all of Reich's ideas militates against acceptance of dance therapy into the mainstream of psychiatric treatment. This is unfortunate, since dance therapy may be useful in the treatment of many conditions, including body image disturbances.

HOLISTIC TREATMENT PROGRAMS

Obesity is a complex condition that is notoriously resistant to treatment. Various specialists treat obesity in specialized ways: psychologists use behavior modification, psychoanalysts use long-term intensive psychotherapy, surgeons perform bypass operations, and internists emphasize dietary approaches. It is likely that the most effective treatment plans in the future will be those which incorporate an individualized evaluation and utilize the skills of a wide range of specialists.

An interesting recent development has been the eating disorders clinics which have sprung up across the country, usually as specialty clinics at a university. A major characteristic of these clinics is that they are interdisciplinary efforts with a complete evaluation, including medical history, physical examination, social history, dietary history, and psychiatric evaluation. The best clinics include an internist, psychiatrist, pediatrician, dietician, and psychologist as a minimum staff. Usually research and evaluation of the effectiveness of treatment is an integral part of such programs.

Figure 13.4 illustrates one possible evaluation sequence for an eating

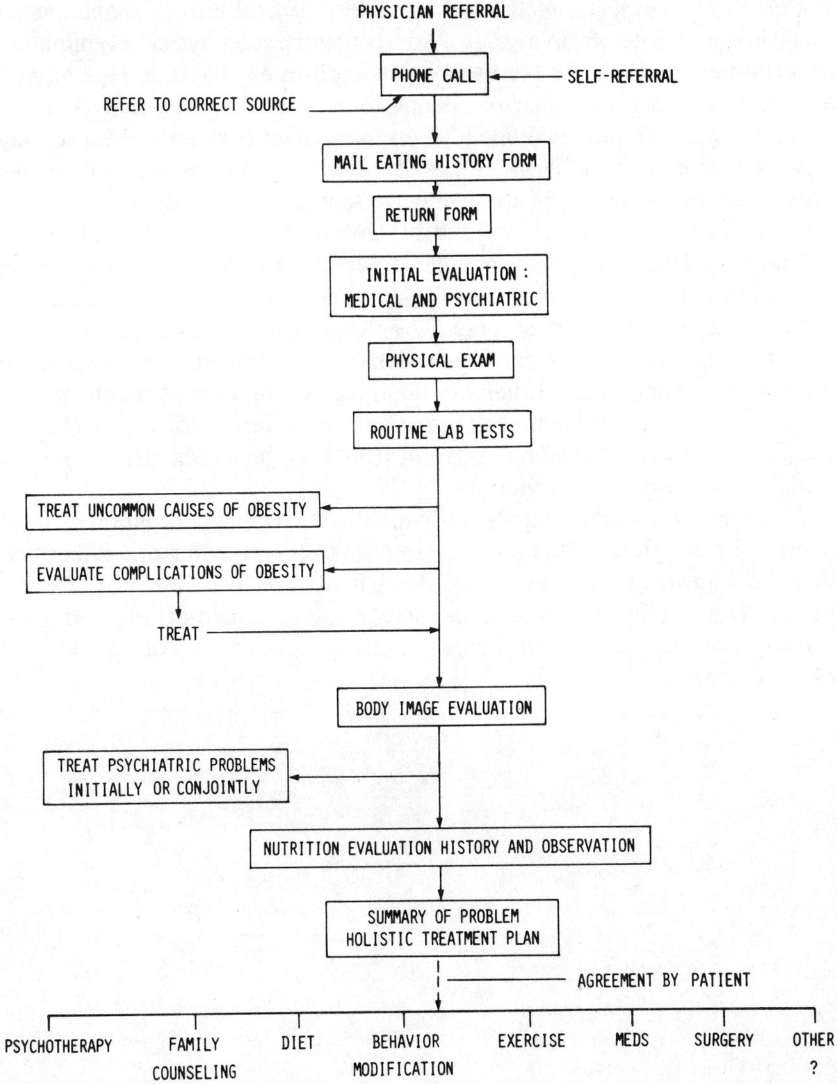

Figure 13.4. Eating disorders clinic: evaluation sequence at the University of South Florida Eating Disorders Clinic.

disorders clinic. After the patient calls the clinic, or is referred to the clinic, he is sent the Stanford Eating Disorders Form. The patient is only seen after completion of this questionnaire, as Agras and colleagues have found it to be an effective screening device. At Stanford[66] there were 374 contacts with the eating disorders clinic and 168 questionnaires were distributed; 101 forms were returned and 87 of these patients were also retained. Since the dropout rate from obesity treatment programs is very high, any method which identifies patients who will continue in treatment is useful.

At the first visit a complete psychiatric and medical history is obtained, a social history elicited from available family members, a physical examination is performed, and routine laboratory tests performed. The rare patient with an uncommon organic cause of his obesity is treated and patients with the sequelae of obesity are evaluated. Then the patient is evaluated for a body image disturbance, usually by a Draw-A-Person test. Those with body image distortions or evidence of moderate or severe psychiatric problems are referred for preliminary or conjoint psychiatric treatment. Then there is a nutritional evaluation which includes observation of the individual during one or more meals in the laboratory. This work-up can usually be completed in two, or at the most three, sessions. The clinical team meets and summarizes their findings including recommendations. Some patients are referred for individual psychotherapy initially in situations where weight loss may trigger serious psychiatric problems. Some patients are referred for psychotherapy with a behavior modification program (this may be either at the clinic or TOPS or Overeaters Anonymous).

In summary, a well designed individualized treatment program is most likely to be helpful to obese patients. Interdisciplinary teamwork will ensure that the knowledge and expertise of all fields are available to the obese person. Other treatment modalities include exercise, medication, and occasionally referral for possible bypass surgery. Appendix 5 lists the current eating disorders clinics.[67]

APPENDIX 4

Food Management Questionnaire

(Reprinted with permission from D. B. Jeffrey and R. C. Katz[14])

Directions: Write the letter (a), (b), or (c) in the column that most represents your food habits.

(a) (b) (c)

I. Buying Food

1. Do you usually go to the grocery store (a) without a written food list, (b) with some ideas in your head about what to buy (but no list), (c) with a written food list? c
2. Do you usually buy (a) whatever meets your fancy in the aisles and on the shelves, (b) more than you originally had on your list, (c) from your food list only? c
3. Do you usually shop (a) when you are hungry, (b) whenever you need to, (c) when you are not hungry? b
4. Do you usually purchase (a) unnecessary quantities of most foods, (b) unnecessary quantities of some foods, (c) only moderate quantities of food? c
5. Do you buy mostly (a) high-calorie foods, (b) a combination of high- and low-calorie foods, or (c) low-calorie nutritious foods? c

II. Storing Food

1. Do you usually store food in (a) transparent accessible containers in the refrigerator, (b) whatever is handy, or (c) in opaque (non-see-through) difficult-to-reach containers in the refrigerator? b
2. Do you usually store food in (a) transparent, easy-to-reach containers in the cupboards, (b) whatever is handy, or (c) in opaque difficult-to-reach containers in the cupboards? b
3. Do you (a) usually leave food on the kitchen countertop, in the living room, or in the TV room, (b) sometimes leave food on the kitchen countertop, in the living room, or in the TV room, or (c) almost never leave food on

the kitchen countertop, in the living room, or in the TV room?

III. Preparing Food

1. (a) Do others usually prepare your food, or (b) do you usually prepare your own food?
2. Do you (or others) usually prepare (a) high-calorie meals or (b) low-calorie meals?
3. Do you (or others) usually prepare (a) quantities of food for more than one helping or (b) quantities sufficient for only *one* helping?

IV. Serving Food

1. (a) Do others usually serve your food, or (b) do you usually serve your own food?
2. Do you usually serve (a) more than you need, or (b) a moderate portion?
3. Do you usually serve yourself (a) second portions or (b) only one portion?
4. Do you usually (a) put bowls or food containers on the table or (b) leave them in the kitchen?

V. Eating

1. Do you put (a) a large or (b) a small quantity of food on your spoon or fork?
2. Do you chew your food (a) rapidly or (b) slowly?
3. Do you (a) put one bite of food after another into your mouth or (b) wait between bites?
4. Do you (a) eat so fast you don't have time to enjoy your food or (b) do you eat slowly enough to enjoy it thoroughly?
5. Do you (a) eat all the food in front of you or (b) stop eating when you're full, even though there's food on your plate?

VI. Cleaning-Up

1. After eating do you (a) sit around or (b) leave the table?
2. After finishing the main dish do you (a) leave the leftovers on the table or (b) clear the table before having a cup of coffee or tea?

VII. Snacking

1. Do you snack (a) frequently (say, more than three times daily) or (b) occasionally? a
2. Do you snack (a) large quantities of food (e.g., a sandwich and a piece of cake) or (b) small quantities of food? b
3. Do you snack (a) high-calorie foods (e.g., cookies) or (b) low-calorie foods (e.g., celery and carrots)? b

Total number (a) responses ______

Total number (b) responses ______

Total number (c) responses ______

Add up the number of (b) and (c) responses. 16 or more indicate a good set of food management behaviors.

APPENDIX 5

Directory of Medical Center Weight Control Clinics

(Adapted and reprinted with permission from Behavioral Medicine[67])

Center for Effective Living
Granville Medical Center Bldg.
Weaver Dr., P.O. Box 498
Granville, OH 43023
(614) 587-4734
Contact: Gordon Kimbrell, MD
Established: 1976
Patient preferences: Adults
Hours: By appointment
Fees: $100 for initial evaluation; $15 per group session; $25 per individual session
Minimum commitment: 4 weeks for behavioral evaluation of eating habits; 10–24 treatment sessions (by individual contract)
Primary treatment modality: Behavioral

Center for Optimal growth
50 Severance Circle
Cleveland Heights, OH 44118
(216) 291-1100, ext. 417
Contact: Mary E. Wheeler, PhD
Established: 1975
Patient preferences: Children between 2–18
Hours: Monday–Friday, 9 AM–5 PM
Fees: Contact Center
Minimum commitment: Long-term follow-up
Primary treatment modality: Behavioral

Clinic for Eating Disorders
Dept. of Psychiatry, University of Cincinnati
231 Bethesda Ave.
Cincinnati, OH 45267
(513) 872-5118
Contact: Susan Dyrenforth; Wayne Wooley, PhD
Established: 1974
Patient preferences: Adolescents and Adults
Hours: Monday–Friday, 9 AM–5 PM
Fees: $35 for initial interviews; $35 per session
Minimum commitment: 15 weeks
Primary treatment modality: Behavioral

Correspondence Weight Reduction
University of Southern California
734 W. Adams Blvd.
Los Angeles, CA 90007
(213) 741-2287
Contact: Albert Marston, PhD
Established: 1976
Patient preferences: Adults
Hours: Correspondence program
Fees: $150
Primary treatment modality: Behavioral

Dietary Rehabilitation Clinic
Duke University Medical Center
Health Service Division
Box 2914
Durham, NC 27710
(919) 684-8111
Contact: Suzanne Roberts; Bert Loro, PhD; Sigrid J. Nelius, MD
Established: 1972

Patient preferences: Adults
Hours: Monday–Friday, 8 AM–5 PM
Fees: Contact Clinic
Minimum commitment: 4 weeks
Primary treatment modality: Combined

Dietetic Consult Service
Peter Bent Brigham Hospital
721 Huntington Ave.
Boston, MA 02115
(617) 732-6000
Contact: Wendy Midgley; Helene Fuchs
Established: 1946
Patient preferences: Adolescents and Adults
Hours: Monday–Friday, 9 AM–4 PM
Fees: Contact hospital registration office
Primary treatment modality: Nutritional

Food Habits Management Program
Adult Development Program
University of Washington
Rm. 122, Coach House
4701 24th St., NE
Seattle, WA 98105
(206) 543-0936
Contact: Julie Waltz; Cornelius Bakker, MD
Established: 1972
Patient preferences: Adolescents and Adults
Hours: Monday–Friday, 8:30 AM–4 PM
Fees: Contact Program
Minimum commitment: 6–16 weeks, depending on treatment program
Primary treatment modality: Combined

Frances Stern Nutrition Center
185 Harrison Ave.
Boston, MA 02111
(617) 956-5273
Contact: Johanna Dwyer, PhD
Established: 1918
Patient preferences: All ages
Hours: Monday–Friday,
Fees: Contact Center
Minimum commitment: Individual
Primary treatment modality: Nutritional

Heart Health for Diet and Weight Control
Stanford Heart Disease Prevention Program
Stanford University Medical Center
Stanford, CA 94305
(415) 327-2873
Contact: Susan Wengert
Established: 1977
Client preferences: Adults
Hours: Evenings
Fees: Contact Program
Primary treatment modality: Educational

Institute for Behavioral Education
1000 Valley Forge Circle
Suite 105
King of Prussia, PA 19406
(215) 783-0150
Contact: Henry A. Jordan, MD; Leonard Levitz, MD
Established: 1971
Patient preferences: Adults
Hours: Wednesday–Thursday, 9 AM–5 PM
Fees: $575
Minimum commitment: 5 months
Primary treatment modality: Behavioral

Methodist Hospital Weight Control Program
6516 Bertner
Mail Station M.S. 121
Houston, TX 77030
(713) 790-2166
Contact: Lynne Scott, MS
Established: 1977
Patient preferences: Adolescents and Adults
Hours: Monday–Thursday, 9 AM–5 PM
Fees: $100
Minimum commitment: 8 weeks
Primary treatment modality: Behavioral

The New Weigh of Life—Behavioral Management for Weight Control
LDS Hospital
325 8th Ave.
Salt Lake City, UT 84143
(801) 350-1731
Contact: Timothy Butler
Established: 1976
Patient preferences: Adults
Hours: Tuesday, Wednesday, Thursday afternoons
Fees: $15 for initial interview; $125 ($25 refundable upon completion of program); $25 per session
Minimum commitment: 1 1/2 yrs.
Primary treatment modality: Behavioral

North Shore University Hospital Obesity Center
Community Drive
Manhasset, NY 11030
(516) 562-4635
Contact: Ruth Waldbaum, MD
Established: 1975
Patient preferences: Children and Adolescents
Hours: Thursday afternoons
Fees: $20 per session for private patients; scaled down for clinic patients
Primary treatment modality: Behavioral

Nutritional Clinic
Massachusetts General Hospital
Fruit St.
Boston, MA 02144
(617) 726-2779
Contact: Alma Blake
Established: 1974
Patient preferences: Adults
Hours: Monday–Friday, 9 AM–5 PM
Fees: Contact Clinic
Primary treatment modality: Behavioral

Nutrition and Bariatric Associates
Cedars of Lebanon Hospital
South Bldg., Suite A
1295 NW 14th St.
Miami, FL 33125
(305) 545-7666
Contact: Leonard Haimes, MD
Established: 1976
Patient preferences: All ages
Hours: Tuesday, Wednesday, Thursday, 9 AM–5 PM
Fees: Contact Associates
Minimum commitment: 12 weeks
Primary treatment modality: Combined

University of South Florida Eating Disorders Clinic
Dept. of Psychiatry
College of Medicine
12901 No. 30th St.
Tampa, FL 33612
(813) 974-4242
Contact: Pauline S. Powers, M.D.
Established: 1979
Patient preferences: Adults and Adolescents
Hours: Tuesday afternoons
Fees: Contact clinic
Minimum commitment: Individual
Primary treatment modality: Combined

Vanderbilt Weight Management Program
Dept. of Psychology
Vanderbilt University
Nashville, TN 37240
(615) 322-2874
Contact: Martin Katahn, PhD; John Pleas, PhD
Established: 1976
Patient preferences: Adults (for intensive clinical program, patients must be at least 50 pounds overweight)
Hours: Depends on program selected
Fees: Depends on program selected
Programs: 1. Educational program; 10–16 week commitment; $65. 2. Weight management specialist training; 9 months commitment and one year's work in field; contact Dr. Katahn for fee schedule. 3. Intensive clinical program; 6 months commitment; $650.00
Primary treatment modality: Combined

The Weight Control Center of the Obesity Research Center
St. Luke's Hospital Center
411 W. 114th St., Suite 2D
New York, NY 10025
(212) 870-1743
Contact: Andrea G. Denison, RN; Robert Bernstein, MD
Established: 1977
Patient preferences: Adolescents and Adults
Hours: Monday–Friday, 9 AM–5 PM
Fees: Contact Center
Minimum commitment: Individual
Primary treatment modality: Combined

Weight Management Clinic
Medical University of South Carolina
171 Ashley Ave.
Charleston, SC 29403
(803) 792-2971
Contact: Hal Currey
Established: 1974
Patient preferences: Adolescents and Adults
Hours: Wednesday afternoons
Fees: $100.00
Minimum commitment: 12 weeks
Primary treatment modality: Behavioral

References

1. Rand CS, Stunkard AJ: Psychoanalysis and obesity. J Am Acad Psychoanal 5: 459–497, 1977.
2. Bruch H: Eating Disorders: Obesity, Anorexia Nervosa and the Person Within. New York, Basic Books, 1973.
3. Schachter S, Goldman R, Gordon A: Effects of fear, food deprivation, and obesity on eating. J Pers Soc Psychol 10: 91–97, 1968.
4. Teitelbaum P, Campbell BA: Ingestion patterns in hyperphagic and normal rats. J Comp Physiol Psychol 51: 135–141, 1958.
5. Stunkard A, Koch C: The interpretation of gastric motility. I. Apparent bias in the reports of hunger by obese persons. Arch Gen Psychiatry 11: 74–82, 1964.
6. Nisbett RE: Determinants of food intake in human obesity. Science 159: 1254–1255, 1968.
7. Schachter S, cited in Stunkard AJ: From explanation to action in psychosomatic medicine: the case of obesity. Psychosom Med 37: 195–236, 1975.
8. Johnson WG: The effect of prior taste and food visibility on the food directed instrumental performance of obese individuals. Unpublished doctoral dissertation, Catholic Univ of America, 1970, cited in Schachter S: Some extraordinary facts about obese humans and rats. Am Psychol 26: 129–144, 1971.
9. Schachter S: Some extraordinary facts about obese humans and rats. Am Psychol 26: 129–144, 1971.
10. Nisbett R, Kanouse D: Obesity, food deprivation and supermarket shopping behavior. J Pers Soc Psychol 12: 289–294, 1969.
11. Wooley SC: Physiologic versus cognitive factors in short-term regulation in the obese and non-obese. Psychosom Med 34: 62–68, 1972.
12. Stunkard AJ: From explanation to action in psychosomatic medicine: the case of obesity. Psychosom Med 37: 195–236, 1975.
13. Kazdin AE: Self-monitoring and behavior change. In: Self-Control: Power to the Person. Mahoney MJ, Thoresen CE (eds). Monterey, Brooks/Cole, 1974, cited in Stunkard AJ: From explanation to action in psychosomatic medicine: the case of obesity. Psychosom Med 37: 195–236, 1975.
14. Jeffrey DB, Katz RC: Take It Off and Keep It Off. Englewood Cliffs, NJ, Prentice-Hall, Inc, 1977.
15. Brightwell DR: New Eating Behavior: Practical Management of Obesity. I. Physician's Guide to Behavior Therapy in Treating Obesity. New York, Penwalt Corp, 1975.
16. Smiciklas-Wright H, D'Augelli AR: Preliminary prevention for overweight: preschool eating patterns (PEP) program. J Am Diet Assoc 72: 626–629, 1978.
17. Mahoney MJ: Fat fiction. Behav Ther 6: 416–418, 1975.
18. Stuart RB, Davis B: Slim Chance in a Fat World. Champaign, Ill, Research Press Co, 1972, pp 66–98.
19. Schachter S, Rodin J (eds): Obese Humans and Rats. Potomac, MD, Lawrence Erlbaum Assoc, 1974, cited in Milich RS: A critical analysis of Schachter's externality theory of obesity. J Abnorm Psychol 84: 586–588, 1975.
20. Mahoney MJ: Self-reward and self-monitoring techniques for weight control. Behav Ther 5: 48–57, 1974.
21. Brightwell DR: Treating obesity with behavior modification. Postgrad Med 55: 52–58, 1974.
22. Brownell KD, Stunkard AJ: Behavioral treatment of obesity in children. Am J Dis Child 132: 403–412, 1978.
23. Jacobson E: Progressive Relaxation. Chicago, Univ of Chicago Press, 1938.
24. Birk L: Behavior therapy and behavioral psychotherapy. In: Harvard Guide to Modern Psychiatry. Nicholi AM Jr (ed). Cambridge, Belknap Press of Harvard Univ Press, 1978, p 441.
25. Wolpe J: Psychotherapy by Reciprocal Inhibition. Stanford, Stanford Univ Press, 1958, cited in Birk L: Behavior therapy and behavioral psychotherapy. In: Harvard Guide to Modern Psychiatry. Nicholi AM Jr (ed). Cambridge, Belknap Press of Harvard Univ Press, 1978, p 446.
26. Lazarus AA: Behavior Therapy and Beyond. New York, McGraw-Hill, 1971.

27. Mahoney MJ, Mahoney K: Treatment of obesity: a clinical exploration. In: Obesity: Behavioral Approaches to Dietary Management. Williams BJ, Martin S, Foreyt JP (eds). New York, Brunner/Mazel, 1976, pp 30–39.
28. Beck A: Cognitive therapy: nature and relation to behavior therapy. Behav Ther 1: 184–200, 1970.
29. Stunkard AJ, McLaren-Hume M: The results of treatment of obesity: a review of the literature and report of a series. Arch Intern Med 103: 79–85, 1959.
30. Stuart RB: Behavioral control of overeating. Beh Res Ther 5: 357–365, 1967.
31. Harris MB: Self-directed program for weight control: a pilot study. J Abnorm Psychol 74: 263–270, 1969.
32. Penick SB, Filion R, Fox S, Stunkard AJ: Behavior modification in the treatment of obesity. Psychosom Med 33: 49–55, 1971.
33. Currey H, Malcolm R, Riddle E, Schachte M: Behavioral treatment of obesity: limitations and results with the chronically obese. JAMA 237: 2829–2831, 1977.
34. Musante GJ: The behavioral approach to the management of obesity. Cont Ed 7: 24–31, 1977.
35. Stunkard AJ, Penick SB: Behavior modification in the treatment of obesity: the problem of maintaining weight loss. Arch Gen Psychiatry 36: 801–806, 1979.
36. Brightwell DR, Sloan CL: Long-term results of behavior therapy for obesity. Behav Ther 8: 898–905, 1977.
37. Ashby WA, Wilson GT: Behavior therapy for obesity: booster sessions and long term maintenance of weight loss. Behav Res Ther 15: 451–463, 1977.
38. Kingsley RG, Wilson GT: Behavior therapy for obesity: a comparative investigation of long term efficacy. J Consult Clin Psychol 45: 288–298, 1977.
39. Revinus TM, Drummond T, Combrinck-Graham L: A group behavior treatment program for overweight children: results of a pilot study. Pediatr Adolescent Endocrinol 1: 55–61, 1976.
40. Kingsley RG, Shapiro J: A comparison of three behavioral programs for the control of obesity in children. Behav Ther 8: 30–36, 1977.
41. Foreyt JP, Kennedy WA: Treatment of overweight by aversion therapy. Behav Res Ther 9: 29–34, 1971.
42. Ley P, Bradshaw PW, Kincey JA, et al: Psychological variables in the control of obesity. In: Obesity Symposium. Burland WL, Samuel PD, Yudkins J (eds). Edinburgh, Churchill Livingston, 1974, pp 316–337.
43. Powers PS, Holland P, Miller C: Transswitching: classical conditioning in the treatment of obesity. In preparation 1979.
44. Kimmel HD, Ray RL: Transswitching: conditioning with tonic and phasic stimuli. J Exp Psychol (Gen) 107: 187–205, 1978.
45. Winkelstein LB: Hypnosis, diet, and weight reduction. NY State J Med 59: 1751–1756, 1959.
46. Joaquin AH: Brief group treatment of obesity through ancillary self-hypnosis. Am J Clin Hypnosis 19: 231–234, 1977.
47. London AJ, Schreiber ED: A controlled study of the effects of group discussions and an anorexiant in outpatient treatment of obesity. Ann Intern Med 65: 80–92, 1966.
48. Munves ED: Dietetic interview or group discussion-decision in reducing. J Am Diet Assoc 29: 1197–1203, 1953.
49. Bowser LJ, Trulson MF, Bowling RC, Stare FJ: Methods of reducing: group therapy vs individual clinic interview. J Am Diet Assoc 29: 1193–1196, 1953.
50. Holt H, Winick C: Group psychotherapy with obese women. Arch Gen Psychiatry 5: 156–168, 1961.
51. Bray GA: The Obese Patient. Philadelphia, WB Saunders, 1976, p 329.
52. Stunkard AJ, Levine H, Fox, S: The management of obesity: patient self-help and medical treatment. Arch Intern Med 125: 1067–1072, 1970.
53. Stunkard AJ: The success of TOPS, a self-help group. Postgrad Med 51: 143–147, 1972.
54. Garb JR, Stunkard AJ: A further assessment of the effectiveness of TOPS in the control of obesity. Arch Intern Med 134: 716–720, 1974.
55. Wagonfeld S, Wolowitz HM: Obesity and the self-help group: a look at TOPS. Am J Psychiatry 125: 145–148, 1968.

56. Levitz LS, Stunkard AJ: A therapeutic coalition for obesity: behavior modification and patient self-help. Am J Psychiatry 131: 423–427, 1974.
57. Overeaters Anonymous: A program for compulsive eaters. World Service Office, 2190 190th St, Torrance, CA 90504.
58. Cuthbertson DP: The effect of massage on the metabolism of normal individuals. Q J Med 1: 387–400, 1932.
59. Kalb SW: The fallacy of massage in the treatment of obesity. J Med Soc NJ 41: 406–407, 1944.
60. Aerobic Dancing, Inc, c/o J Sorensen, 38325 Fitzgerald Circle, Freemont, CA. 94536.
61. Minuchin S, Rosman BL, Baker L: Psychosomatic Families: Anorexia Nervosa in Context. Cambridge, Harvard Univ Press, 1978.
62. Jordan HA, Levitz LS: Behavior modification in the treatment of childhood obesity. Curr Concepts Nutr 3: 141–150, 1975.
63. Brownell K: Family intervention and drug treatments. Presentation at 132nd Annual Meeting American Psychiatric Assoc, May 16, 1979, Chicago, Ill.
64. Smallwood JC: Dance-movement therapy: Current Psychiatric Therapies, Vol 14. Masserman JH (ed). New York, Grune & Stratton, Inc, 1974.
65. Elkind D: Wilhelm Reich. In: Comprehensive Textbook of Psychiatry II. Freedman AM, Kaplan HI, Sadock BJ (eds). Baltimore, Williams & Wilkins, 1975, pp 650–654.
66. Agras WS, Ferguson JM, Greaves C, et al: A clinical and research questionnaire for obese patients. In: Obesity: Behavioral Approaches to Dietary Management. Williams BJ, Martin S, Foreyt JP (eds). New York, Brunner/Mazel Inc, 1976, pp 168–176.
67. Directory of medical vender weight control clinics. Behav Med, July 1978, p 44.

CHAPTER

14

Prevention

Although prevention of disease has never been as popular as treatment, in the last decade two major findings have captured the attention of the practicing physician. The increasing incidence of severe coronary artery disease and the elucidation of the major risk factors in several broad epidemiological studies have clearly indicated the urgent need for preventive measures. The fact that atherosclerotic heart disease is often silent until a fatal myocardial infarction highlights the need for early identification of the patient at risk, before clinical presentation of disease.

A risk factor is defined as a personal characteristic which is associated with an excess rate of development of disease. In the Framingham study,[1] a broadly-based longitudinal prospective epidemiological study, several risk factors for coronary artery disease have been identified, including cigarette smoking, hypertension, diabetes, Type A personality, high cholesterol levels, and probably obesity. Although obesity *per se* is apparently not a potent risk factor,[2] obesity does predispose to hypertension, diabetes, and hypercholesterolemia, conditions which increase the likelihood of coronary heart disease dramatically. The Western life style with a high lipid, high sodium, high calorie diet, and decreased activity levels appears to be responsible for the rising incidence of both atherosclerosis and obesity. Furthermore, the origins of the risk factors are probably in childhood. Autopsies of casualties in the Korean War[3] showed relatively advanced atherosclerotic changes in the vessels of even young men in their late teens and early 20's. Changes in the coronary arteries of children aged 5 have been considered by some to be pre-atheromatous.[4] Thus, the antecedents of atherosclerosis probably begin in childhood and may continue undetected until the occurrence of a serious or fatal clinical event. These findings have stimulated interest in preventive measures, including changes in infant feeding and childhood eating patterns. Pediatricians probably have the greatest opportunity and responsibility for the initiation of good nutrition habits that may prevent the most prevalent degenerative diseases. Kannel[1] goes so far as to say that "a heart attack or stroke by age 50 may be regarded as a failure of the pediatrician."

The second major finding that has stimulated interest in the prevention of obesity is the fat cell proliferation theory. This theory posits that there are critical periods during which fat cells increase in number and that an increase in adipose tissue at any other period is solely due to hypertrophy of existing fat cells. Furthermore, the number of fat cells present after these critical periods are believed to remain constant and reduction in adipose tissue occurs only by a decrease in the size of the existing fat cells. The implication for prevention is that if adipocyte proliferation can be kept within normal limits during the critical periods in childhood and adolescence, obesity in adulthood may be prevented. There are several problems with this theory which have been outlined earlier, but its major advantage has been its stimulus to research and education, particularly in the area of prevention. Many of the recommendations predicated on this theory are sound, but their value may be for reasons other than the adipocyte proliferation theory. Breast milk has been highly recommended during the first 4 to 6 months, partly to prevent overnutrition during the postulated childhood critical period of adipose cell multiplication. The result may be to decrease obesity, but the reason could be because some characteristic of breast milk is necessary for the development of the neuroendocrine satiety mechanism. Hall[5] notes that breast milk changes in composition from the beginning to the end of an individual feeding and postulates that this change may trigger a decrease in food intake.

PRIMARY, SECONDARY, AND TERTIARY PREVENTION

The classical division of prevention into primary, secondary, and tertiary is readily applicable to obesity. Primary prevention focuses on diminishing the incidence of new cases in a population over a period of time by counteracting the forces that produce the illness or condition. The goal of primary prevention is to decrease the risk of the population in general, and the individual is seen as representative of the issues confronting an entire population group. In the case of obesity, the major trends that increase obesity include overfeeding in infancy and childhood, an increasingly sedentary life style, and commercial pressures to increase consumption of food. Primary prevention programs designed to counteract these influences include education regarding the value of breast-feeding and exercise programs in the schools. Certain nutritional groups are attempting by legal means to limit television commercials that foster poor nutrition habits in youngsters; this activity is a primary prevention measure.

Secondary prevention aims to reduce the disability rate of obesity by lowering the prevalence of established cases of obesity. Prevalence is the number of cases of obesity at any given time as distinct from incidence, which is the number of new cases of obesity occurring during a certain time period. Secondary prevention attempts to decrease prevalence of obesity and primary prevention aims to decrease the incidence of obesity. There are two major aspects of secondary prevention: early identification of obesity and improved treatment. Periodic weighing of infants is one method of identifying the onset of obesity early. The search for improved treatment methods, notably behavior modification, is another aspect of secondary prevention. Identification of new cases of obesity will probably improve rapidly as physicians, pediatricians in particular, become more aware of the hazards of obesity and the tendency of obese children to become obese adults[6] (Fig 14.1). It seems unlikely that the current treatment modalities will dramatically decrease the prevalence of obesity. New methods are urgently needed.

Tertiary prevention includes efforts designed to reduce the residual effects of obesity and the complications of obesity, including hypertension, diabetes, and atherosclerosis. Programs that are designed to rehabilitate stroke victims or coronary patients are examples of tertiary prevention.

The prevalence of obesity is so widespread and the incidence increasing so rapidly, that one patient remarked "we will soon be in the majority." In view of the deleterious consequences of obesity, it is imperative that efforts be directed to all three areas of prevention, but particularly primary prevention. The following discussion highlights current preventive approaches and suggests possible avenues for further research and action.

PRIMARY PREVENTION

Antepartum Measures

Primary preventive measures for obesity are needed during pregnancy. The adipocyte proliferation theory posits that the first critical period of fat cell multiplication begins during the third trimester and extends into the first year of life. Overnutrition during the third trimester might result in an increased number of fat cells and predispose to obesity. The evidence for this idea is scanty, but suggestive (see Chapter 3). Measures that result in an adequate, but not excessive, weight gain during pregnancy would be a primary preventive measure. However, most attempts to limit the weight gain of pregnant women have not met with great success. Kilay[7] says, "It is rather simple to tell a woman she is gaining weight too fast in pregnancy. Such statements are medically worthless and destructive to the doctor-patient relationship, and cause a woman to restrict rather than modify her caloric intake." Instead, he advises educating the woman about proper nutrition and assisting her in making a suitable modification of her diet. Food intake

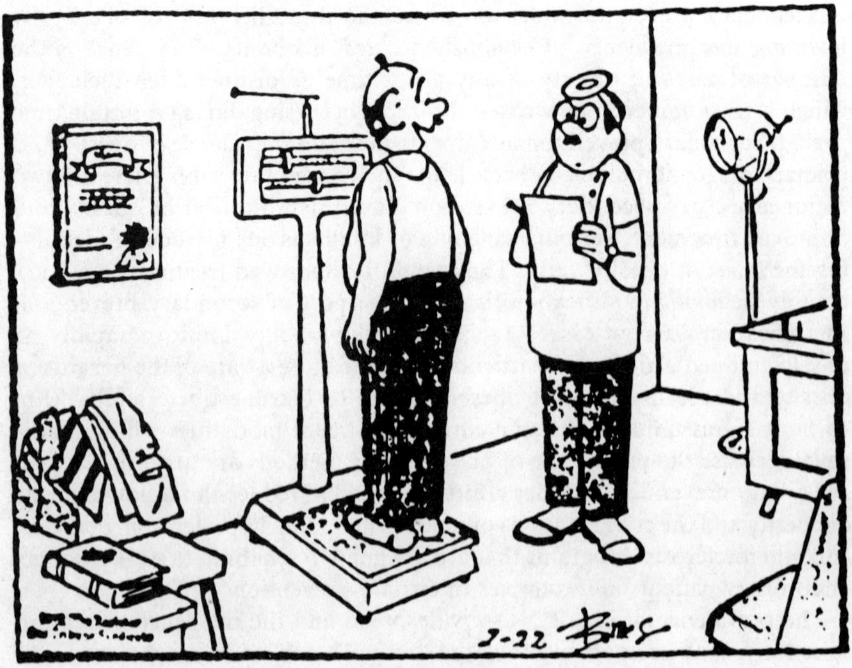

"Can I help it if I never lost my baby fat?"

Figure 14.1. Infantile obesity usually persists. (Reprinted with permission from the Register and Tribune Syndicate, Inc.)

diaries that help pinpoint the situations in which overeating occurs can be helpful for the pregnant woman. Also many women erroneously believe that exercise is prohibited during pregnancy, and a marked alteration in physical activity may result in excessive weight gain. Advising the woman about prudent exercise is another preventive measure. There are also anecdotal reports from many obese women that excessive weight gain during pregnancy was never lost, and there are a few epidemiological studies that suggest that women who have borne several children are more likely to weigh more for height and age than nulliparous women.

Infancy

Nutrition during the first year may have lifelong impact. Protein calorie malnutrition, which occurs in widespread areas of the world, may inhibit brain development in a way that can never be later corrected with adequate nutrition since myelinization, which requires adequate protein, occurs during a circumscribed period in early life. Similarly, it is thought that the first year of life may be part of a critical period of adipocyte multiplication and overnutrition may result in an increased complement of fat cells. Preventive measures include breast-feeding and delayed introduction of solid foods. Breast-fed babies are less likely to be obese, and the composition of humanized cow's milk does not duplicate breast milk, which contains a number of species specific immunoglobulins. Furthermore, the process of breast-feeding promotes a positive mother-child relationship. La Leche Organization has done much to promote breast-feeding and has been much more knowledgable than many physicians in anticipating and managing problems with breast-feeding. The medical profession might support such organizations as a primary preventive measure against obesity.

Nutritionists, who are often the last professionals to be consulted for advice about infant feeding, have noted that a number of factors militate against breast-feeding.[8] The nursing staff is often ill-informed about breast-feeding and may encourage bottle-feeding in a variety of ways. One woman who had been obese in adolescence with a subsequent continuing battle with obesity decided to nurse her baby, in part to prevent excessive weight gain and an increased number of fat cells. At her first attempt to breast-feed, the baby did not immediately suck and the nurses said, "That baby looks puny, is not going to suck and will need bottle-feeding." Not surprisingly, the mother was frightened by what proved to be a quite inaccurate statement and strong reassurance was needed when the mother tried to breast-feed the next time. The nursing staff needs further education about the value of breast-feeding and must be able to instruct the mother and assist her if any difficulties occur. It is the rare mother who is unable to breast-feed and even less common for a normal infant to obtain inadequate nutrition by breast-feeding. Education of the nursing staff is an example of primary prevention and might best be done by a nutritionist or a well-informed pediatrician.

With increasing education of physicians and nutritionists, delaying introduction of solid foods may be easier. Semi-solids should not be given until at least the 4th month of life and are not necessary until 6 months. In Sweden the use of solid food has been simplified by labeling jars with a number which refers to the earliest month in which the food should be introduced. In the United States there are strong commercial pressures to use prepared infant feedings, which are often less nutritious and more expensive than those which can be prepared at home. Several primary preventive measures might be helpful, including legislation limiting salt and sugar content of some of these baby foods, and labels advising against use before the 4th month.

The effectiveness of preventive programs in infancy is only now being evaluated. Pisacano et al.[9] studied two groups of children. The control group of 40 children were infants seen in 1964 and fed a conventional diet of formula for 3 months, followed by whole cow's milk and monthly additions of baby foods, an egg a day, custards, and puddings. The test group consisted of 80 children who followed "The Prudent Diet." This diet allows cereal and unsweetened fruit before age 3 months and periodic introduction of other foods low in sugar and salt in prescribed amounts. Of the infants fed the standard 1964 diet 34.1% were overweight at 3 months compared to 25% fed "The Prudent Diet." More importantly, however, by age 3 years the control group still had a prevalence of 25.5% overweight compared to 1.28% in the test group. This study was conducted by a group of busy pediatricians and suggests that primary preventive measures can be relatively easily incorporated into an office practice. One problem with this study is that solid foods were introduced earlier than would be currently recommended. However, the study was started in 1970 and at that time cereals and fruits were introduced earlier.

Energy expenditure of infants has been a serious consideration in the Soviet Union for years.[6] A gymnastic is used which includes a massage and gentle passive movement and is prescribed for normal infants as well as many sick, even undernourished, babies. Massage is recommended after 1 month and passive exercise after 2 months. Similarly, in Germany in 1955, Kaiser[10] wrote a book entitled *Suckling Gymnastiks.* In the United States, exercise may be encouraged by the use of various crib toys which move and amuse the baby (and parents) and encourage the baby to exercise. In some warmer areas of the country, babies are taught to swim during the 1st year of life. Some other devices such as the "jumper," "sling" ("baby bouncer"), and the "seated" walker may also encourage physical activity in the infant. Mayer[11] has shown that even in infancy some babies are more placid than others and this disposition may contribute to the development of obesity. In a sedentary society, measures that increase physical activity, beginning even at a very early age, may serve to prevent obesity.

Childhood

During childhood, lifelong eating and exercise patterns are established. The child first models his eating behavior after that of his family, and during the school years his peers dramatically influence food intake. Although childhood, at least until age 8 or 9, is thought to be a quiescent period for adipose cell replication, obesity may begin during this age span and may even result in an abnormal increase in adipose cell multiplication. More important, however, is the fact that nutrition patterns are usually firmly entrenched by the end of childhood. A child may eat well-balanced meals with a few low-calorie snacks, or may habitually consume high-fat and high-carbohydrate meals and snacks. Although physicians, nutritionists, and educators have long advocated balanced meals that incorporate some foods from all of the basic food groups, usually a strict health education model has been used that has proven ineffective. Recently, primary prevention programs have been started; these aim at systematic intervention in customary eating patterns. Since information alone has little impact on ingrained behavioral patterns, these programs have incorporated the behavior modification paradigm for prevention of obesity.

PEP Program

The Preschool Eating Patterns (PEP) program described by Smiciklas-Wright and D'Augelli[12] is designed to improve the eating habits of normal children with the parents acting as the agent of change. The goal of the PEP program is to foster a "thin eating style" which includes leisurely eating, moderate-sized portions, eating when hungry rather than in response to situational cues, and slow chewing. This program is available to any family with preschool-age children that wishes to incorporate health-related eating and activity patterns into their family life style. Groups composed of four sets of parents met weekly for 5 weeks for 2 to 3 hours with two teachers, one a nutritionist and one a behavioral science specialist. The parents were taught to pinpoint specific behavioral changes they thought were needed, and they assisted in designing a strategy to incorporate the change into the family system. Reinforcement was used to strengthen better eating habits. This project is a novel attempt to utilize some of the effective behavioral techniques in a preventive program. Unfortunately, the report does not indicate how effective the measures were in producing change. It may be helpful to teach a "thin eating style," but the implication is that there is an "obese eating style," and this notion is probably incorrect. Nonetheless, this program is a significant step forward in utilizing current knowledge to prevent obesity.

Other Preventive Programs for Children

Behavioral scientists and nutritionists have begun to collaborate in designing preventive programs. Herbert-Jackson and Risey[13] have studied the food preferences of preschool age children in an attempt to guide them to more nutritious choices. These investigators studied children between the ages of 1 and 3 who were making the transition from an infant to an adult diet and presented them with more than 100 food items low in sugar, salt, preservatives, and saturated fats. The foods were ranked in the order of acceptance by the children and menus were compiled which met the youngsters' nutrient needs and were also acceptable. This technique avoids some of the traditional difficulties encountered in attempting to motivate children to eat balanced nutritious meals.

In the last few years, several well-written books that have become available provide techniques for helping interested parents modify the eating habits of their children and prevent later obesity. Jeffrey and Katz[14] have prepared a readable accurate book entitled *Take It Off and Keep It Off*, which has an outstanding chapter entitled "Improving Your Child's Eating Habits: Prevention at Its Best." There are three major steps to improving eating habits: identification of the maladaptive behavior, selection of realistic alternatives, and finally reinforcement for change to better eating habits. Table 14.1 lists several of the ways that children learn to overeat. The authors make the point that learning is not a one-way process. Children may learn to equate

Table 14.1
How children learn to overeat (Reprinted with permission from D. B. Jeffrey and R. C. Katz: Take It Off and Keep It Off. Prentice-Hall, Inc., Englewood Cliffs, NJ, 1977, p 233.)

1. Millions of dollars are spent annually on television, newspapers, and magazine advertisements to tempt and encourage children to eat high-calorie food.
2. Access to fattening foods is made easy by buying them and keeping them around the house.
3. Too many junk foods are given as snacks. They soon become expected and preferred over more nutritious foods.
4. Too much time is spent in sedentary activities such as TV viewing. Too little positive instruction and encouragement is given for active play, regular exercise, and family sports.
5. Children are admonished to eat every bite. They are told to hurry up and eat, because others are waiting or the food will get cold. They are sometimes led to believe that if they don't clean their plates, they will hurt their parents' feelings or not grow big and strong. On top of this, more than one child has been made to feel guilty for *not* eating by moralistic spiels about the starvation that abounds in other countries.
6. Food is used to tranquilize children when they become upset or discouraged. They learn that food can make them feel better or relieve their emotional sorrows. They also learn that one way to obtain extra food is to become upset and demand it.
7. Food, especially sweets, is used to reward good behavior. It may become a symbol of parental love, satisfaction, or special accomplishment.
8. The same foods are used to pacify children when they become rambunctious or bored. For parents this can be an expedient way of getting the kids out of their hair.
9. Special outings to the zoo, the park, and the movies become occasions to overindulge in fattening treats, candies, ice cream, and hot dogs. As time goes on, the outings may not be much fun without the eating (which is probably as true for many of us adults as well).
10. Nutritious but perhaps less palatable foods are made to appear as necessary evils, while rich desserts become a cause for celebration and fanfare. The underlying message is that only the rich foods should be eaten whenever the opportunity arises.
11. The net effect of all these experiences is that young children learn to eat many of the wrong foods. They also learn to consume more than they need for normal growth and activities. In the words of one popular song, they become "Junk Food Junkies."

food with affection or find that food relieves emotional sorrows, but the parent who observes that candy or snacks calm a child or result in a smile usually finds this response very reinforcing and is more likely to offer food the next time the child is distraught. The behavioral methods described by Jeffrey and Katz are applicable not only to children who are overweight but also can easily be adapted for use in families who do not have obese children and wish to prevent future problems.

Some school age children develop obesity following an emotional trauma or period of enforced bedrest. Divorce, death of a parent, hospitalization, illness of a parent, or birth of a sibling have all been identified as precipitating events. Primary preventive measures for obesity must aim at identifying these children and providing counseling at school or elsewhere before the onset of obesity. Family physicians or pediatricians are probably in the best position to identify these stresses and intervene either by providing supportive therapy for the child or referring the child for psychotherapy. If a lengthy hospitalization is needed, the physician should check periodically over the next several months for marked changes in growth.

Adolescence

Obesity in adolescence is not only difficult to treat once it occurs but may result in a permanent body image disturbance. According to the adipocyte proliferation theory a second critical period of adipose cell division occurs just before or during adolescence and therefore measures that prevent teenage obesity might obviate the possibility of an increased complement of fat cells in adult life. Although the evidence for this critical period of fat cell multiplication is scanty, prevention of obesity during this age period is important. The attitudinal aspect of body image may be "imprinted" during adolescence; obese youngsters are often the target of peer criticism and may develop a negative attitude toward their appearance which is retained even if weight is lost. Prevention of obesity during the teenage years decreases the likelihood of a lifelong battle with obesity. In patients who are already obese, the physician still has an opportunity to prevent a body image disturbance. Many families are unaware of the impact of derogatory remarks made to an obese youngster and are often willing to modify their comments. An informed empathic physician can enlist the family's cooperation and may be able to prevent the development of a body image disturbance.

Significant emotional events in adolescence can also result in obesity. Recognition of the underlying stress will result in referral for appropriate psychiatric intervention. The following case illustrates the tragedy which can occur when this is not done:

Marilyn, a 24-year-old single woman who is 5 feet 9 inches tall and weighs 100 pounds, came to the clinic with the complaint of recurrent vomiting, amenorrhea, inability to gain weight and compulsive handling of food. She reported a normal weight until age 14 when her parents divorced and she gradually began to gain weight until she was 200 pounds at age 17. She says she was sad and angry at her parents' separation and began to eat to assuage her unhappiness. She tried a variety of diets and finally went to a surgeon who wired her jaws shut to prevent any food intake except fluids. She lost weight precipitously down to 130 pounds at which time the wires were removed. She continued to be dissatisfied with her appearance and decided to induce vomiting to lose even more weight. She gradually lost down to 100 pounds and became preoccupied with food, weight, and vomiting. She had periodic binges in which she would consume huge quantities of food and feel repentant afterwards. She thought she was fat despite clear visual evidence to the contrary. The diagnosis of anorexia nervosa was made, but although both mother and patient said they were desperate for her to gain weight, they refused hospitalization and treatment.

This patient is an example of failure of prevention. At age 14, a clear precipitating event occurred and the patient's gradual weight gain over several years was the symptom of the underlying conflict. An astute family physician keeping periodic weight tables might have detected the onset of obesity and referred her for psychiatric treatment. Clearly the treatment of her obesity with jaw-wiring was inappropriate because the cause of her obesity was not ameliorated. Attempts at decreasing residual disability in this patient have thus far been unsuccessful.

Since inactivity may be one cause of adolescent obesity, programs designed to increase the activity of a normal weight teenager or those at risk (e.g., adolescents with one or both parents who are obese) might be effective primary prevention measures. One famous study of obese teenagers showed that they actually exercised less than their slender peers, even when playing volleyball or other ostensibly strenuous acitvity.[15] It is possible, of course, that inactivity is the consequence rather than the cause of their obesity, but it is not likely. Seltzer and Mayer[16] introduced an exercise program into a public school for obese elementary and junior high school students and found that the group, in general, lost weight. Although this is really a secondary preventive measure (because the children involved were already obese) a curricular change in physical education in all schools might decrease the tendency toward obesity.

Prevention of Obesity in Adulthood

Adults who have not been obese as children are less likely to be obese later in life, but they are not immune. Recent studies of important life events have suggested that during particularly stressful life periods, obesity may be more likely to start. For men, marriage, the birth of children, and important career milestones are significant life events that may trigger conflict and result in obesity. The significant life events for women have been more thoroughly studied and include marriage, childbirth, and menopause. Obesity is more likely to follow each of these events and therefore careful attention to insidious weight gain at these times may prevent later intractable obesity. During pregnancy, most women are under careful medical scrutiny and excessive weight gain is usually detected. The obstetrician who offers careful well-informed nutritional counseling to the pregnant woman may be able to prevent future obesity in both mother and child.

Although there are normally no periods of adipose cell multiplication during adult life, some investigators have postulated that certain stimuli may initiate an abnormal period of fat cell division.[17] Thus far, this idea has not been proven but might account for the occasional adult patient who gains excessive weight in adulthood. Identification of the stimuli that serve to trigger this sequence of events would be the first step in a primary prevention program.

Resistance to Primary Prevention Programs

There are several reasons why prevention of obesity has thus far been a dismal failure. First, both the public and the medical profession are more interested in treatment than in primary prevention. Government agencies and private individuals are willing to fund enormous tertiary prevention programs. For example, the Coronary Care Units in Tampa are well staffed, well insured, and are the focus of much research and education. Cardiologists and cardiac surgeons who treat patients with the ravages of atherosclerosis are among the most prestigious physicians in the nation. Programs aimed at increasing the exercise level of the nation's teenagers or decreasing the advertisement of high-fat, high-carbohydrate foods on children's television shows receive but a lukewarm endorsement from physicians and patients alike.

Second, there is group resistance to any change that challenges long-established cultural beliefs and habits. Sometimes the proposed change threatens, or seems to threaten, the power, prestige, or economic security of certain special segments in society. Many of the proposed preventive measures threaten the economic welfare of certain food maufacturers. The underlying philosophy of increased consumption and a rising gross national product is in opposition to programs that foster a decrease in food consumption at all ages. Delaying the introduction of solid foods might prevent infantile obesity, but will be costly to the powerful billion-dollar baby food industry. Resistance can thus be expected from this segment of the food industry. Some nutritional groups have introduced legislation to limit advertisements for high-calorie, high-fat junk foods during children's television shows; thus far, little progress has been made, as the producers of these products have a vested economic stake in increasing sales, even if consumption of these foods may be partly responsible for the dramatic rise in obesity.

Group resistance to proposed changes may take the form of anxiety or hostility, the true sources of which are unconscious. Marmor and colleagues[18] have noted that good health is linked in the unconscious with the basic needs for security, survival, and mastery, and ill health is associated with fears of body disintegration, dissolution, and death. In early development, certain factors are related to health or illness; e.g., what goes into the mouth is strongly related to good or evil. Children are told, "Eat this . . . it is good for you" or "Don't put that in your mouth . . . it will make you sick." Health and security become associated with eating foods that are "pure," or "wholesome," and sickness, insecurity, and death are associated with eating "impure" or "poisonous" food. Thus, asking a large group to change a deeply ingrained cultural food habit is a threat to the security, safety, and intactness of its members. If a food once believed to be pure and wholesome is found in fact to be hazardous to health, simple re-educative measures will not suffice. Since much of the opposition arises from unconscious conflict, it is not surprising that appeal to reason often fails to sway the opposition; e.g., cane sugar was once considered a pure and wholesome food (and this belief is still exploited by advertisements for "pure" cane sugar) but is now thought to provide only empty calories and promote obesity and dental caries. Despite nutritional warnings, however, large groups of children continue to consume large quantities of cane sugar. Advertisements that depict healthy happy youngsters chewing cane sugar in Hawaii effectively link health and sugar consumption, even if this link is made unconsciously.

Group resistance to change is usually greater if the proposed change is rapid or its proponents enthusiastic. Generally, the more time allowed for education and preparation of the group, the less likely there is to be vociferous resistance. Also, if there is much heated rhetoric or debate on the topic, group resistance may increase. Marmor notes that there are a few very vocal groups that are involved over and over again in opposition to widely disparate health programs. These individuals are those in whom the association between traditional health and security and well-being are rigidly ingrained and not available for analysis. These individuals are at the polar end of the general, more flexible, cultural connection between security and various health habits. These extremists may be found opposing programs as different as mental health bills, fluoridation projects, ecology plans, or food additives.

By the same token, resistance to change is not all bad and scientific conservatism has probably prevented premature introduction of many unproven ideas. In terms of obesity, it is unfortunate that there was not more resistance to bottle-feeding or the early introduction of solid foods. Bottle-feeding is actually a colossal cultural experiment of the last 50 years, the full consequences of which are still not known. A more conservative attitude might have been advantageous.

Finally, family physicians and pediatricians who are the first line of defense in preventing obesity, may have inaccurate or incomplete nutritional knowledge to educate their patients. Milton and Fox[19] report a survey of the attitudes and practices of Nebraska physicians in the field of infant feeding and nutrition. The more important items from their questionnaire are summarized in Table 14.2, but generally the study revealed that many of these physicians had outdated or erroneous information about infant nutrition. Although most (73%) agreed that preventive measures against obesity should be taken during the first few months, 40% of the respondents thought that adding solid foods early helped the babies sleep through the night, and 16% of the physicians did not believe that fat cell number may be determined by infant feeding practices. In general, although there was evidence that a sizable number of physicians remained ignorant about some of the major

Table 14.2
Nutritional knowledge of physicians (Adapted and reprinted with permission from Milton and Fox,[19] p 417)

Statement	Response				
	Strongly Disagree	Disagree	Undecided	Agree	Strongly Agree
It is not necessary to take preventive measures against obesity during the first few months of life.	44.7	28.8	4.1	12.9	8.8
Overfeeding infants may encourage a habit of overeating which is carried into later life.	2.4	3.5	9.4	37.6	47.1
Breast-fed babies tend to be heavier than bottle-fed babies.	12.4	53.5	25.9	7.1	1.2
Healthy babies require some sugar or other concentrated sweets for energy.	24.1	46.5	11.2	12.4	4.1
One advantage of adding solid food to the diet very early is that it helps the baby sleep through the night.	13.5	28.2	16.5	37.6	2.9
Maintaining low serum cholesterol levels in childhood is of little importance in reducing the incidence of heart disease as adults.	15.3	40.6	31.2	10.0	2.4
One advantage of breast feeding is that the mother does not observe how much the infant has eaten.	10.0	41.2	25.3	20.0	2.9

current tenets of infant nutrition, the majority were relatively well informed. However, one major practice regarding infant nutrition that runs counter to current knowledge is introduction of solid foods. Most of these physicians recommended that cereal be introduced at 1.5 months, yet no solid foods are needed until 4 to 6 months.

In summary, there are several reasons why primary preventive programs for obesity have not yet achieved optimal effectiveness. First, there is always group resistance to change, sometimes based on rational scientific conservatism and sometimes based on anxiety which has its origin in the unconscious. In addition, medicine has traditionally been more interested in treatment than prevention, and this attitude is largely reflected in a society that offers prestige and economic support to tertiary treatment programs. Finally, physicians are not yet fully informed about nutrition, and practice is not always consonant with current nutritional data.

SECONDARY PREVENTION

Secondary prevention measures include early identification of obesity and rapid effective treatment once obesity is diagnosed. Early identification programs are now underway in many parts of the country for infants and preschool age children. Since most young children are seen periodically by their pediatricians and are usually weighed and measured for height, the onset of obesity can usually be easily identified. As physicians begin to realize that a fat baby or child is more likely to be a fat adult, youngsters who grow too rapidly in weight will be identified. During infancy, changes in feeding are usually simple once the child is recognized as overweight. School-age children are seen less often by their physicians, but are captive in school most of the day throughout the year; screening programs in the schools may be the best way to identify obese school-age children. Improved nutritional offerings at the school cafeteria and in vending machines may help prevent or alleviate obesity. Exercise programs have been demonstrated effective in treating obesity in pre-teen and teenage children. In adolescence, the obese child is often identified after large amounts of weight have been gained and treatment is often ineffective. As noted in Chapter 11, the treatment of choice for these youngsters is often an exercise program rather than a reducing diet.

In the last 10 years, there has been a surge of interest in developing methods for early identification of obesity and quantifying the extent of obesity. These methods include triceps skinfold measures, ultrasound, and various height-weight measures. Although there are still large gaps in our knowledge, the normal fat content for individuals at all ages is gradually being determined. Inexpensive, accurate methods for quantifying the extent of obesity will greatly aid in the early identification of patients who are just developing obesity.

Once the obese youngster or adult has been identified, treatment measures are instituted; these may include diet, exercise, behavior modification, drugs, or bypass surgery. With the exception of bypass surgery, none is effective for even half of the patients identified. Most of the patients who enter treatment will either drop out or fail to lose significant amounts of weight, or if they do lose weight, they will usually regain the lost weight. Despite this pessimistic finding regarding the effectiveness of the secondary prevention of obesity, it is important to note that some patients do lose weight and maintain that loss for years. Our efforts may be best directed toward identifying those patients who are likely to be successful in certain treatment programs. Only recently have concerted efforts been made for providing comprehensive individualized treatment programs for obese patients and these efforts may provide better results.

In the case of some of the other eating disorders, strides are being made toward early identification of patients. There is an Association for Anorexia Nervosa and Associated Diseases (ANAD)[20] which attempts to disseminate information about treatment of anorexia nervosa patients in the hope that early intervention will decrease the high mortality and morbidity rate of these patients. A self-help group called the Anorexia Nervosa Aid Society, Inc.,[21] has been formed to provide services and programs for anyone with anorexia nervosa and to aid in the education, research, cure, and prevention of this illness.

TERTIARY PREVENTION

Unfortunately, primary and secondary prevention for obesity often fail, and many patients remain obese and develop hypertension, diabetes, carbohydrate intolerance, or atherosclerosis. These diseases have very high morbidity and mortality rates and may collectively account for 40–50% of the deaths in the United States. Much physician time and hospital occupancy is accounted for by these conditions which often become dramatically symptomatic during middle life. Tertiary treatment programs are designed to ameliorate the effects of the disease which cannot be cured. Although a patient may have atherosclerotic heart disease, treatment is aimed at increasing his functional capacity as much as possible through diet, exercise, medication, and sometimes cardiovascular surgery. Hypertension may result in cardiac or brain damage that is permanent, even if the individual loses weight and becomes normotensive. Thus, tertiary prevention, at best, may leave major residual defects and often is completely ineffective.

SUMMARY

In conclusion, programs aimed at preventing obesity are likely to have great future impact on some of the major diseases of our time—atherosclerosis, hypertension, and diabetes. Not only is established obesity very difficult to treat, but some of the obesity-related diseases may be irreversible even after weight loss. Secondary prevention entails early case identification, often by the pediatrician, and comprehensive holistic treatment programs for obese individuals. Tertiary treatment of the obesity-related diseases is least effective. Yet, it is the method in which our society and the medical profession invest the most time, money, and enthusiasm.

References

1. Kannel WB: Coronary risk factors. II. Prospects for prevention of atherosclerosis in the young. Aust NZ J Med 6: 410–419, 1976.
2. Turner RW: Perspectives in coronary prevention. Postgrad Med J 54: 141–148, 1978.
3. Enos W, Holmes R, Beyer J: Coronary disease among United States soldiers killed in action in Korea. JAMA 152: 1090–1093, 1953.
4. Osborn G: Stages in Development of Coronary Disease Observed From 1500 Young Subjects. Editions du centre national de la recherche scientifique, Paris, Anatole-France, cited in Turner RW: Perspectives in coronary prevention. Postgrad Med 54: 141–145, 1978.
5. Hall B: Changing composition of human milk and early development of an appetite control. Lancet 1: 779–781, 1975.
6. Jelliffe DB, Jelliffe EFP: Fat babies: Prevalence, perils and prevention. Environ Child Health Monogr 41: 123–159, 1975.
7. Kilay DZ: Dysfunctional antepartum nutrition. J Reprod Med 7: 251–256, 1971.
8. Barlow DH, Tillotson JL: Behavioral science and nutrition: a new perspective. J Am Diet Assoc 72: 368–371, 1978.
9. Pisacano JC, Lichter H, Ritter J, Siegal AP: An attempt at prevention of obesity in infancy. Pediatrics 61: 360–364, 1978.
10. Kaiser W: "Sauglins gymnastik" (Suckling gymnastics). Heidelberg, Von Defloff, Neumann, Heuride, 1955.
11. Mayer J: The fat baby. Postgrad Med 44: 277–278, 1968.
12. Smiciklas-Wright H, D'Augelli AR: Primary prevention for overweight: preschool eating patterns (PEP) program. J Am Diet Assoc 72: 626–629, 1978.
13. Herbert-Jackson E, Risey TR: Behavioral nutrition: consumption of foods of the future by toddlers. J Appl Behav Anal, in press, cited in Barlow DH, Tillotson JL: Behavioral science and nutrition: a new perspective. J Am Diet Assoc 72: 368–371, 1978.
14. Jeffrey DB, Katz RC: Take It Off and Keep It Off. Englewood Cliffs, NJ, Prentice-Hall, 1977, pp 229–264.
15. Bullen B, Reed RB, Mayer J: Physical activity of obese and non-obese adolescent girls appraised by motion picture sampling. Am J Clin Nutr 14: 211–223, 1964.
16. Seltzer CC, Mayer J: An effective weight control program in a public school system. Am J Public Health 60: 679–689, 1970.
17. Hirsch J, Batchelor B: Adipose tissue cellularity in human obesity. Clin Endocrinol Metab 5: 299–311, 1976.
18. Marmor J, Bernard VW, Ottenberg P: Psychodynamics of group opposition to health programs. Am J Orthopsychiatry 30: 330–345, 1960.
19. Milton SE, Fox HM: Nebraska physicians' attitudes and practices in the field of infant feeding and nutrition. J Am Diet Assoc 73: 416–419, 1978.
20. Anorexia Nervosa and Associated Diseases (ANAD): Suite 2020, 550 Frontage Rd. Northfield, IL 60093. Phone 312-831-3438.
21. Anorexia Nervosa Aid Society, Inc.: 101 Cedar Lane, Teaneck, NJ 07666. Phone 201-836-1800.

Index

J

K

L

Q

R

S

T

U

V

W

Y

Z